Rapid Perioperative Care

Rapid Perioperative Care

Paul Wicker MSc, PGCE, BSc, RGN, RMN
Visiting Professor
First Hospital of Nanjing, China;
Fellow of the Higher Education Academy

Sara Dalby MSc, BSc (Hons), RGN, Dip HE
Surgical Care Practitioner
Aintree University Hospital Trust;
Associate Lecturer
Edge Hill University;
Winston Churchill Fellow

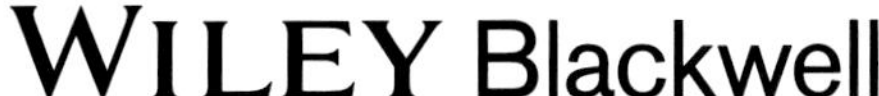

This edition first published 2017 © 2017 by John Wiley and Sons, Ltd

Registered office: John Wiley & Sons, Ltd, The Atrium, Southern Gate, Chichester, West Sussex, PO19 8SQ, UK

Editorial offices: 9600 Garsington Road, Oxford, OX4 2DQ, UK
The Atrium, Southern Gate, Chichester, West Sussex, PO19 8SQ, UK
111 River Street, Hoboken, NJ 07030-5774, USA

For details of our global editorial offices, for customer services and for information about how to apply for permission to reuse the copyright material in this book please see our website at www.wiley.com/wiley-blackwell

Library of Congress Cataloging-in-Publication Data
[to come, includes 9781119121237]

A catalogue record for this book is available from the British Library.

Wiley also publishes its books in a variety of electronic formats. Some content that appears in print may not be available in electronic books.

Cover image: © Paul Wicker

1 2017

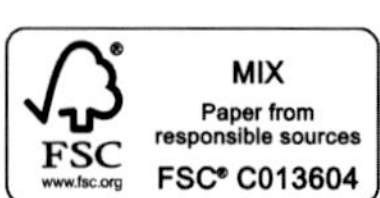

Contents

Section 3 Surgical Specialities, 129

Sara Dalby

Section 4 Surgical Scrub Skills, 191

Sara Dalby

Section 5 Surgical Assisting, 257

Sara Dalby

Preface

This book has been written by C. Paul Wicker and Sara Dalby for perioperative practitioners (students, nurses and ODPs) and junior doctors who work in anaesthetics, surgery and recovery. This *Rapid* series book covers a wide range of subjects related to perioperative practice and perioperative care, and each chapter is relatively short and concise so that practitioners can read the chapter efficiently and effectively, which will encourage them to learn how to undertake tasks and actions within the operating department. This book will provide practitioners with detailed knowledge and understanding of many aspects of perioperative practice which will support them in their work in clinical practice and enable them to deliver the best possible care to all perioperative patients.

This book will use a structured approach to perioperative care, starting with an introduction to the perioperative environment, anaesthetics, surgery and recovery, and critical care for patients who have serious health problems.

The first section is called 'Preoperative Preparation' which covers areas such as roles of theatre practitioners, preoperative assessment checklists, perioperative equipment, medication and several other chapters. This is an important area for junior theatre practitioners so that they know how to prepare the operating room prior to the patient arriving.

The second section is called 'Anaesthesia' and is related to anaesthetic procedures, which are very important to patients because, basically, anaesthesia maintains their homeostasis and physiological status during surgical procedures. Chapters include checking anaesthetic equipment, general and local anaesthesia, rapid sequence induction, airway management and so on. The purpose of anaesthesia is to keep the patient unconscious during the surgical procedure, and maintain oxygenation, blood pressure, pulse, and fluid levels throughout the surgery. The use of anaesthetic drugs also helps to prevent postoperative pain and can help prevent problems such as low blood pressure or malignant hyperthermia.

The next three sections are related to surgery – 'Surgical Specialities', 'Surgical Scrub Skills' and 'Surgical Assisting'. The first two sections cover many areas of surgery, including all aspects of surgery such as vascular, breast, orthopaedics, laparoscopic and colorectal surgery, as well as skin preparation, electrosurgery, wound healing, dressings, haemostasis and so on. These two sections cover most surgical specialities and also all aspects of actions taken during surgery by both the surgeons and the scrub practitioner. The final section on surgery covers the actions taken by surgical assistants, including legal issues, suture materials, wound closure, camera holding, retraction and so on. This chapter will provide you with detailed information about the role of the surgical assistant, which will help you to understand fully the ability to assist surgeons, for those practitioners who have undertaken appropriate first assistant training.

The sixth section is called 'Recovery' and is related to recovery care of patients. Chapters include recovery room design, patient handover, monitoring, assessment, medications, bleeding problems and so on. When the patient enters the recovery room, he or she recovers from the anaesthesia and surgery. Recovery practitioners monitor patients carefully to ensure they don't suffer side effects and do recover from their anaesthesia and surgery safely. Monitoring includes respiration, breathing, blood loss, temperature, blood pressure, pulse and so on. Patients may also need supervising in case of postoperative problems caused by anaesthetic drugs, for example anxiety or delirium.

Postoperative problems include many areas such as postoperative pain, nausea and vomiting, electrolyte imbalance, low fluid balance, low blood pressure, malignant hyperthermia and so on. These problems may be resolved by recovery staff or may need an anaesthetist's or surgeon's actions. The 13 chapters regarding recovery should provide you with a good level of knowledge and skills in regards to caring for postoperative patients.

The final section is about 'Perioperative Critical Care' which covers areas such as management of critically ill patients, hypothermia, hyperthermia, deep vein thrombosis, latex allergies, pressure ulcers, diabetes, anaemia, morbidly obese patients and others. Critical care of patients is important and urgent when they are suffering from serious illnesses or conditions, and so these 13 chapters cover many areas which will be of interest to you when you need to deal with these patient conditions.

This *Rapid* series book on perioperative care will provide theatre practitioners with short, detailed and concise information about many aspects of their role. This will be useful for trained staff and for students and will help to ensure patient safety and effective working.

Enjoy this book and we hope that you like it!

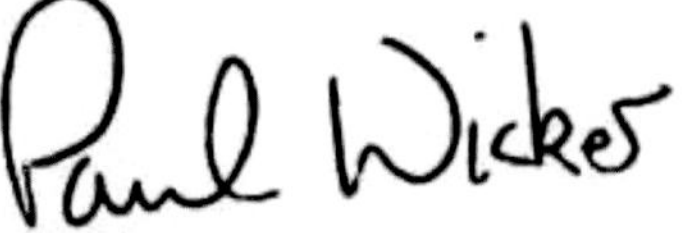
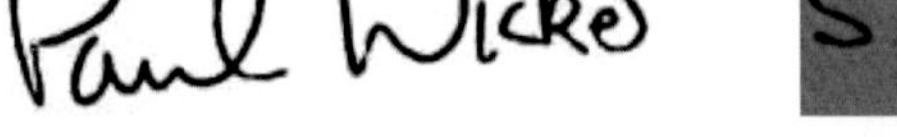
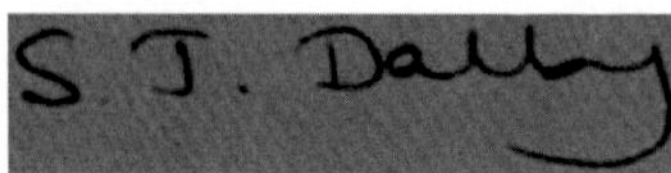

Paul Wicker **Sara Dalby**

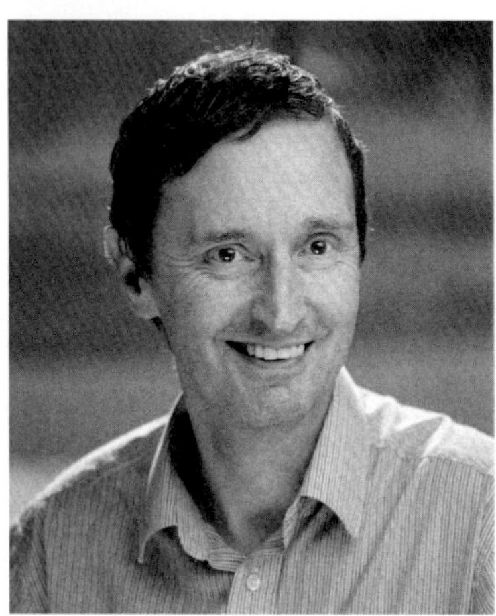

Acknowledgements

Sara Dalby and myself have asked many people to review the chapters to ensure they are written correctly and clearly. This has taken some time to undertake; however, all chapters have been reviewed and updated which has been of great benefit to us both.

The reviewers who have checked over all the chapters which Paul Wicker has written include Africa Bocos (my wife), Rachel Simpson, Ashley Wooding, Helen Lowes, Laura Rowe and Natalie Lockhart. These reviewers are all qualified operating department practitioners, and they have read through the chapters thoroughly in order to ensure they are correct and well written. Some of the chapters were updated which has helped me in ensuring the chapters are read easily and contain the correct information. Paul Wicker gives his best and sincerest thanks to these reviewers for all the work they have done in updating my chapters.

Sara Dalby also asked several reviewers to look at all the chapters she has written in regards to surgery to ensure the chapters are accurate and concise. Sara would like to thank all these reviewers for their help and assistance, and their knowledge and skills in reading the chapters and updating them.

These people include:

Jill Mordaunt, Practice Education Manager
Jennie Grainger, Registrar General Surgery with Specialist Interest in Coloproctology
Elizabeth Clark, Consultant Anaesthetist
Kaylie Hughes, Speciality Registrar Urology
Tim Gilbert, Core Surgical Trainee General Surgery
Dave Ormesher, Speciality Registrar Vascular Surgery
Laura Ormesher, Speciality Registrar Obstetrics and Gynaecology
Claire Morris, Speciality Leader Orthopaedics and Trauma
Zoe Panayi, Senior House Officer General Surgery
Elizabeth Kane, Core Surgical Trainee General Surgery
Helen Bermingham, Core Surgical Trainee General Surgery
Andrew McAvoy, Speciality Registrar Colorectal Surgery
Kristen Daniels, Physician Assistant Plastic Surgery

Photos have kindly been provided by Aintree University Hospital, Liverpool Womens Hospital, and from the Cadaveric Workshop at University of South Manchester.

Finally, we would also want to thank Karen Moore and James Watson for their help in developing our book from John Wiley & Sons Limited, and for their help and support in getting this book published.

Kind regards to all.

Paul Wicker
Sara Dalby

Abbreviations

AAA	abdominal aortic aneurysm
AAGBI	Association of Anaesthetists of Great Britain and Ireland
ABG	arterial blood gas
ACL	anterior cruciate ligament (knee)
ACS	acute coronary syndrome
AF	atrial fibrillation
ARDS	adult respiratory distress syndrome
ARF	acute renal failure, acute rheumatic fever
AV	arteriovenous or arterial-venous
AVR	aortic valve replacement
BMD	bone mass density
BMI	body mass index
BMR	basic metabolic rate
BNF	British National Formulary
BP	blood pressure
C	centigrade, Celsius
C/S	caesarean section
CABG	coronary artery bypass graft
CAD	coronary artery disease
CBD	common bile duct
CBF	cerebral blood flow
CEA	carotid endarterectomy (vascular surgery)
CF	cystic fibrosis
CHD	congenital heart disease
CHF	chronic heart failure
CNS	central nervous system
CO_2	carbon dioxide
COPD	chronic obstructive pulmonary disease
CPAP	continuous positive airway pressure
CPR	cardiopulmonary resuscitation
CT	computed tomography
CV	cardiovascular
CVC	central venous catheter
CVD	cardiovascular disease
CXR	chest x-ray
DCU	Day Case Unit
DoH	Department of Health
DIC	disseminated intravascular coagulation

DL	direct laryngoscopy
DOB	date of birth
DVT	deep vein thrombosis
ECF	extracellular fluid
ECG	electrocardiogram; electrocardiography
ECT	electroconvulsive therapy
EEG	electroencephalography
ET	endotracheal
ETT	endotracheal tube
F	Fahrenheit
FEF	forced expiratory flow
fem-fem	femoral-to-femoral bypass (vascular surgery)
fem-pop	femoro-popliteal bypass (vascular surgery)
FFP	fresh frozen plasma
GA	general anaesthesia
GU	genitourinary
H&P	history and physical examination
H_2O	water
HA	haemolytic anaemia
HAV	hepatitis A virus
Hb	haemoglobin
HBV	hepatitis B virus
HCPC	Health and Care Professions Council
HCV	hepatitis C virus
HR	heart rate
I&D	incision and drainage
ICF	intracellular fluid
ICP	intracranial pressure
IHD	ischaemic heart disease
IM	intramuscular
IP	inpatient
IPPV	intermittent positive pressure ventilation
ISF	interstitial fluid
IV	intravenous
IVC	inferior vena cava
IVF	in vitro fertilization
IVIG	intravenous immune globulin
K	potassium
kg	kilogram
L	litre
LIH	left inguinal hernia
LMA	laryngeal mask airway

LV	left ventricular
MD	muscular dystrophy
MH	malignant hyperthermia
MI	myocardial infarction
ML	millilitre
mol	mole
MS	multiple sclerosis
MVR	mitral valve replacement
NG	nasogastric
NICE	National Institute for Health and Care Excellence
NM	neuromuscular
NPSA	National Patient Safety Agency
NSAID	nonsteroidal anti-inflammatory drug
O_2	oxygen
ODP	operating department practice, operating department practitioner
OPD	outpatient department
P	pulse
Pa	Pascal
PaCO2	arterial carbon dioxide partial pressure (measured from a blood gas sample)
PACU	post-anaesthesia care unit
PAH	pulmonary arterial hypertension
PaO2	arterial oxygen partial pressure (measured from a blood gas sample)
PAP	pulmonary artery pressure
PAWCP	pulmonary artery wedge capillary pressure
pCO_2	partial pressure of carbon dioxide
PE	pulmonary embolism
PEEP	positive end expiratory pressure
PKD	polycystic kidney disease
PNS	peripheral nervous system
pO_2	partial pressure of oxygen
PONV	postoperative nausea and vomiting
RA	right atrium
RBC	red blood cell
RCT	randomised controlled trial
RHD	rheumatic heart disease
RSI	rapid sequence induction
SaO_2	saturation level of arterial oxyhaemoglobin
SBO	small bowel obstruction
SIRS	systemic inflammatory response syndrome
SOB	shortness of breath
SpO_2	oxygen saturation measured by a pulse oximeter

SVA	supraventricular arrhythmia
SVT	supraventricular tachycardia
T	temperature
TAH	total abdominal hysterectomy
TB	tuberculosis
TBI	traumatic brain injury
TGA	transient global amnesia
TIA	transient ischaemic attack
TIMI	thrombolysis in myocardial infarction
TIVA	total intravenous anaesthesia
TURP	transurethral resection of prostate
TVR	tricuspid valve replacement
TVV	tricuspid valve valvuloplasty (valve repair)
UA	urinalysis
UE	upper extremity
UFH	unfractionated heparin
UO	urine output
URI	upper respiratory infection
UTI	urinary tract infection
VCO_2	carbon dioxide production
VF	ventricular fibrillation
VHD	valvular heart disease
VO_2	oxygen consumption
VS	vital signs
VT	ventricular tachycardia
WB	whole blood
WBC	white blood cell

SECTION 1

Preoperative Preparation

Paul Wicker

1 The Role of the Anaesthetic Practitioner

An anaesthetic practitioner is an essential member of the operating department team working alongside anaesthetists, surgeons, practitioners and healthcare support workers to ensure that anaesthesia for the patient is as safe and effective as possible. Anaesthetic practitioners provide high standards of patient care and skilled support alongside the other members of the perioperative team during the perioperative phases before, during and after surgery (Fynes *et al.* 2014). It is also essential that they continue with updates and attend current in-house training to maintain their skills and knowledge.

The role of the anaesthetic practitioner has nationally agreed standards and levels of practice, implemented by the Royal College of Anaesthetists (RCA 2006). An anaesthetic practitioner's roles are also covered by the College of Operating Department Practitioners and the Health Care Professions Council. Hospital regulations manage these standards appropriately and are implemented within a nationally recognised framework (Fynes *et al.* 2014).

The roles and responsibilities of anaesthetic practitioners include working by themselves to prepare equipment and providing care for the patient, as well as offering support to the anaesthetist during all stages of anaesthesia (Fynes *et al.* 2014). The main roles and responsibilities of the anaesthetic practitioner include:

- To deliver psychological and emotional support to the patient
- To check the anaesthetic machine
- To prepare the anaesthetic equipment
- To support the patient throughout the stages of anaesthesia
- To support the anaesthetist during anaesthesia
- To understand responsibility and accountability for the patient during anaesthesia, including patient documentation, for example the consent form and the World Health Organization (WHO) Surgical Safety Checklist.

Preanaesthetic phase

The anaesthetic practitioner assists the patient before surgery and provides individualised care. This will include supporting the patient by reducing anxiety, placing blood pressure cuffs, connecting electrocardiograph (ECG) electrodes and pulse oximeters, and preparing IV fluids and anaesthetic drugs (NHS Modernisation Agency 2005). The practitioner will also communicate effectively within the team to pass on problems, issues or any past adverse events, such as when catheterising patients and when preparing and assisting in the safe insertion of invasive physiological monitoring such as central venous pressure (CVP) lines and arterial lines.

The anaesthetic practitioner is also able to support the patient if he or she has any concerns. For example, most patients fear anaesthesia, because of fearing the risk of waking

Rapid Perioperative Care, First Edition. Paul Wicker and Sara Dalby.

up too early or not waking up following surgical procedures. Many patients ask, 'Will I wake up alright after surgery?' and then become anxious if they don't receive a reply. One of the main roles is therefore to provide psychological support, which is something that practitioners can do on a face-to-face basis. This may include discussing problems, offering reassurance to the patient to let them know they are monitored safely, ensuring the patient is comfortable, talking to the patient and reassuring the patient throughout their time in theatre (Fynes *et al.* 2014).

The anaesthetic practitioner will also undertake roles which will also involve many clinical skills, such as preparing a wide range of specialist equipment and drugs (Copley 2006). This includes:

- Testing anaesthetic machines
- Preparing anaesthetic equipment (AAGBI 2012)
- Preparing intravenous equipment
- Making devices available to safely secure the patient's airway during anaesthesia
- Ensuring drugs such as propofol, local anaesthetics, anaesthetic gases and so on are available
- Knowledge of the different operating tables, including positioning equipment, clamps and pressure-relieving devices.

Anaesthesia

There are three parts to anaesthesia:

1. *Induction*: This is when the patient goes to sleep using anaesthetic drugs.
2. *Maintenance*: This is maintaining the anaesthetic during surgery.
3. *Reversal*: This is wakening the patient up by stopping the administration of drugs and anaesthetic gases, or by using specialist drugs to revive the patient (Goodman & Spry 2014).

Responsibility of the practitioner for the care of the patient throughout the stages of anaesthesia is vitally important (Fynes *et al.* 2014). The practitioner is responsible for ensuring the patient is positioned correctly to maintain safety and comfort, to ensure pressure areas are supported, and also to provide maximum access during the operative procedure. The practitioner also needs to follow legal and ethical considerations, and ensure that they are following the Health and Care Professions Council (HCPC) regulations and guidelines.

Checking the anaesthetic machine

Making sure the anaesthetic machine is working correctly is an essential part of the anaesthetic practitioner's role, in collaboration with the anaesthetist. Knowing 'how' it works is of course equally important (Goodman & Spry 2014). During induction of anaesthesia, the patient is at one of the most vulnerable points in his or her perioperative care. Equipment error can therefore put the patient at high risk of harm, for example through airway obstruction, circulatory problems, reduced blood oxygenation or even death, because of errors such as flow reversal though the back bar on the anaesthetic machine (Smith *et al.* 2007).

Practitioners should check the anaesthetic machines by using the Association of Anaesthetists of Great Britain and Northern Ireland checklist (AAGBI 2012) and the manufacturer's manual as guides to ensure the machine is safe to use. There is a joint responsibility between the anaesthetist and anaesthetic assistant for ensuring the correct functioning of anaesthetic equipment before patient use. Often, the anaesthetic assistant will assemble and check the equipment in preparation for the anaesthetist, who then ensures that he or she has the correct equipment for the anaesthetic procedure. The assistant's role is therefore to support the anaesthetist, check the equipment and ensure the patient's safety (Wicker & Smith 2008).

Errors during anaesthesia have often been associated with lack of proper equipment checks. However, checking an anaesthetic machine using a checklist can lead to a reduction of incidents. Patient safety can be increased by the use of the checklist for checking new anaesthetic machines which can highlight faults during their manufacture. For example, wrong assembly of the anaesthetic machine can lead to errors such as high dosages of volatile agents. The use of a checklist also needs to be carried out when equipment is returned from servicing – it cannot be guaranteed that a serviced or brand-new anaesthetic machine is working perfectly. A thorough check will therefore ensure the equipment has been returned in a working condition and is ready for use. However, it is not the ultimate responsibility of the anaesthetic practitioner to ensure the anaesthetic machine is in perfect working order; it is the anaesthetist who carries the main responsibility. Nonetheless, practitioners have a duty of care to identify and report any faults and are also responsible for their actions, including recordkeeping of anaesthetic machine checks (Fynes *et al.* 2014).

Monitoring responsibilities

The anaesthetic practitioner's responsibility is to attach two ECG electrodes to the patient's upper left and right-sided chest, and one ECG electrode to the lower left side of the chest, before anaesthesia so heart rate and rhythm are monitored by the ECG monitor during induction of anaesthesia. There are many other areas to monitor, and three of the most important are blood pressure, oxygen saturation and temperature.

Non-invasive blood pressure (NIBP) measurement

NIBP is measured by using a blood pressure cuff which is fastened around the arm or leg. The air tube is then attached to the monitor which inflates and deflates the cuff according to the time settings. The blood pressure reading is displayed on the monitor and registers the systolic, mean and diastolic pressures. Normally, the monitor records all measurements over time and provides a trend to indicate when the blood pressure has risen or fallen. Invasive blood pressure monitoring equipment is also used to provide a continuous record of blood pressure. This normally works by connecting a monitor to a transducer which in turn is connected to an intra-arterial line (O'Neill 2010).

Attaching the blood pressure cuff around the patient's arm monitors blood pressure and will ensure that blood pressure is maintained at the correct level. Anaesthetic drugs can reduce or increase blood pressure because of vasoconstriction, vasodilation or effects on the heart, so it is important that blood pressure is constantly monitored.

Pulse oximeters

A pulse oximeter measures the patient's oxygen saturation in their blood. Normal oxygen saturation is between 95 and 100%; anything less than 95% is seen as causing problems for the patient. Patients with chronic obstructive pulmonary disease (COPD) may also suffer from hypoxia. The pulse oximeter is normally attached to a finger, but it can also be attached to an earlobe or toe. The light source in the probe passes through the tissue, and the patient's oxygen concentration is measured via the absorption of the light, then recorded on the monitoring screen (O'Neill 2010). The light is detected by light sensors and is altered by the levels of oxyhaemoglobin and deoxyhaemoglobin. The pulse oximeter should be regularly checked to ensure that it is correctly placed on the extremity and also that circulation at that point is not impaired. Constantly observing the patient's oxygen levels is essential during anaesthesia, and using a pulse oximeter is one of the most important monitors used during anaesthesia as it can help to identify patient problems associated with low oxygen levels (Valdez-Lowe *et al.* 2009).

Conclusion

Anaesthetic practitioners have the potential to contribute to team working, and this results in enhancing patient care and patient access, improving operating room capacity and reducing cancellations and waiting times. Practitioners can also enhance the learning experiences of anaesthetic trainees and other junior anaesthetic practitioners.

2 The Role of the Surgical Practitioner

The surgical practitioner role includes preparing the operating room, scrubbing and circulating as well as contributing to the WHO checklist (see Chapter 7). Scrubbing involves working within the sterile field to assist the surgeon and being responsible for delivery of instruments and equipment. The circulator, or runner, provides the link between the scrub nurse and the non-sterile areas outside the surgical field. Circulators are also able to provide equipment needed for the surgical team such as sutures, swabs or prostheses. Circulating staff also assist in preparing the patient for surgery. This includes moving the patient onto the operating table, exposing the surgical site and connecting the patient to equipment that is necessary for surgery, such as the electrosurgery machine or suction machine. As the surgical team are unable to leave the operating table during surgery, the circulator provides communication between the surgical team and the rest of the theatre department, wards or laboratories (Conway *et al.* 2014).

Scrub practitioners are operating department practitioners (ODPs) or post registration nurses. ODPs are now more common in the operating room because the BSc (Hons) ODP programmes educate and train practitioners in all three roles in the operating department – anaesthetics, surgery and recovery. Preregistration nurses often observe in operating departments as they may not have the skills and knowledge needed to work in anaesthesia or surgery. Following their qualification, nurses may undertake CPD modules in anaesthesia, surgery and recovery to gain the necessary perioperative skills and knowledge.

Scrub practitioners need an understanding of operating room procedures, including the instruments and equipment needed for surgery, and must remain calm and clear-headed, even when under pressure because of, for example, urgent surgery. Practitioners communicate well when working with surgeons and aiding them during the surgery (Wicker & Nightingale 2010).

Surgical practitioners provide patient care before, during and after surgical procedures. Surgical practitioners must therefore be registered by the HCPC or Nursing & Midwifery Council (NMC), and have the necessary surgical expertise. When scrub practitioners assist the surgeon, it can be demanding, challenging and sometimes exciting, but circulating practitioners are also essential to provide support to the surgical team.

Scrub practitioners

The role of scrub practitioners is to ensure the best, safest and most effective care for the patient by supporting and aiding surgeons during the surgical procedure (Smith 2005). To undertake this role, they must have knowledge and skills related to patient care, anatomy and physiology, surgery, and the instruments and equipment needed for the procedure. Experienced scrub practitioners prepare equipment and instruments before the start of surgery and support the surgeon throughout the procedure. Inexperienced

Rapid Perioperative Care, First Edition. Paul Wicker and Sara Dalby.

scrub practitioners, however, need support from mentors or colleagues during surgery as inefficiency may lead to delays or serious errors with instrument handling and use.

Before surgery

Surgical practitioners clean and prepare the operating room before surgery, including organising instruments and equipment for surgery. Scrub practitioners preserve the sterile environment by scrubbing hands and arms with betadine or chlorhexidine, and putting on suitable sterile surgical garments which include a gown, mask and gloves (Gruendemann & Fernsebner 1995). The scrub practitioner will prepare, check the function of and count the instruments and equipment before the patient arrives in the operating room to ensure everything is ready for the surgeon to commence surgery. The surgical practitioner will ask the circulator to show them the consent form with the correct procedure and patient identification number. The circulator will also identify any patient allergies and the correct equipment, for example if they are operating on a specific limb that needs left or right-sided tools.

When the surgeons arrive and start surgical scrubbing, the circulating practitioners may help them don their gown and gloves before exposing the patient for the surgical procedure.

During surgery

The main role of the scrub practitioner during surgery is to provide a quick, safe and effective procedure by selecting and passing instruments and swabs ready for the surgeon to receive. The practitioner may also support the surgeon during surgery by cutting sutures or other minor tasks (Smith 2005). Scrub practitioners must have knowledge and understanding of the surgical procedure, the patient's anatomy and the instruments which are required for specific procedures so they can quickly pass them over to the surgeon (Conway 2014). The scrub practitioner also needs to watch the procedure carefully to prepare instruments in advance. The practitioner should also retrieve instruments that the surgeon has stopped using, as these can sometimes fall off the operating table onto the floor. Also important is the need to keep track of any samples of tissues, as the surgeon can hand out many samples from different parts of the surgical site in quick succession, which must be kept separate. The scrub practitioner will then clean the instruments after use and place each instrument back in its place on the instrument trolley. If required, the scrub practitioner will ask for other instruments or items from the circulating practitioners.

After surgery

Scrub practitioners count all instruments, sponges, swabs and other tools and verbally communicate to the surgeon in regards to the count once surgery is completed. It is essential that swabs are counted so that they are not left inside the patient (D'Lima 2014). Scrub practitioners then remove instruments and equipment from the operating area, assist the surgeon in applying a dressing to the surgical site and accompany the patient to the recovery area to inform recovery staff of the procedure, dressings, suction drains and so on (Wicker & Nightingale 2010). Scrub practitioners also complete necessary documentation about the surgery in the surgical record book and input relevant information into the computer.

Circulating practitioners

Circulating practitioners create and preserve a clean and sterile operating room environment in preparation for treating patients before surgery. Having a clean and safe environment will promote health for staff and prevent patients from acquiring infections following surgery (Goodman & Spry 2014). Perioperative practitioners may also undertake pre and

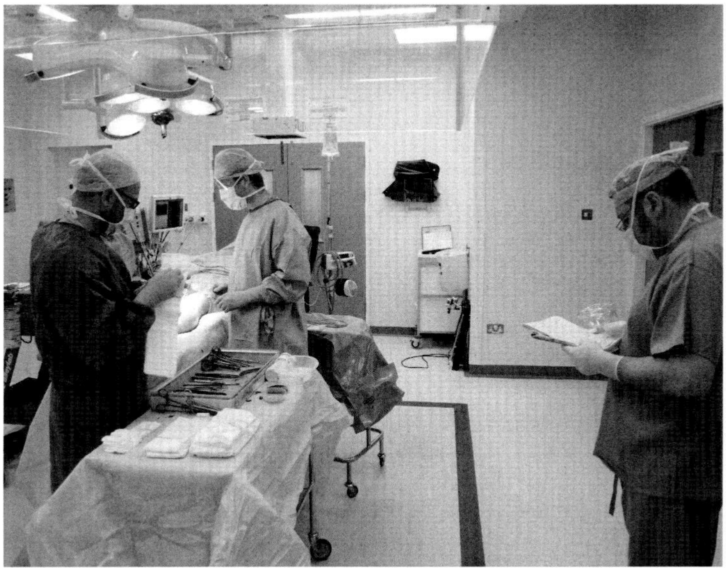

Photo 1 Carrying out the WHO checklist. Courtesy of Aintree Hospital, Liverpool

postoperative assessments of patients, and it is also important that they support, care and educate patients about their surgical treatment before and after surgery.

The circulating practitioner is also responsible for setting up the operating room before a surgical procedure gets underway (Goodman & Spry 2014). This role includes checking disposables, such as pads, swabs and sutures; laying out instrument trays; preparing equipment, such as diathermy and suction machines; and preparing any other equipment needed. The circulating practitioner also checks all equipment needed during the procedure to verify that it is functioning properly. When the patient arrives in the OR, the circulating practitioner usually verifies the patient's identity and necessary consent forms. This includes showing the consent to the surgical practitioner, and then reviewing the site and nature of the procedure with the surgeon (Goodman & Spry 2014).

Theatre practitioners clean and maintain the operating room and inform the surgical team of anything that may be contaminated before the start of surgery. They are also responsible for opening sterile packages, so the surgical team may easily access the sterile equipment without becoming contaminated (Goodman & Spry 2014). However, they must always avoid touching the sterile field, for example the instrument trolley or the drapes covering the patient, because they do not scrub or wear sterile gloves or a gown. The circulating practitioners and other members of the surgical team also position the patient correctly and safely on the operating table. The circulating practitioner connects any necessary equipment, such as suction and diathermy, and liaises with the surgeon about his or her needs. During the operation, the circulating practitioner provides the surgical team with sterile fluids and medications as required and renews the surgical team's supplies if they need more sterile drapes or instruments. Each member of the surgical team has specific personal responsibilities, including maintaining an overview of the patient's condition. For example, if an arm or leg accidently falls off the operating table, then this is one of the circulating practitioner's responsibilities to prevent it from happening, or to replace the arm or leg in a safe position (Wicker & Nightingale 2010).

Outside of surgery, perioperative practitioners also play a role in patient care before and after procedures, including the initiation of the WHO checklist (Photo 1). Before surgery, a practitioner draws up the patient's plan of care and spends time to document and record any allergies or other health-related issues. After surgery, theatre practitioners complete the WHO checklist and patient care plan, and the circulating practitioner helps the scrub practitioner and other staff to clean the room and prepare it for the next surgical procedure (Wicker & Nightingale 2010).

3 The Role of the Recovery Practitioner

The three perioperative roles in the operating department are anaesthetic, surgery and recovery practitioners. The recovery practitioner is seen as an autonomous practitioner because anaesthetic and surgical practitioners assist medical staff, but recovery practitioners work mostly on their own initiative and with each other. Hospitals have a clear separation between the recovery unit and the operating room because the patient has completed anaesthesia and surgery on entry to the recovery room, or PACU (post-anaesthesia care unit). Although the recovery room is still seen to be part of the patient's perioperative experience, theatre and recovery practitioners remain two separate groups of staff. While recovery practitioners do understand anaesthesia and surgery, they are more focussed on the postoperative care of patients and their recovery from their anaesthetic and surgical procedures. In some situations, however, theatre practitioners may be asked to work in all areas of the operating department.

The role of practitioners in recovery

The role of recovery practitioners involves one-to-one care of patients who have undergone a procedure under general, regional or local anaesthetic (Hatfield & Tronson 2009). Patients in recovery range from small elective cases to complicated emergency procedures, and post-operative care varies in individuality and depth of skills, knowledge and experience needed to afford the best possible care (Alfaro 2013).

The skills undertaken by postoperative practitioners in the recovery area are complex and include the following:

- Managing the patient's airway (Alfaro 2013)
- Pain management
- High-quality patient care
- Knowledge of anatomy and physiology, as well as recognising symptoms such as shock or internal bleeding
- Monitoring pulse rate, respiratory rate, oxygen saturation, temperature and blood pressure (Hatfield & Tronson 2009)
- Care of wounds and dressings
- Helping with mobility
- Adequate blood circulation
- Fluid and electrolyte maintenance
- Treating nausea and vomiting
- Providing verbal support and reassurance to patients
- Documenting observations, consciousness, drugs, pain levels and so on
- Providing information to ward staff during handover of patient.

Rapid Perioperative Care, First Edition. Paul Wicker and Sara Dalby.

Admission to recovery

In some hospitals, the recovery practitioner will enter the operating room and escort the patient to recovery alongside the anaesthetist and the scrub practitioner. The recovery practitioner must ensure the correct equipment is available for the patient, including an oxygen cylinder attached to the trolley and connected to the patient using a Hudson mask, and an anaesthetic circuit for an intubated patient (AAGBI 2013). There should also be a suction unit in case the patient vomits during the transfer to the recovery area.

On admission to recovery, the recovery practitioner will receive information from the scrub practitioner about surgery and the anaesthetist about the patient's status following anaesthesia and the medicines which have been administered, as well as further medication which may be required (Hatfield & Tronson 2009). Examples of the scrub practitioner's handover include:

- The surgical procedure
- The wound closure, dressings and surgical drains
- Confirmation of the presence (or not) of a urinary catheter
- Issues about pressure sores, pain, disabilities and so on
- Allergies
- Local anaesthetic drugs that have been in use.

The anaesthetist will also cover all areas including:

- The patient's name and the type of anaesthesia used
- Any relevant medical history, for example diabetes or dementia
- Analgesia administered during surgery and the patient's needs post anaesthesia
- Fluid and electrolyte balance and any need for further IV fluids.

The anaesthetist will also support the recovery practitioner for a short time in recovery. This will include assessing the patient to ensure he or she is breathing regularly, airways are intact, oxygen saturation is stable, circulation is stable (blood pressure and pulse) and the patient is recovering safely (Alfaro 2013). The anaesthetist will also stay with the patient if there are any continuing problems.

Initial assessment of a patient

On arrival in recovery, the oxygen tube is transferred to the oxygen supply attached to the wall. The oxygen delivered will depend on the patient's level of consciousness at the discretion of the anaesthetist (AAGBI 2013). O_2 flow is monitored using the flow meter which is attached to the wall. The fraction of inspired oxygen (FiO_2) inhaled by the patient is lower than the flow rate. For example, a flow rate of 5 L per minute normally delivers approximately 0.4 L per minute to the patient, depending on the methods of delivery, including different masks or nasal cannula.

Once the patient is receiving an acceptable quantity of oxygen, he or she will then be connected to monitors, including:

- *ECG monitor*: monitors pulse, rate and rhythm
- *Blood pressure*: automatic blood pressure cuff attached to upper arm
- *Oxygen saturation*: pulse oximeter
- *Respiratory rate*: normally, a maximum of 12–20 breaths per minute
- *Temperature*: These measurements should be recorded regularly.

Other monitors may also be required depending on the surgery undertaken and the physiological status of the patient.

Sometimes, a patient is admitted to recovery with an endotracheal tube (ET) tube still in place. If this is the case, the anaesthetist will need equipment to remove the ET tube once the patient wakes up, for example by using suction, a face mask and a syringe to remove air from the cuff of the ET tube. This is also undertaken by recovery staff in some hospitals where training has been undertaken.

Under most circumstances, an ABCDE approach is used to assess patients during their recovery (Hatfield & Tronson 2009). This assessment consists of:

A = Airway
B = Breathing
C = Circulation
D = Disability
E = Exposure.

Practitioners use this method of assessment continuously while the patient is in the recovery room to ensure safe patient care. Care for patients, however, depends upon the needs of the patient and the procedures they have undergone, and so care is individualised depending on their needs (AAGBI 2013). For example, surgery on limbs will need consistent monitoring of circulation, sensations felt by the patient, and their ability to move fingers or toes.

Documentation needs to be completed and recorded clearly, accurately and concisely to ensure that records are kept of the patient's recovery period. Recovery charts differ between hospitals, but most contain the following basic items:

- The time the patient entered the unit
- Vital signs
- Drugs given, including dose and route
- Unexpected events, such as vomiting or sudden onset of pain
- Specific postoperative instructions (e.g. oxygen therapy for the ward)
- Records are signed and dated by the recovery practitioner.

Discharge of patient

Normally following an hour in the recovery room, if the patient has recovered fully then they are discharged (Hatfield & Tronson 2009). Sometimes patients may be discharged within 20 min, especially those undergoing day surgery or minor surgery. However, they must meet the minimum criteria, dependent on their state of health and the hospital regulations:

- Maintaining the patient's airway
- Stable blood pressure, pulse and rhythm
- Conscious and able to uphold a 5-sec head lift
- Oxygen saturation greater than 95%
- No pain, nausea or vomiting
- Clean, dry and warm
- All documentation is completed and signed.

The recovery practitioner prepares the patient for returning to the ward and contacts ward staff to come and collect the patient. In some circumstances, however, the recovery practitioner may return the patient to their ward if ward staff are not available. Once the ward nurse arrives, the recovery practitioner will hand over all the relevant documentation and verbally communicate to the ward nurse of the anaesthetic and surgical procedures. Also the practitioner will hand over postoperative instructions given by the anaesthetist, the analgesia which the patient has received and the vital sign recordings taken in the recovery room. The ward nurse will then accept that the patient is ready to be handed over, sign the form and escort the patient safely back to the ward.

4 Preoperative Assessment of Perioperative Patients

Introduction

Pre-assessment of perioperative patients is essential to prepare patients for anaesthesia, surgery and recovery, and to ensure that they understand the anaesthetic and surgical procedures, as well as their postoperative recovery period. This role can be carried out by operating department practitioners and nurses. Practitioners also need to understand the physiological status of the patient so they can communicate this information to perioperative staff (including anaesthetists, surgeons and perioperative practitioners) and inform them of any patient issues. This chapter covers preoperative assessment, planning and education, and reducing intraoperative and postoperative complications.

Ensuring that surgical patients are prepared prior to surgery increases their safety and improves their surgical outcomes. Practitioners become involved in preoperative patient care because of their capacity to assess the individual needs of a patient before anaesthesia and surgery (Holmes 2005).

The perioperative patient is subject to many stressors that can induce anxiety, for example:

- Threats to their sense of identity
- Fear of dying or not waking up
- Fear of the surgical procedure
- Delay in surgery or change of anaesthetists.

Practitioners can help the patient during these times because of their knowledge and skills, as well as their work with other professional colleagues within both the ward and the operating department. Practitioners therefore carry out preoperative assessment, education and care as necessary parts of the patient's treatment (Goodman & Spry 2014). Pre-assessment clinics also support the multidisciplinary team in undertaking preoperative medical and patient assessments.

Preoperative preparation

Care plans for patients are a key part of today's care for perioperative patients (Table 4.1, 'Care planning'). Several key elements of care planning may involve:

- *Preoperative education*: Including communication with the patient and information regarding anaesthesia, surgical procedure, pain relief, surgical techniques, preoperative actions, postoperative analgesia, postoperative vomiting and postoperative exercises (Wicker 2010).
- *Preoperative assessment*: Including status of elderly patients, concurrent illnesses, physiological status of the patient and injuries that trauma patients may have suffered.

Rapid Perioperative Care, First Edition. Paul Wicker and Sara Dalby.

Table 4.1 Care planning

Hospitals develop individualised care plans which help practitioners deliver the care required in an organised and effective way. The assessment process for preoperative and postoperative care often involves the following stages.

Assessment on entry to the ward

Patient details:

- Name:
- Patient number:
- Surgical procedure:
- Ward:
- Verification of operative site:

Walking to the operating department:

- Has the patient taken sedation on admission:
- Does the patient have a history of instability:
- Does the patient have a history of dizziness:
- Does the patient need a mobility aid to walk:

Baseline observations:

- Pulse:
- Blood pressure:
- Urine output:
- Height:
- Respiration rate:
- Temperature:
- Weight:
- Waterlow Score:
- Hearing aid:
- Skin integrity:

Ward preoperative checklist (immediately before the patient leaves the ward for surgery)

Confirm the following:

Patient details:
Consent form:
Allergies:
Intended surgical site verified and marked:
Blood results are valid and recorded:
ECG recorded:
Fasted as per hospital guidelines:
Pre-medication given:
Anticoagulants given:
Contact lenses and jewellery removed:
Dentures removed:
Caps crowns or bridges present:
Makeup and nail varnish removed:
Pacemaker in situ:
Patient placed on trolley safely:
Pregnancy test:

Signature of ward nurse:

Operating theatre reception confirmations

Blood results are valid and completed:
Ward preop care planning checklist completed:
Confirm patient's details:
Consent form present and completed:
Allergies:

Signature of theatre practitioner:

Further comments:

(continued overleaf)

Table 4.1 (*continued*)

Postoperative checklist
Care assessment on admission to recovery
Airway support:
- None
- Oral
- Nasal tube
- Endotracheal tube
- Laryngeal mask
- Tracheostomy

Breathing:
- Respiration rate and quality:
- Oxygen levels:
  - Venti masks
  - Ventilator
  - Nasal specs
  - Breathing circuit
  - Temperature
  - Oxygen saturation

Circulation:
- Arterial line inserted:
- Central venous pressure lines:
- Skin or mucous membrane:
  - Flushed
  - Pale
  - Cyanosis
  - Pink
  - Warm
  - Dry
  - Cool
  - Moist
  - Clammy

Intravenous therapies – specify:
Bladder irrigation – specify:
Other:
Comments:

Recovery Room Observations
CVP:
Temperature:
SpO_2:
- Litres per minute:

Blood pressure:
Pulse:
Respiration:
Pupil reactions to light:
Muscle tone (ability to move limbs):
Wound condition:
Drains:
Peripheral perfusion:
Other observations:

Perioperative drugs given to the patient:
- Fentanyl plus local anaesthetic:
- Spinal anaesthetic:
- Plain local anaesthetic:
- Other analgesics:
- Anti-emetics:

(*continued overleaf*)

Table 4.1 (*continued*)

Recovery room care given:
Progress and actions taken:

Recovery evaluation and handover information:
All information given to ward nurse on discharge of patient, including:

- Airways
- Respiration
- Cardiovascular status
- Medications given
- Comfort and safety
- Wound management
- Fluid management
- Anaesthetic and surgical procedures
- Time of discharge from recovery.

- *Informed consent*: Including information about the anaesthesia and surgery before completion of the consent form. The consent policies and procedures of the hospital, underpinned by legal practices, help to ensure patient safety and involve the patient in their proposed treatment and care (Wicker 2015).
- *Patient preparation before surgery*: Including confirmation of preoperative fasting guidelines, not smoking, use of DVT (deep venous thrombosis) stockings, use of patient gown and hat, and confirmation of patient details on the wristband (Goodman & Spry 2014).
- *Discharge planning*: This happens either before or after surgery, depending on the length of the patient's stay. Discharge planning should cover such areas as pain relief, mobilisation exercises, dressing changes, postoperative drugs and identifying and managing possible postoperative complications.

Reducing postoperative complications

There are several postoperative complications which can occur following surgery and anaesthesia, and preoperative assessment and planning can help to prevent these complications from happening. Actions also need to be undertaken by recovery practitioners when patients suffer from postoperative complications during recovery.

Respiratory care

Practitioners undertake preoperative airway assessment (Sweitzer 2008) by assessing the patient's airway and breathing patterns and any problems which the patient identifies. Practitioners will also support anaesthetists by reducing the risk of intraoperative airway problems, achieving best airway management and recording information for intraoperative use (Sweitzer 2008).

- Pre-assessment of respiratory function lessens the risk of chest infection following surgery.
- Assess the patient's respiration, for example breathing rate, sputum and secretions, cardiovascular status and pulse oximetry.
- Direct patients should be instructed not to smoke before or after surgery.
- Drug therapy, such as antibiotics or bronchial dilators, may be given preoperatively.
- Teach the patient breathing exercises and good positioning when in bed (Wicker 2015).

Joint stiffness

Patients who have stiff joints may need support during surgery (Wicker 2010); for example, a stiff neck makes intubation difficult. It is also painful for a patient with a stiff hip to be placed in the lithotomy position, and an arm placed on an arm board, especially if the arm is pushed towards the head, may damage the brachial plexus (Wicker 2010).

- Pre-assessment and understanding of a patient's joints which are stiff or damaged are important before surgery.
- Practitioners who pre-assess patients should inform perioperative staff about patients who have stiff joints to prevent harm during surgery.

Urinary problems

Urinary tract infection can lead to prolonged postoperative recovery due to discomfort and surgical complications (Berger 2005). Education is necessary about the need to maintain good fluid intake and follow medical orders on fluid balance. Maintaining postoperative fluid intake is also important to prevent further urinary and renal problems (Goodman & Spry 2014).

- Preoperatively, catheters need to be inserted carefully, following agreed sterile techniques to prevent colonisation postoperatively.
- Patients require information in regards to maintaining good fluid intake and following medical orders on fluid balance to prevent further urinary and renal problems (Wicker 2015).
- Pre and postoperative assessment and recording of urine output must also be undertaken.

Pressure sores

The presence of pressure sores results in an extended stay in hospital and causes distress to patients (Schultz 2005).

Practitioners can use pressure sore assessment scales, the most common being the updated Waterlow Scale (Waterlow 1985), to assess risk factors for developing pressure sores. If the patient receives a high score, then this is an indication of the potential for skin damage and ward nurses need to carry out suitable preventive measures to protect the patient (Wicker 2015).

- Pre-assessment of the patient's likelihood of developing pressure sores is important to prevent patient harm.
- Pressure sores occur because of excessive pressure leading to reduced blood supply and tissue hypoxia.
- Patients at risk include the elderly, patients undergoing long surgical procedures, patients with concurrent illness and poor health, and those with reduced mobility.
- Risk factors in assessment scales include age, gender, smoking history, nutritional status, mobility, build, medication, incontinence, existing vascular diseases and proposed duration of the surgical procedure.
- Pressure-relieving devices and techniques include a low-pressure mattress and frequent changes of position while on the ward.
- The perioperative team should be informed of the need for the patient to be protected during surgery by using gel pads and careful positioning.

Deep venous thrombosis

DVT can affect between 15 and 40% of perioperative patients undergoing general surgery (Mood & Tang 2009). Pre-assessment of the risk of DVT will provide the patient with suitable treatment before and during surgery (Nelson *et al.* 2008) (Table 4.2).

DVT assessment tools often contain several risk factors, including age, body mass, mobility, trauma risk, disease and type of surgical intervention (Wicker 2015). Patients at risk of DVTs are identified in low, medium or high-risk categories, and treatment given may

Table 4.2 Deep venous thrombosis

Practitioners can pre-assess factors contributing to DVT development and minimise the risks to the patient during surgery. Reduce the likelihood of DVT by:

- Pre-assessing the patient for the possibility of developing DVT
- Encouraging the patient to wear GCS before surgery
- Avoiding abnormal leg positioning
- Avoiding extreme degrees of leg rotation
- Performing passive limb exercises if required
- Encouraging movement if the patient is confined to a bed
- Encouraging walking if the patient is fit to do so
- Placing a patient susceptible to DVT in a leg-up position to encourage venous drainage
- Avoiding placing the patient in a limb-down position to reduce the risk of lower limb oedema leading to venous stagnation and vascular damage
- Ensuring the patient at risk of DVT receives heparin and warfarin, aspirin, dextran or other anticoagulants.

include graduated compression stockings (GCS), heparin or intermittent pneumatic compression therapy (IPCT) (Nelson *et al.* 2008, Mood & Tang 2009). Most wards now have protocols in place for DVT prophylaxis to help protect patients from this condition.

- Preoperative assessment of blood circulation can help to reduce the incidence of DVT and pulmonary embolism.
- Reasons leading to DVT include endothelial damage to blood vessels, long periods of immobility leading to venous stagnation; medication which affects clotting mechanisms (e.g. contraceptive pills), dehydration, pregnancy and nephritic syndrome.
- Treatment to prevent DVT can include:
  - *Low risk*: GCS
  - *Moderate risk*: GCS plus low-dose heparin
  - *High risk*: GCS, adjusted dose of heparin and IPCT.

Nausea and vomiting

Preoperative assessment of patients can identify patients who are susceptible to PONV (postoperative nausea and vomiting), since PONV occurs in many surgical patients (Wicker & Cox 2010). PONV is treated with anti-emetics which antagonise the various neurotransmitter systems which cause nausea and vomiting. Careful pre-assessment of the likelihood of nausea and vomiting occurring will also help ensure the patient receives effective treatment (Wicker & Cox 2010). For example, a previous episode of PONV can highlight the need to include a preoperative anti-emetic.

- Preoperative assessment of patients can identify patients who are susceptible to PONV.
- Patient education is important as many patients believe that nausea and vomiting are caused by anaesthesia.
- Risk factors that can cause PONV include extreme anxiety, faulty preoperative fasting and a history of seasickness or motion sickness.
- PONV can result in aspiration of stomach contents into the lungs, damage to wound sites caused by straining, and electrolyte imbalances (Wicker 2015).
- PONV is treated by using anti-emetics, such as haloperidol, ondansetron, metoclopramide and cyclizine. Acupuncture can also be used in certain circumstances.
- PONV can also be treated by reducing anxiety through communication with the patient and by alleviating pain.

Pain

Assessing and educating patients about pain relief and the use of analgesics will support patients following surgery (Wicker & Cox 2010). Practitioners need to inform patients about the approaches to pain treatment and the support that they can offer following surgery to reduce pain (Wicker & Cox 2010).

Acute Pain Services (APS) educate patients and ward nurses about pain management. APS also provide preoperative and postoperative information and care for patients, including patient-controlled analgesia and epidural infusions.

- Practitioners should inform patients preoperatively about the approaches to pain treatment and the support that they can offer following surgery, to reduce patient anxiety and postoperative pain.
- Medical drugs may be given to the patient postoperatively at the discretion of the anaesthetist. Pain killers can include opiates, NSAIDS (nonsteroidal anti-inflammatory drugs) and other drugs (Wicker 2015).
- APS can also provide preoperative and postoperative information and care for patients.

5 Perioperative Patient Care

The word *perioperative* refers to the patient's total surgical experience which includes the pre-, intra- and postoperative phases, from the time the patient arrives in reception to the time they leave the recovery area.

Preoperative visiting

Preoperative visiting has been available for many years, although the recent changes in the NHS and a fall in perioperative staff has made this more difficult to carry out. However, in the past both ODPs and nurses from operating theatres would carry out preoperative visiting to assess, identify and de-stress patients before they arrived in the operating department. Research over the years has shown that visiting patients can improve their overall care in the operating theatre, thereby reducing potential problems. Preoperative visits enable practitioners to develop a care pathway plan prior to the patient arriving in the department (Wicker & O'Neill 2010). Even today, some hospitals recommend preoperative visiting in order to reduce patient anxiety regarding the proposed treatment and to demonstrate high levels of patient care and safety.

In the modern NHS, patients often stay in hospital for less time, and most patients are admitted for surgery less than 24 h before surgery starts. Day surgery patients are also increasing, and they usually arrive and leave on the same day.

Because of the decrease in patient time and the decrease in staffing, preoperative visits by theatre staff would still contribute to the continuity of care. However, pre-admission/assessment clinics are now common in most hospitals and help to prepare the patient for surgery (Phillips 2004). It is therefore essential that there is good communication between preadmission clinics and the perioperative staff to ensure the patient's individual needs are identified and met.

Patient preparation

Preparing the perioperative environment starts before the patient arrives. Information is recovered by the theatre staff from the operating theatre list, which is provided daily before scheduled elective surgical lists. The theatre list provides the patient's name, age, gender and planned procedure, enabling practitioners to prepare the operating room (OR) to provide a safe environment (Goodman & Spry 2014). For example, this will involve (Wicker & O'Neill 2010):

- Preparing the correct airway equipment
- Preparing the operating table and positioning equipment
- Preparing equipment to offset patient allergies, for example a latex allergy
- Pressure area care, for example heel supports, shoulder roll, gel mattress or head ring
- Preparing equipment for immobility problems, for example stiff legs or arms
- Preparing for hearing problems, for example if the patient is undergoing local anaesthetic
- Reviewing the medical history, for example preparing drugs to prevent postoperative vomiting.

Rapid Perioperative Care, First Edition. Paul Wicker and Sara Dalby.

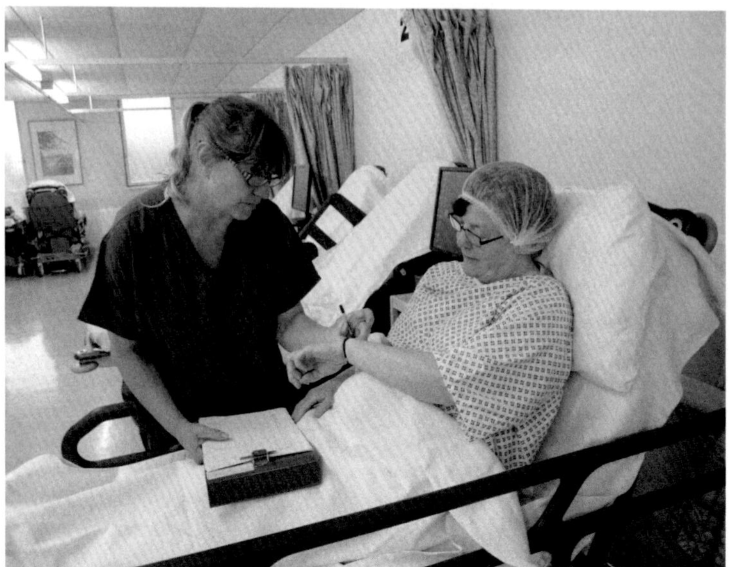

Photo 2 Admitting a patient to the operating department. Source: Courtesy of Liverpool Women's Hospital

Several other issues will also be covered if needed by the patient (Goodman & Spry 2014).

The patient will be escorted to the reception area in the operating department by a porter and a ward nurse. The ward staff will check the validity of the patient's identity, consent form, patient notes and patient care plan (Photo 2). The patient can be transported towards the operating department by using a wheelchair, trolley or bed or by walking. The patient is admitted to the reception area and is checked by the reception staff to ensure all their information is correct, which enables staff to provide the best possible care. An elderly patient may have dementia or be confused, and may need further explanations and reassurance. The patient will be greeted by name, and then the practitioner will introduce themselves to the patient. A preoperative checklist is always completed, following hospital regulations to ensure the correct operation is carried out (Wicker & O'Neill 2010). The patient is always treated with privacy, dignity and respect to cultural, religious, ethnic and racial beliefs.

Care during anaesthesia

The anaesthetic practitioner prepares the anaesthetic room, anaesthetic machines and other anaesthetic equipment to provide safe care during anaesthesia (Wicker & O'Neill 2010). This will include:

- Checking the anaesthetic machine
- Checking intubation equipment
- Preparing anaesthetic drugs (Griffiths 2000)
- Checking oxygen supplies
- Checking suction equipment
- Preparing monitors as needed
- Preparing IV fluids and giving sets.

The anaesthetic practitioner must follow the anaesthetist's needs and display knowledge, skills and understanding about anaesthesia (Goodman & Spry 2014). The practitioner also needs to support the patient, including offering:

- Amiable communication, sometimes including humour
- Comfort and dignity for the patient
- Reassurance and discussion about anaesthesia and surgery
- Consideration of the needs of the patient.

Patients may be anxious on entry to the anaesthetic room, which may inhibit communication. It is therefore useful to talk to the patient and reassure them about the procedures that are going to take place (Harris 2015). It is always useful to have a practitioner in the room to spend time with the patient while the anaesthetic practitioner continues with preparing equipment for the anaesthetist.

When the anaesthetist arrives and anaesthesia is induced, all personnel in the anaesthetic room should be calm and quiet to minimise disruption or disturbance for the patient, which will help the patient maintain a calm state of mind (Griffiths 2000, Harris 2015). During anaesthesia, the anaesthetic practitioner will observe and monitor the patient's wellbeing, and assist the surgical team to position the patient safely.

Intraoperative care

The surgical team needs to assess, identify, control, monitor, reduce and evaluate risks to improve the quality of care delivered by using the WHO surgical safety checklist (Goodman & Spry 2014). During surgery, the patient is vulnerable and is reliant on the surgical team to ensure support and care, and that the surgery and anaesthesia are carried out safely and effectively.

Examples of clinical risks include:

- Patient positioning
- Infections
- Deep venous thrombosis (DVT)
- Hypothermia or hyperthermia
- Inappropriate use of equipment.

Many more risks are possible, which is why the WHO surgical safety checklist is now compulsory in every operating theatre to reduce the chances of harm to the patient.

Other examples of patient issues during the intraoperative phase include the following (Goodman & Spry 2014).

Patient positioning

- Avoiding nerve and joint injury
- Avoiding shearing, friction burns and damage to tissues
- Avoiding ischaemia and pressure sores from developing
- Avoiding radial nerve injury, if the arm is left hanging over the edge of the operating table
- Avoiding ulnar and fibular nerve injury due to compression or pressure.

Deep venous thrombosis

- DVT occurs because of haemostasis, vessel wall trauma and increased coagulation caused by anaesthetic drugs or physiological status of the patient.
- DVT prophylaxis includes the use of graduated compression stockings, low-molecular-weight heparin and intermittent pneumatic compression devices (Rothrock 2007).

Inadvertent hypothermia

Hypothermia happens in many patients because of the cool air and the light clothing worn, as well as the effects of anaesthetic drugs and surgical procedures. Hypothermia becomes a problem if the patient's temperature drops below 36 °C (Rothrock 2007). If the patient is hypothermic, the following areas need to be considered (Wicker & O'Neill 2010):

- Regular temperature monitoring must be carried out on all surgical patients.
- Operating room temperature should be a minimum of 21 °C.
- IV fluids should be warmed.
- The patient should have a warm blanket or Bear Hugger and be kept covered before surgery.
- Very young or very old patients may develop hypothermia.
- Long surgical procedures can result in hypothermia.
- Lack of mobility and shivering can reduce temperature.
- Anaesthetic drugs can lead to vasoconstriction, causing cold in the peripheries, or vasodilation which can lead to decrease of core body heat.
- Detrimental effects include bleeding, infection and increased stay in recovery (Goodman & Spry 2014, Rothrock 2007).

There are many other risks associated with patients during surgery; these include handling of instruments, swab and instrument counts, leaving instruments or objects inside wounds, diathermy burns, pressure sores and others (Rothrock 2007). Therefore, it is essential that the WHO checklist is carried out and the surgical team monitors the patient constantly to uphold their safety.

Transferring the patient to recovery

Following completion of the surgery, surgical practitioners undertake the last part of the WHO surgical safety checklist (WHO 2009) and complete the care plan accordingly, detailing, for example:

- The surgical procedure
- Patient's surgical positioning
- Use of diathermy
- Patient monitoring
- Confirmation of the needle, swab and instrument counts
- Method of skin closure
- Presence of any drains or catheters (WHO 2009).

The patient is normally extubated in the operating room, and gently woken up before being transferred to the recovery room. After the patient has left the operating room, the staff will then clean and tidy the OR and prepare for the arrival of the next patient.

Postoperative care

Recovery practitioners care for and assess the patient postoperatively to prevent potential complications and to ensure the patient's wellbeing until they are fully recovered. The recovery room is normally staffed by nurses and ODPs, who are expected to deal quickly and efficiently with any problems which the patient develops. Recovery practitioners manage the patient's care autonomously, although they would request assistance from anaesthetists and surgeons only when needed in urgent or emergency situations (Goodman & Spry 2014).

Practitioners prepare for each patient before the patient's arrival to ensure that equipment and drugs are available, including resuscitation equipment, airway equipment, oxygen and suction devices, monitoring equipment, patient warming equipment, analgesic pumps and so on (Reed 2003).

Transfer from the operating room to the recovery room happens once the anaesthetist is satisfied that the patient's condition is stable. On arrival in recovery, the patient's care is transferred to the recovery practitioner. The recovery practitioner then carries out immediate assessment of the patient, focussing on airway, breathing and circulation, as well as the patient's vital signs, wound site, comfort and safety.

The main areas for recovery practitioners to consider initially include the following.

Airway management

- The airway must be patent, clear of blood and mucous.
- Assess ventilation; in case of problems, insert a guedal or laryngeal mask airway.
- Assess the patient's position to optimise ventilation.
- Commence oxygen therapy immediately via an oxygen mask or nasal cannula. Usually, this is at 40%.
- Attach a pulse oximeter to a finger or ear lobe to monitor oxygen saturation.
- Continue to monitor the patient constantly until the patient recovers from the anaesthetic or surgery (Goodman & Spry 2014).

Breathing

- Ensure normal chest movements, and check on inhalations and exhalations.
- Check causes of noisy breathing, and take suitable actions.
- Check causes of silent breathing or no inhalations or exhalations.
- Check for peripheral cyanosis, for example lips or nailbeds.
- Check the respiratory rate.

Circulation

Once the airway has been established as being satisfactory, then blood pressure and pulse will be monitored (Wicker & O'Neill 2010). Assessment of appropriate blood circulation includes the presence of a conscious state, as well as normal skin temperature, pulse and blood pressure, which provide an indication that circulation is normal and is perfusing all organs (Rothrock 2007). Checking the blood pressure against the preoperative blood pressure, and the blood pressure in theatre, gives a good indication that the blood pressure is at a normal range for each individual patient.

- Inspect wounds and drains for evidence of bleeding.
- Check oxygen levels using a pulse oximeter and checking peripheries for cyanosis.

Once the initial assessment of airway, breathing and circulation has been completed, the recovery practitioner will discuss the information given about the patient with the anaesthetist and the theatre practitioner (Reed 2003). The discussion will include:

- Past medical history
- The surgical procedure
- Any issues with vital signs
- Drugs given to the patient, including analgesics and sedatives
- Any blood loss
- Type and amount of intravenous infusions
- Presence of any catheters and drains
- Any errors that occurred during the surgery and any potential postoperative problems.

The anaesthetist will also discuss specific postoperative instructions for each patient, including analgesics, oxygen therapy and monitoring requirements (Rothrock 2007).

Following the discussion, the recovery practitioner will continue to undertake further patient assessments (Reed 2003), including:

- Checking the patient's consciousness level
- Identifying reflexes or movements
- Checking for need for intravenous infusions, including type and rate of delivery
- Recognising pain in the patient by using a pain-scoring chart, and taking actions to reduce pain and discomfort
- Reducing postoperative nausea and vomiting to relieve the patient of discomfort and problems such as excessive bleeding, pain, and pulmonary and cardiovascular complications
- Filling of wound drains
- Filling of urine bags using urinary catheters, including colour, drainage and amount
- Completing observations, such as observing monitors of temperature, pulse and blood pressure; checking wound site; preventing pressure sores and so on.

The recovery practitioner must always record the postoperative assessment and observations in the patient's documentation to ensure that any actions taken are recorded in case of future problems; this record thereby provides a detailed record of their care and interventions undertaken by healthcare professionals (Goodman & Spry 2014). Waking up from the anaesthetic can also be a frightening experience for the patient because of bright lights, noises, different surroundings, confusion and disorientation caused by the anaesthetic drugs. The recovery practitioner can help reduce anxiety by reassuring the patient, speaking with and supporting the patient by letting him or her know where they are, what is happening and how problems are being solved (Reed 2003). It is also important that practitioners preserve confidentiality, privacy, dignity and respect for the patient.

Discharge of the patient back to the ward

The length of time the patient stays in the recovery room depends on the type of anaesthetic, the surgical procedure and any postoperative recovery issues. Discharge is allowed once the patient has fully recovered and has been assessed for the level of consciousness, respiration, circulation, pain control, haemostasis and wound care (Reed 2003). All written and recorded information is given to the ward nurse, and information is also given about the patient's physiological status. Discharge criteria are also met on the patient's intracranial pressure. The ward nurse will then take on the responsibility for the patient's postoperative care on the return to the ward.

Throughout the perioperative experience, practitioners should always have the patient's best interests in the forefront of their minds and be the patient's advocate at all times.

6 Operating Theatre Attire and Personal Protective Equipment

Operating theatre attire usually includes tops, trousers, hats, socks and clogs. Personal protective equipment (PPE), which protects staff from cross-infection or cross-contamination, includes gowns, gloves, masks, aprons, eye protection and disposable, fluid-resistant shoe covers. PPE is made available to personnel to reduce the risk of exposure to infection during surgery (Goodman & Spry 2014). Hospital guidelines usually identify the need to wear PPE during surgical procedures, and so normally certain items of PPE would always be used during surgical cases. PPE, including masks, gowns and shoe covers, must be removed before leaving the operating room. If shoe covers are not worn, then shoes covered in blood, body fluids or pus must be removed and washed before leaving the operating room.

Protective eyewear is used during surgery to prevent splashes in the eyes, by substances such as blood, tissues, body fluids, infected materials or faeces. It is advisable for the surgical team to wear masks with full face shields, or alternatively glasses or goggles (Goodman & Spry 2014). Normal eyeglasses are not considered to be a safe form of protection as they will often allow splashes to enter the eye, leading to a potential for cross-infection problems for the surgeon or the surgical team.

All individuals who enter the operating department must wear designated surgical attire (DOH 2010). This attire is worn only once at the beginning of the shift and then sent for cleaning to a laundry service when leaving the facility. If a practitioner needs to leave the operating department to go to a ward or other department, then either cover gowns should be used, or outside attire worn instead. Moving outside the operating department in normal surgical attire is not considered to be appropriate or standard practice, according to hospital regulations, to prevent the exposure of patients and practitioners to cross-infection. Practitioners should also change theatre scrubs if they become soiled, especially if there is need for the practitioner to move to another theatre and a different surgical procedure (DOH 2010). For example, if a practitioner participated in vascular surgery in the morning, and then moves to general surgery in the afternoon, he or she should change theatre scrubs because of the risk of cross-contamination transfer of the microorganisms from the previous operating room to the next operating room.

Practitioners working in the operating room would include the following attire for the purpose of self-protection:

1. Disposable surgical caps which cover hair, or hoods which also cover facial hair such as beards or moustaches and prevent hair or dandruff from falling into the patient's wound area.
2. Scrub trousers and tops which are found in changing rooms and have been cleaned and laundered. Tops may be tucked into the pants to prevent skin scales being released into the air. Surgical attire that becomes contaminated with blood or body fluids must be changed as soon as possible to prevent infection.

Rapid Perioperative Care, First Edition. Paul Wicker and Sara Dalby.

3. Jackets are useful to keep circulating staff warm if the operating room is below normal temperature of around 21 °C.
4. Disposable shoe covers are worn in some operating rooms, but often they are not worn as removing them can lead to infection on the hands. If they are worn, then they must be changed when visibly contaminated and removed before leaving the operating room.
5. Surgical clogs or shoes need to be clean and offer protection from injury. They normally have no holes or perforations along with a low heel and non-skid soles.
6. Surgical masks are always worn during major surgical procedures or when the scrub practitioner is starting to set up for a sterile procedure. A new facemask should be used for each new surgical procedure. The face masks should also not be hung around the neck or placed in pockets after they have been used; they should be disposed of carefully (Wicker & O'Neil 2010).

Jewellery, such as earrings, bracelets or necklaces, are not normally allowed in operating rooms as they could come loose and drop into the patient's wound or be permanently lost (Wicker & O'Neil 2010). Jewellery should therefore be kept confined in the practitioner's dressing cupboard or in their scrub attire. Rings and watches may be allowed, depending on hospital regulations, but they must always be removed before surgical hand scrubs. A necklace may be worn if it is not viewable and is confined within the scrub attire. Small earrings may be acceptable for circulating staff but they should be kept under the cap, especially when surgical procedures are being performed.

It is also important that perfume, aftershave or any strong odour (such as sweating armpits) that is considered offensive to patients or interferes with employees' roles should not be allowed. Any visitors, guests or company representatives who enter the operating room must also follow the hospital's surgical attire policy. Identification badges are normally worn by all operating room staff, and they must be pinned to the surgical attire top, and be visible and safe for patients. Nail polish should not be worn by scrub practitioners or circulating practitioners in the theatre area (NICE 2013). Practitioners undertaking direct patient contact must also keep nails less than ¼ inch long and not wear artificial nails or nail extenders to prevent harm to the patient (NICE 2008).

All surgical practitioners working in the operating room have the authority and responsibility to monitor proper surgical attire compliance in case staff do not wear the correct attire or PPE. In some hospitals, different colours hats and scrubs are worn for practitioners undertaking different roles, or if levels of experience are different, for example in students and qualified and senior practitioners. Any issues that arise must be corrected immediately, and if there are further problems then they need reporting to the theatre manager or supervisor. Noncompliance with attire and PPE may result in disciplinary action being taken by the theatre manager.

7 Surgical Safety Checklist

The WHO Surgical Safety Checklist (SSCL) was developed in 2008 (PSF 2015), with a goal to reduce the number of deaths and patient complications through surgical intervention. It is also to improve the safety of surgery, and it produces a framework to enable hospitals to augment patient safety. Most hospitals now use the WHO SSCL and develop policies to make sure it is used properly. The WHO SSCL has also been updated over the years and is now much more efficient and effective (NPSA 2009). Managers, such as Chief of Surgery, Matrons, General Managers and lead practitioners, now have the responsibility to ensure that staff undertake the SSCL in the correct manner, and also look into incidents or 'never events'. The SSCL is used for all patients, and the completed checklist is retained in the patient's notes. Failure of staff to follow the SSCL may result in disciplinary actions.

The structure of the SSCL provides a standard set of checklists, which often varies between hospitals and may include:

- Pre and post-surgery briefing
- SIGN IN before Anaesthesia
- 'Stop before you block' – for regional anaesthesia
- The TIME OUT Pause before surgery starts
- Sign Out.

Team brief

While all theatre practitioners learn technical and nontechnical skills, it is the nontechnical skills, for example poor communication or poor teamwork, which account for most adverse clinical events. A gathering of the team to discuss the pre-list briefing before the theatre list starts helps to enhance the team's knowledge and understanding of the surgical list and enables healthcare practitioners to have a greater understanding of actions required for patient care (Hunter & Finney 2011).

The team briefing involves some of the following actions:

- Staff discuss the actions needed for all surgical patients before the operating list starts.
- The brief is updated if there are any changes, for example consultant surgeons leave the operating room or new patients are added to the list.
- All members of the anaesthetic, surgical and theatre teams are included in the brief.
- The lead practitioner normally leads the discussion and identifies the key areas for discussion.
- The brief covers main issues such as health of the patient, type of anaesthetic required, the surgical procedure, moving and handling, patient positioning, equipment required and so on.

Pre-anaesthetic SIGN IN

The SIGN IN section of the WHO checklist is carried out by the anaesthetist and the anaesthetic practitioner before anaesthesia starts for every patient. The SIGN IN questions and

Rapid Perioperative Care, First Edition. Paul Wicker and Sara Dalby.

checks on the WHO SSCL are read aloud by the anaesthetic practitioner and confirmed by the anaesthetist (NPSA 2009). When the anaesthetist delivers a local anaesthetic, he or she confirms the site for delivery of the local anaesthetic by referring to the operating list, the consent form and the site marking on the patient. Other checks for the SIGN IN may include:

- Checking the patient for potential risk factors such as allergies, airway problems, cardiac problems and so on
- Risk of blood loss during surgery
- Checking of anaesthetic machine
- Preparation of instruments and equipment
- Preparation of anaesthetic drugs
- Confirmation of surgical site marking.

TIME OUT

The TIME OUT phase happens before surgery starts to confirm the correct patient is present, the correct procedure and the correct site for surgery (Hunter & Finney 2011). All staff must stop and listen when the TIME OUT is being discussed to give their full attention and understanding.

The surgeon undertaking the surgery initiates the TIME OUT and asks a theatre practitioner to read the TIME OUT section of the SSCL form aloud (WHO 2013). Issues include:

- Checking the identity of the patient against the medical notes and the patient's wristband
- Confirming the consent form is signed and dated
- Confirming the checks are correct
- If there are any problems, any member of the theatre team should raise a concern and confirm issues such as identity, correct consent, correct site, correct surgery and so on.

SIGN OUT

On completion of surgery and before the patient and members of the team leave the operating theatre, the final SIGN OUT is read verbally and the checklist completed (Haynes *et al.* 2009).

- The theatre practitioner confirms with the team the name of the procedure recorded for the patient. This happens because the procedure may have changed during the operation, so any updates must be described by the surgical team.
- Practitioners must confirm that instruments, swabs and sharps counts are correct, following local hospital policy. This prevents missing or retained swabs and instruments being left inside the patient.
- Practitioners must ensure that specimens are correctly labelled. This is important as false labelling can result in false results for the patient, or potential mix-ups with other patients.
- Highlighting any equipment problems ensures the removal of faulty equipment from the operating theatre and new equipment installed.
- Any key concerns for the patient during recovery are identified by the Surgeon, Anaesthetist and Registered Practitioner, including for example postoperative pain, nausea, vomiting, harm to joints, pressure sores and so on. The team will carry out a review of the postoperative recovery plan, focussing issues that might affect the patient.

Conclusion

Using the SSCL helps to address important safety concerns for the patient, enabling all members of the surgical team to focus on the patient and the procedure. This enables the surgical team to proceed confidently with the surgical procedure, delivering excellent patient care and preventing complications (NPSA 2009). The use of the SSCL also promotes team building and brings the theatre team closer together, enabling them to understand what each member of the team is doing throughout the day, and supporting good communication (Cvetic 2011). However, there are still issues in some hospitals when they don't carry out the WHO checklist effectively.

The checklist may be modified to suit the particular clinical area, for example orthopaedics is totally different from cardiothoracic surgery. However, important safety checks should not be changed and will assist the theatre team to comply with every element of the checklist. Specific clinical placement areas may also need to add other safety checks for specific procedures (Hunter *et al.* 2011).

It is important the WHO safety checklist is utilised effectively for each and every patient, as this will reduce errors and patient harm. Failure to use the WHO SSCL may result in 'never events' happening, patient injury and possible harm to staff. The SSCL has been proven to reduce anaesthetic and surgical errors, and enhance the overall safety of the patient (Cvetic, 2011).

The SSCL gives the practitioner the opportunity to document everything they have implemented for each individual patient, for example ensuring pressure-relieving devices are in place. If there was ever any doubt about the care delivered to the patient, the checklist can then be referred to and discussed with the staff.

8 Teaching Students How to Use Operating Theatre Equipment

The purpose of this chapter is to show how ODP students are taught in simulated clinical skills areas within their university.

Equipment in the operating room is expensive and complex, with many different types of equipment available depending on the surgery taking place. It is therefore essential that perioperative students have knowledge and understanding of all perioperative equipment they use, and follow local policies on cleaning, checking and preparing equipment before its use. This ensures it is fully working and reduces the risk of harm to patients or staff.

Tutors are responsible for ensuring that students follow the Health and Safety at Work Regulations, and ensuring that policies are in place which state the correct use and maintenance of equipment. Tutors also teach students how to ensure that there are planned maintenance programmes in place to ensure all equipment is safe and ready to use. The student's responsibilities, while being trained, will include checking recording equipment and following local policies as well as national guidelines. A major consideration for all operating theatre practitioners is that if they are not familiar with a particular piece of equipment, then they should not use it or set it up. For this reason, all students need to be adequately trained and educated in order to reduce the risk of harm to themselves and their patients.

Anaesthetic equipment

Checking anaesthetic equipment before starting anaesthesia helps to avoid critical incidents. The anaesthetic machine is checked by the tutor, who informs students of the methods used for checking the anaesthetic machine. In hospitals, though, the anaesthetist will have the responsibility for ensuring that the anaesthetic machine is fully operational. The main components of an anaesthetic machine will include:

- *Ventilators*: These enable breathing for the patients.
- *Vaporisers*: These contain anaesthetic solutions used for inhaling into the patient's lungs.
- *Scavenger systems*: This is used to gather gas after it is exhaled from the patient and is ejected from the operating room.
- *Flow control valves and meters*: These measure the amount of gases being inhaled by the patients.
- *Gas supply, via pipelines or cylinders*: These contain anaesthetic gases such as oxygen and nitrous oxide.
- *Patient monitors*: These measure the patient's ECG rhythm, pulse rate, blood pressure, respiration rate, oxygen saturation and temperature.

Every piece of equipment is checked thoroughly by using the settings on the anaesthetic machine and by testing them so that they work correctly.

Rapid Perioperative Care, First Edition. Paul Wicker and Sara Dalby.

Total intravenous anaesthesia may also be used in place of general anaesthetics. Tutors will teach students about the use of drug agents such as propofol, alfentanil and remifentanil which are used as they have rapid anaesthetic and pain-killing effects on the patient. Students will be shown how drugs are injected into the patient at a particular rate or as a bolus by using a syringe pump. The syringe must fit securely in the clamp on the syringe pump, and the battery needs to be checked to ensure it is fully charged. These drugs are only used in hospitals; however, students are informed of the dosage and the use of the drugs in clinical simulation areas.

Tutors will also show students how to extract secretions or vomit from the patient's airway using suction catheters. They should be checked to ensure they are working, they are at the right setting and the tube and suction catheter are connected.

Students are also taught how to monitor equipment which provides continual assessment of the patient during anaesthesia. Monitors include pulse oximetry, non-invasive blood pressure monitors, temperature gauges, capnography and electrocardiography. Monitors need to be tested for alarm settings, frequency of recordings and cycling times.

Surgical equipment

Tutors also teach students about the use of surgical equipment which are in use during surgery, all of which need to be checked before the start of surgery to ensure they are clean, in working condition and ready to use.

Electrosurgical generators exist in most operating rooms as they are the best way to reduce bleeding and also to cut tissues. However, it is also one of the most dangerous pieces of equipment as it can potentially burn patient tissues. Before the start of surgery, it is important to examine, test and set up all electrosurgical equipment. Electrosurgery is taught during classroom sessions, and pieces of meat (e.g. pork) are used to identify how electrosurgery works.

A piece of equipment called a pulse lavage can irrigate wounds using 0.9% saline or water. Normally, it is high power and can therefore cause splashing around the wound. Tutors and students will therefore wear visors and preferably masks if they are within the vicinity of this machine when in use. The devices can be either electrical or air powered. In all cases, equipment needs to be checked to ensure it is intact and operational.

Principles of the swab and instrument count (SIC)

Tutors will teach students about starting the SIC along with the circulating practitioner. The scrub and circulating practitioners carry out the count appropriately and ensure that all instruments and equipment are properly managed.

Students will be shown how to carry out SICs before the surgery starts, during surgery if a cavity is closed (e.g. the bladder), before the start of wound closure and after surgery finishes. During surgery, there is usually a minimum of three counts, and for minor surgery (e.g. removing a sebaceous cyst) a minimum of two counts. Circulating students will record SICs on whiteboards on the wall of the operating room. The board is used so that all staff can see the counts if required. There is no national policy for recording counts; however, each hospital or clinical skills area needs to have its own system. The local policy should detail how items such as swabs, needles, clips, patties and so on are recorded, and how items such as swabs are accounted for when discarded or taken away from the surgical procedure.

The students will be shown how to carry out SICs routinely, according to policies, normally in the sequence of swabs, sharps, other items (e.g. sutures, slings and patties) and finally instruments and instrument trays. The students will be told to count items first at the site of surgery, then on the mayo table and finally on the instrument trolley, thereby ensuring that items do not get counted twice.

In a hospital with a real patient, if a swab does get lost and cannot be found, then the patient should be x-rayed to detect the x-ray-detectable marker on the swab. If carried out while the wound is open, then the swab can be located and removed; if carried out after the wound has closed, then further surgery will be required.

Surgical instruments or items occasionally drop off the operating table because of faulty placement or being knocked off the table. If this happens, they should be placed within sight of the student, perhaps in a bowl or near the swab board, to include them in the count. No items used during the procedure should be removed from the operating theatre until the final check is complete. The reason for this is that a needle or swab can get mixed up with a drape or sheet, and if removed from theatre it cannot then be accounted for. If a SIC check is incorrect, then the practitioner must inform the surgeon immediately.

Checking swabs and other items

Students will carry out the swab check in the following way:

1. Before the start of the procedure, count all swabs and packs in bundles of five and record on the swab board.
2. Count and record other items, such as blades, sutures and needles, on the swab board.
3. Undertake counts before, during and after the procedure, and whenever an item becomes lost.
4. Discard any swabs with problems, such as missing x-ray strips or missing swabs from within packets, and remove from the operating room before surgery starts.
5. During surgery, open individual swabs and packs and show to the circulating practitioner to verify that it is only one swab, and not two swabs stuck together.
6. Count swabs and packs during the procedure, and discard into a swab disposal system. This may be a swab rack with plastic pockets, or a plastic bag which is tied up and placed in a basin.
7. Record swabs inserted into body cavities on the swab board.
8. Carry out SICs when closing a cavity, when closing the wound and once surgery is finished.
9. Verify and record correct swab checks using the Surgical Safety Checklist and the patient care plan.

Basic surgical instruments

Tutors inform students about basic surgical instruments used in most surgical procedures. Instruments are classified according to their purpose, including actions such as cutting and dissecting, grasping and holding, clamping and occluding, exposing and retracting, suturing and stapling, suctioning and aspirating, micro-instrumentation and powered surgical instruments. The student when scrubbed up will be told to be responsible for counting all instruments before and after the surgery, careful handling of instruments, protecting sharp ends of instruments and laying out instruments on the trolley in preparation for surgery. The student will be told about the names of the instruments, their intended purpose and when the surgeon requires them, and how to pass them to the surgeon in a safe and effective manner. Students will also need to clean instruments during surgery and pack them safely after surgery finishes to maintain their working condition.

Types of instruments

Cutting and dissecting: Surgeons normally carry out cutting and dissecting with scalpels as a first step in surgery. The most common scalpels are numbers 10, 11, 15, 20 and 23. Scalpel blades attach to Bard Parker handles and are either handed to the surgeon in a kidney dish or placed in his hand. The student will hold the handle between the thumb and forefinger, with the blade under the practitioner's palm, and then place it in the surgeon's hand, handle first. The number 10 and 20 blades are the most commonly used for cutting almost everything, including skin, fat, muscles and nerves. Vascular surgeons often use an 11 blade, and plastic and paediatric surgeons often use a 15 blade. Surgeons also use scissors for cutting tissues, including curved and straight mayo scissors which are able to cut tough tissues, for example ligaments, and curved Metzenbaum scissors which cut delicate tissues. Suture scissors are used to cut sutures or items such as tapes, dressings or swabs. Other instruments used for cutting and dissecting include reusable surgical knives, bone cutters, biopsy forceps, punches, curettes, snares and blunt dissectors.

Grasping and holding: Toothed forceps, for example Lanes tissue forceps, are useful for holding tough tissues such as skin, ligaments or muscles. Non-toothed forceps can hold delicate tissues, such as blood vessels and nerves, which may rip easily. Allis forceps and Babcock forceps are held in the same way as scissors, but the ends have broad metallic prongs which can grip onto tissues such as skin or visceral organs without too much pressure. Babcock forceps are designed to hold onto bowel tissues, whereas Allis forceps are designed to hold onto skin flaps, peritoneum or small blood vessels. Orthopaedic surgeons use bone holders to hold bones together, or to manipulate broken bones. Backhaus towel clips are rarely used, and are designed to hold drapes together or to attach instruments or tubes.

Clamping and occluding: Artery forceps clamp blood vessels so surgeons can cut and tie them without the loss of blood. Surgeons also use them to hold and manipulate tissues. Artery forceps include Mosquito forceps, which are very small; Dunhill, Spencer Wells or Criles forceps (medium); and Mayo forceps, which are large. Kocher forceps are similar to Mayo forceps but contain a tooth at the tip of the blades which can grab onto tissues and hold them tightly. Surgeons use non-crushing intestinal clamps to close the ends of the intestine after it has been cut or dissected. The grip is light but firm, and the serrations within the blades of the clamp flow from the handle to the tip. Vascular clamps of various sizes from very small to very large are similar and are also non-crushing.

Exposing and retracting: Many types of retractors exist. The Balfour retractor is large and is used during a laparotomy to hold open the abdominal wall so the surgeon can see the organs inside. These retractors help in visualisation of the operative field and help to prevent trauma to other tissues. Langenbecks retractors, which are L-shaped, are used to hold wounds open by hand. Farabeuf retractors have a long flat blade with L-shaped bends on each end which hold and retract deep tissues. The Travers and Weitlaner retractors are self-retaining retractors which lock into position and hold wounds open while grasping onto the tissue edges with curved prongs. Surgeons also use various hooks to retract skin edges, such as skin hooks and bone hooks. Some of these hooks are sharp, while others are blunt and cause less trauma to tissues. Senn retractors and cat's paws retractors are small and help to retract skin in minor surgery. These retractors have either an L-shaped end or a curved and slightly sharp end that looks like a cat's paw.

Suturing and stapling: Sutures are attached to needle holders. The tips often have tungsten carbide jaws with cross-hatched serrations to hold the needle firmly to eliminate twisting or turning of the needle and to prevent damaging it. Mayo's needle holders are commonly used as they are simple and sturdy instruments. Bowel staplers are used for anastomosing ends of bowel. They are usually single use and come in various shapes and sizes. Staples can often be loaded onto the ends of the staple devices more than once per use. Skin staples are also single use and are in the shape of a 'gun'. The surgeon presses the skin stapler on the skin and then presses the trigger to release the staple into the skin.

Suctioning and aspirating: Suction devices remove blood and fluids to give a clear view of the surgical field, and they help to monitor blood loss. They are often used in intermediate or major operations, for example in a laparotomy where fluid is poured into the abdomen to clean the abdominal contents following surgery. There are various types, sizes and shapes of suction device used, including Yankaur suckers, which are used mostly for superficial wound suctioning, and for suction of the mouth and throat. The Frazier sucker is small and narrow and is used in neurosurgery, spinal, max-fax or minor orthopaedic surgery, where there is little fluid. The Poole abdominal suction device is long, with suction holes along its length, and is used for removing large amounts of fluid.

Powered surgical instruments: There is a vast array of electrically powered instruments, the most common of which are drills, burrs, saws, reamers and abraders. These are often used in orthopaedics for several uses, including cutting bone, drilling holes for screws and reaming the inside of bone shafts to enable the insertion of nails.

After being taught by tutors in clinical simulation areas in the university, students will have basic information to help them understand the role of the scrub practitioner during surgery in hospitals. This is essential to ensure that patients are kept safe and secure when undergoing surgical procedures.

9 Perioperative Equipment

Operating rooms contain specialised equipment which supports patients throughout their anaesthetic and surgical procedures. The operating room equipment is normally very expensive, depending on the types of equipment needed for anaesthesia and surgery taking place. Practitioners need to follow the Health and Safety at Work Regulations (HSE 1999) to ensure the equipment is upheld regularly and used correctly and safely. Practitioners need to have the knowledge and understanding about how perioperative equipment is used, and they also need to follow local and national policies on cleaning, checking and preparing equipment before the patient arrives. All perioperative practitioners should be trained and educated about the safe use of equipment, which is essential to ensure it is fully functional and minimises the risk of harm to patients or staff (AFPP 2011). Theatre managers are normally responsible for making sure that equipment is stored correctly and maintained by the company from where it was purchased, in line with company recommendations and policies.

Initial equipment checks

The most efficient way to check equipment before the patient arrives is to use a checklist which identifies the checks in order to document and rectify any errors. The checklist will include sections such as selecting correct equipment, identifying any faults, calibrating equipment, testing equipment, cleaning and so on. Electrical equipment and sterile equipment that is packaged also need to be checked and authenticated before use.

Operating room equipment

When the anaesthetised patient is brought into the operating room, the anaesthetic monitoring equipment is normally located at the head of the operating table. The anaesthetist can then monitor the patient's status during surgery. Operating rooms have specialised equipment, depending on the methods by which anaesthesia and surgery are performed. This can include equipment such as respiratory monitors, cardiac monitors, resuscitative devices, patient monitors and diagnostic tools. There are usually many more different types of equipment available in every operating room.

Anaesthetic equipment

Practitioners undertake pre-checks of anaesthetic equipment to prevent harm to the patient. The anaesthetic machine is checked by the anaesthetist and the anaesthetic assistant to ensure that it is safe and has passed the self-check and leak test to ensure it is ready and fit for use (AAGBI 2012). An anaesthetic machine contains the following pieces of equipment:

- Ventilators
- Vaporisers

Rapid Perioperative Care, First Edition. Paul Wicker and Sara Dalby.

- Scavenger systems
- Flow control valves and meters
- Gas supply – via pipelines or cylinders
- Pressure regulators.

Monitoring equipment provides continual assessment of the patient during anaesthesia and includes:

- Pulse oximetry – tests the pulse and oxygenation
- Non-invasive blood pressure monitors
- Temperature gauges
- Capnography
- Electrocardiography (ECG).

Monitors are tested for alarm settings, frequency of recordings and cycling times (DH 2013).

Equipment for resuscitation

The equipment used for emergency resuscitation can include the following devices, dependent on the type of anaesthesia, the type of surgery or the operating department in use:

- Heart–lung bypass machine:
  - Also named a cardiopulmonary bypass pump
  - Used during cardiothoracic surgery; provides oxygen and blood circulation during heart or lung surgery
  - Provides oxygen and removes carbon dioxide from the blood
  - Enables circulation of blood around the body without the heart beating.
- Ventilator (or respirator):
  - Provides pulmonary ventilation by using a breathing circuit, gas supply, heating/humidification mechanism, monitors and alarms
  - Regulates the volume, pressure and flow of respiration.
- Infusion pump
  - A device that delivers fluids intravenously or through an epidural catheter.
  - They deliver continuous anaesthesia, drugs and blood infusions to the patient.
- Resuscitation trolley
  - A moveable cart containing emergency resuscitation equipment
  - Emergency equipment includes a defibrillator, airway intubation devices, resuscitation bag/mask and medication box.
  - Resuscitation carts are located in the operating department for easy accessibility.
- Intra-aortic balloon pump
  - This device helps reduce the heart's workload and helps blood flow to the coronary arteries.
  - Used for patients with angina, myocardial infarction or other cardiac complications.
  - A catheter is inserted into the aorta with a balloon on the end, and it can then display heart rate, blood pressure and ECG readings on the monitor.

Patient-monitoring equipment

The equipment used for patient monitoring includes the following:

- Physiological monitoring systems
  - The patient-monitoring systems monitor patients' physiological parameters continuously by using electrodes or sensors which are connected to the patient.

  - Areas monitored include electrical activity of the heart using an ECG machine, cardiac output, blood pressure, body temperature, respiratory rate, and arterial haemoglobin, oxygen saturation and carbon dioxide levels.
- Pulse oximeter
  - Uses infrared light to measure the amount of oxygen in the blood
  - The pulse oximeter sensor is clipped to the patient's fingers, toes or ear lobes.
  - The monitor also records the level of arterial oxygen saturation in the patient's blood.
- Intracranial pressure monitor (usually in neurosurgery or emergency theatres)
  - Measures and records the pressure of fluid in the brain
  - Used often for patients with head trauma or other conditions affecting the brain
  - Intracranial pressure monitors are inserted into the brain and record levels using sensors.

Surgical equipment

Surgery requires the use of many different types of equipment, and in every case they need to be checked before surgery to make sure they are working and in good condition (Goodman & Spry 2014). Some of the surgical equipment includes:

- Electrosurgical generators (diathermy)
  - Used to reduce bleeding and to cut tissues
  - Can cause accidental burns to patients
  - The generator needs to be examined and tested before the start of the operating list (Cunnington 2006).
- Pulse lavage
  - Used to irrigate wounds using 0.9% saline or water
  - Staff should wear visors and masks for safety, in order to prevent splashing in eyes or the mouth.
  - The device pumps water by using an electrical or air-powered device.
- Visual display units
  - Laparoscopic procedures are monitored by surgeons using video display units.
  - All equipment needs to be checked before surgery.
    - Checking and preparing all laparoscopic equipment
    - Preparing irrigation fluids
    - Checking gas supplies for insufflation
    - Testing the video display unit
    - Testing suction units.
  - Light cables need to work effectively to ensure the inside of the patient's body is easily viewed (Wicker & O'Neill 2010).

Practitioners must be trained thoroughly to ensure that all the equipment is ready and safe for use (DH 2013).

Other operating room equipment

There are many other items of operating room equipment used, depending on the needs of the patient or the surgery and anaesthesia being performed (Goodman & Spry 2014). These include items such as:

- Urinary (Foley) catheters to drain urine during surgery
- Arterial and central venous line catheters to monitor blood pressure
- Swan–Ganz catheters to monitor the function of the heart and record the amount of fluid in the heart

- Chest and endotracheal tubes
- Microscopes
- Robotic technology
- Monitoring electrodes which can monitor nerve conduction
- Tourniquet machines
- Cement mixers (used in orthopaedics).

Conclusion

Checking equipment prior to the patient arriving is essential to ensure that all equipment is working perfectly. If equipment is not checked prior to use, then there may be issues which can lead to the patient suffering from various causes. Teaching and learning of staff in regards to equipment are therefore required to help them understand how the equipment works.

10 Managing Perioperative Medication

Introduction

Many patients who undergo surgery also take medications regularly, normally because of other issues or conditions outside their surgical needs (Kennedy *et al.* 2000). Surgeons and anaesthetists must ask patients about the medication they are taking and decide whether it should be continued until the point of surgery. Sometimes this is not the case, and patients may be asked to stop taking particular medications. There is little research about the use of medications during perioperative care, normally because surgeons and anaesthetists work in specialities and their recommendations vary considerably (Kroenke *et al.* 1998).

However, several papers in the literature have identified the need to either stop or resume medications, depending on the status of the patient and the delivery of anaesthesia and surgery (Saber 2006, Spell 2001). Practitioners, because they spend time caring for patients too, need to know how drugs interact and how they can cause harm to patients.

This chapter focusses on some drugs which are known to have effects during perioperative care, including interacting with anaesthetic drugs as well as with medications given during surgery.

Principles of managing medication

Before anaesthesia or surgery, both the anaesthetist and surgeon will discuss medication issues with the patient, and the patient's past history of taking medications, which may be verified by the patient's GP. This will include medications such as prescribed drugs, herbal medicines, alcohol, nicotine and any illicit drugs such as cocaine or ecstasy (Visala & Macpherson 2012). Essential medications that support the life of the patient, especially in the elderly, may be continued throughout the perioperative period, if feasible, based on the judgement of the doctors (Saber 2006).

However, if any medications are known to cause anaesthetic or surgical complications, then they should be withdrawn before surgery and only administered once the patient has fully recovered. Sometimes drugs taken at home can interact with drugs taken during surgery or anaesthesia, leading to further problems. It is also possible that drugs taken orally before anaesthesia may not be absorbed in the gastrointestinal system because of problems due to poor blood supply, oedema or the action of other medications (Saber 2006).

Perioperative medications

Cardiovascular drugs

Beta blockers help to reduce ischaemia by decreasing oxygen demand in the myocardial muscles, and there is also an increase in catecholamines which can help to prevent arrhythmias. Patients who regularly take beta blockers because of angina run the risk of ischaemia if beta blockers are withdrawn during their perioperative experience, leading to the risk of

Rapid Perioperative Care, First Edition. Paul Wicker and Sara Dalby.

bradycardia, hypotension, morbidity or mortality (Shammash *et al.* 2001). Patients who regularly take beta blockers should therefore normally continue taking them during surgery and throughout their stay in hospital to prevent complications. If the patient cannot take oral beta blockers, it is possible to use intravenous methods such as metoprolol, propranolol and labetalol (Visala & Macpherson 2012). However, patients who are taking a nonselective beta blocker (e.g. propranolol) do not need to switch to a selective beta blocker perioperatively.

Diuretics

Diuretics may cause hypokalaemia and hypovolaemia during the perioperative phase. Hypokalaemia may increase the risk of perioperative arrhythmia, increase the effects of muscle relaxants and provoke paralytic ileus (Saber 2006). Anaesthetists also need to monitor fluid balance and potassium levels, in case of hypovolaemia, if diuretics are given during surgery.

Diuretics are potentially capable of causing hypokalaemia and hypovolaemia during the perioperative phase. Anaesthetists must closely monitor fluid balance and potassium levels when administering diuretics to a patient to prevent hypokalaemia (low potassium), which may increase the risk of perioperative arrhythmias, increase the effects of muscle relaxants and provoke paralytic ileus (Saber 2006). And hypovolaemia (dehydration/blood volume) can cause hypovolaemic shock, kidney failure, seizures and death. It is recommended that the patient has a urinary catheter in situ prior to the start of the surgical procedure in order to monitor urine output.

Anaesthetic agents can also cause systemic vasodilatation, resulting in hypotension in patients who have been given diuretics which reduce their fluid balance. Therefore, it appears that diuretics should be stopped before elective surgery (Kroenke *et al.* 1998). However, if diuretics need to be given to the patient, improved fluid balance can be gained by providing intravenous fluids during surgery.

Gastrointestinal drugs

The stress that patients undergo during surgery can increase the risk of damage to the gastric mucosa. This can be reduced by using H2 blockers or proton pump inhibitors perioperatively, and luckily they do not interact much with anaesthetic agents. Chemical pneumonitis can occur following aspiration of the stomach contents. However, H2 blockers and proton pump inhibitors reduce the possibility of gastric aspiration during anaesthesia by decreasing gastric volume and raising gastric fluid pH (Visala & Macpherson 2012).

Because of the benefits of H2 blockers and proton pump inhibitors, it is best to keep patients on these drugs perioperatively (Visala & Macpherson 2012). Patients who cannot take oral medications can use H2 blockers and proton pump inhibitors intravenously, which are less expensive than oral drugs.

Pulmonary drugs

Reducing the risk of postoperative pulmonary complications in patients with asthma and chronic obstructive pulmonary disease can be managed by using inhaled beta agonists and anticholinergic drugs. These drugs include beta agonists such as albuterol, metaproterenol, salmeterol and formoterol, and anticholinergics such as ipratropium and tiotropium (Visala & Macpherson 2012). These drugs should be inhaled before surgery using a nebulizer or ventilator, and then continue to be used as needed during anaesthesia and surgery.

Other drugs which can be used include theophylline, although it is known to cause serious arrhythmias and neurotoxicity in some cases because it may interact with anaesthetic drugs. It is normally decided therefore to discontinue theophylline (which is a drug used in therapy for respiratory diseases, e.g. chronic obstructive pulmonary disease) before surgery and anaesthesia unless it is essential for the patient. If obstructive lung disease is a condition

Table 10.1 Perioperative management of medications

Name of speciality		
Drug actions	**Drug names**	**Actions**
Cardiovascular		
Beta blockers	Metoprolol, atenolol etc.	Continued until and including the day of operation
ACE inhibitors (ACEIs) and angiotensin receptor blockers (ARBs)	Captopril, lisinopril, losartan, candesartan etc.	Discontinued on the day of anaesthesia and surgery
Calcium channel blockers	Nifedipine, diltiazem etc.	Continued until and including the day of the operation
Nitrates	Nitroglycerin, isosorbide etc.	Continued until and including the day of the operation
Alpha-2 agonists	Clonidine	Continued until and including the day of the operation
Pain killer	Aspirin	Discontinued one week prior to the planned operation, unless required
Oral anticoagulants	Warfarin, Coumadin etc.	Discontinued 5 days prior to the planned operation, unless required
Diuretics	Furosemide, hydrochlorothiazide etc.	Discontinued the day of the operation
Cardiac rhythm management medications	Digoxin, beta blockers, quinidine, amiodarone etc.	Continued until and including the day of the operation
Statins	Atorvastatin, simvastatin etc.	Continued until and including the day of the operation
Cholesterol-lowering medications	Statins, niacin, bile–acid resins, fibric acid derivatives, cholesterol absorption inhibitors etc.	Discontinued the day of the operation
Central nervous system medications		
Anticonvulsants	Phenytoin, tegretol etc.	Continued until and including the day of the operation
Antidepressants	Imipramine, sertraline etc.	Continued until and including the day of the operation
Monoamine oxidase inhibitors	Marplan, nardil, sulphate, parnate, emsam etc.	Discontinued 2 full weeks prior to the planned operation
Antianxiety medications	Diazepam, lorazepam etc.	Continued until and including the day of the operation
Antipsychotics	Haloperidol, Risperdal etc.	Continued until and including the day of the operation
Lithium	Lithium	Continued until and including the day of the operation
Anti-Parkinson drugs	Sinemet etc.	Continued until and including the day of the operation
Recreational drugs	Marijuana, cocaine etc.	Discontinued as soon as possible prior to any planned operation
Vitamins and nutritional supplements		
Over-the-counter vitamins	All vitamins	Continued until the day before the planned operation. Vitamin E should be discontinued one week prior to the operation.
Herbal or alternative preparations		Discontinued one week prior to the surgical procedure

(continued overleaf)

Table 10.1 *(continued)*

Pulmonary medications		
Asthma medications	Theophylline, inhaled steroids etc.	Continued until and including the day of the operation
Chronic pulmonary obstructive disease (COPD) medications	Theophylline, ipratropium, inhaled steroids etc.	Continued until and including the day of the operation
Pulmonary hypertension medications	Sildenafil, prostacyclin etc.	Continued until and including the day of the operation
Endocrine		
Oral hypoglycaemics	Insulin, peptides etc.	Taken the day before the operation and discontinued the day of the operation
Thyroid medications	Synthroid, desiccated thyroid, propylthiouracil etc.	Continued until and including the day of the operation
Steroids	Prednisone, cortef etc.	Continued until and including the day of the operation
Oral contraceptives		Continued until and including the day of the operation
Renal		
Renal drugs	Phosphate binders, renal vitamins, iron, erythropoietin etc.	Taken until the day before the operation, but discontinued the day of the operation
Gynaecology and urology		
Prostate medications	Terazosin, tamsulozsin etc.	Continued until and including the day of the operation
Hormonal medications	Adrenal cortical steroids, antiandrogens, antithyroid agents etc.	Continued until and including the day of the operation
Oral contraceptives	Apri, Azurette, Caziant etc.	Continued until and including the day of the operation
Analgesics		
Painkillers	Aspirin, Alka-Seltzer, Bufferin etc.	Discontinued at least one week prior to the planned operation, unless supported by surgeon or anaesthetist
Opiate-containing analgesics	Vicodin, tylox, methadone etc.	Continued until and including the day of the operation
Nonsteroidal anti-inflammatory compounds	Ibuprofen, naproxen etc.	Discontinued at least 5 days prior to the planned operation
Gastrointestinal		
Gastroesophageal reflux medications	Ranitidine, omeprazole etc.	Continued until and including the day of the operation
Anti-emetics	Ondansetron, metoclopramide etc.	Continued until and including the day of the operation

Adapted from University of Michigan (2015), *Perioperative Management of Chronic Medications*. Available at http://med.umich.edu/preopclinic/guidelines/meds_to_stop1.pdf

in the patient, then other drugs such as beta agonists, glucocorticoids and anticholinergic medications may be used.

Glucocorticoids or corticosteroids are used for patients with pulmonary disease. These patients are at risk of adrenal issues if the steroids are withdrawn, particularly if the patient is under stress before anaesthesia and surgery. Glucocorticoids are useful in maintaining optimal lung functions in such patients, and therefore it is likely that they will be continued during the perioperative period (Saber 2006).

Asthma can be controlled using leukotriene inhibitors such as zileuton (Zyflo), zafirlukast (Accolate) and montelukast (Singulair). Even after the treatment stops, they continue to be effective at working on asthma and pulmonary complications for up to three weeks (Reiss *et al.* 1998). It appears that these drugs do not interact with anaesthetic drugs; therefore, they can be continued before and after the patient's perioperative treatment.

Conclusion

Postoperative outcomes are improved when there is excellent medication management during the perioperative phase of the patient's journey. Most medications can be used throughout the perioperative phase; however, some medications will need to be stopped preoperatively, for example diuretics and oral antidiabetics (Hollevoet *et al.* 2011). Oral antidiabetic medication needs to be stopped at a maximum of 48 h prior to surgery, although some drugs can be stopped 12 h before surgery. Insulin, including fast, medium and long-acting insulin, is normally stopped the evening before surgery (Hollevoet *et al.* 2011).

Consultation with the anaesthetist preoperatively is an important part of the patient's pathway to advise and instruct the patient about the procedure, fasting time and medication. This is because the population is now aging, and the number of elderly patients who take various medications is increasing. For example, patients may take herbal medications or food supplements without mentioning it to the anaesthetist or surgeon. These medications may have implications for the patient during anaesthesia and surgery (Saber 2006). Therefore, it is important that the patient informs the anaesthetist and surgeon of any drugs, vitamins or herbal medications that they are currently taking.

This chapter covers only a few of the main medications used, but it highlights the need for management of drugs during the perioperative phase and suggests the medications which should be stopped or carried on preoperatively, or alternatively whether they should be replaced with other drugs. It is also important that the medical staff and practitioners understand the interactions between the drugs taken by the patient and the drugs delivered during perioperative care, and it is vitally important that these drugs must be taken into consideration during the perioperative care of the patient.

11 Interprofessional Learning and Collaboration

Until the early 1990s, anaesthetists, surgeons and perioperative practitioners did not work together as a team. Surgeons did not care about the role of the perioperative practitioner; they just told them what to do and how to do it. Surgeons and anaesthetists often argued, especially if the anaesthetic took a long time leading to delayed surgery. These attitudes, sometimes resulting in 'horizontal violence', developed because professionals lacked understanding of each other's professional roles.

Interprofessional learning (IPL) is now a key part in the delivery of perioperative patient care and is developing in all perioperative professions in the United Kingdom. Surgeons, anaesthetists, Operating Department Practitioners (ODPs) and nurses must work, learn, communicate and be together, rather than criticising and undermining each other (Wicker 2011).

IPL is about sharing learning knowledge and skills, and communicating between professions. When effective communication and sharing skills and knowledge are carried out, then professions are much more likely to work effectively as a team. IPL is about different groups of professionals learning together, and giving professional insight and education into the holistic care of the patient (Wooding 2013). As the staff and students engage with each other, they begin to understand and get insight into each other's priorities, skills and knowledge (Wicker 2011).

Some of the key points currently associated with IPL include improved teamwork, the use of the World Health Organization (WHO) checklist, better communication and, most of all, better patient outcomes.

Providing interprofessional learning

IPL enhances the holistic care of the patient by ensuring that all professional groups are aware of each other's knowledge and skills, and it enables them to work together to provide the best possible patient care (CAIPE 2011).

IPL also aims to:

- Improve communication, problem solving and reflection.
- Improve professional practice by understanding how to work with other professionals.
- Reduce interprofessional conflict by respecting the work of other professionals.
- Increase professional satisfaction by working with other professionals as a team (Quick 2011).

IPL therefore improves patient care by improving communication between professional groups, respecting team members and improving learning knowledge and skills within the team. This is also echoed in several national standards which highlight the need for a team to work together (NMC 2010), to create the value of interprofessional teamwork and collaboration.

Rapid Perioperative Care, First Edition. Paul Wicker and Sara Dalby.

Table 11.1 Advantages and problems with interprofessional learning and working

Advantages of IPL

- Allows qualified staff and students to collaborate with other professions, understand their needs and share goals or actions within a pleasant environment.
- Increases the connections between other healthcare professions and helps to establish better care outcomes for patients.
- Improves patient care by having healthcare professionals interact with and understand the roles of other such professionals, by increasing and developing the knowledge and skills of staff and students in different environments.
- Helps to develop a multidisciplinary team leading to better care for patients.
- Provides the opportunity for students and staff to refer patients to other professions in order to allocate specific individual patient care.
- Improves interprofessional relationships through good communication and interaction with other professions, leading to the overall best patient care.
- Staff and students can learn and develop knowledge and skills from other professions and be able to reflect on the actions they are taking in clinical practice.

Problems with IPL

- IPL can lead to increased complexity for staff and students, which may not be understandable unless the actions suggested are described in full.
- Students may not appreciate the need for collaboration with other professions if the topics being taught are not relevant to their own profession.
- Work for staff and students can increase if collaboration with other professions is needed.
- Students in universities may not have synchronised timetables and may find collaboration difficult with other professions.
- Interprofessional working requires group participation in the clinical area so that staff learn about the activities of other professions. This may not be possible due to workloads. Ineffective communication between professionals can be detrimental for the care of the patient, contributing to delays, missed key information and lack of equipment for the patient's specific needs.

Consequently, perioperative teamwork has become more effective (Wicker 2011), and IPL has become essential for interprofessional teamwork, both nationally and internationally.

IPL for students

Most universities provide IPL for all health professionals and in several different formats. Universities use IPL to help students have a greater understanding of the roles of other professions. So, for example, ODPs and paramedics can work together in some cases, learning about each other's roles and understanding each other's knowledge and skills.

An example of IPL outside of the universities is the Better Training Better Care project funded by Health Education England (HEE 2014). Junior surgeons often work with perioperative practitioners under the guidance of consultant surgeons. This creates effective teamwork between the junior surgeons and the student practitioners who have good knowledge and skills regarding surgery. This leads to better teamwork and greater collaboration.

Student feedback on IPL is usually positive; it includes understanding of other professionals' roles and the importance of communication and interpersonal collaboration. The purpose of IPL is therefore to improve professional practice and widen the scope of all professionals by including it within their own curriculums.

Due to an ageing population and technological advances, the NHS has become much more complex in recent years. This has led to greater demands on NHS staff as well as reductions in staffing and salaries. However, by using IPL, if the team understands the need to work well together, then hopefully better teamwork will develop, leading to optimal patient care.

In the literature over the past few years, IPL has been identified as being beneficial for preparing students to work as part of a team, and also for improving clinical outcomes both in clinical practice and in preregistration programmes, leading to higher standards of professionalism and enhanced practice (Wooding 2013).

Conclusion

WHO now recognises the need for interprofessional collaboration both in higher education and in clinical practice, in order to improve on the global health crisis. Interprofessional working can sometimes be difficult to understand and implement in different countries, especially those areas where training and education are not at a high level. Healthcare workers may believe that they are working interprofessionally with other health workers, whereas they may simply be working by themselves and ignoring other professionals. Collaboration can only occur when two different professionals interact together, understand each other and work together to help a patient. While healthcare workers need to be professional, they also need to understand the need to be interprofessional in order to address challenges in global ill health, and improve the health outcomes for patients (WHO 2010).

As interprofessional practice in perioperative care is now improving, the perioperative team is more aware of the roles of other team members, which has helped to reduce tension and also enhanced communication and collaboration. Interprofessional working has also increased the knowledge and skills within the perioperative team, and has helped everybody to understand the needs of other professions. This has led to all professions learning from each other, and understanding each other, in a positive way. This ultimately leads to enhancing and delivering the best possible care for the patient, and fewer 'never events' happening.

12 Preventing Surgical Site Infection

Surgical site infections (SSIs) were common before the 1900s, when patients and staff could not be protected by gloves, masks, antiseptics or antibiotics. However, SSIs continue to affect patients and sometimes represent 20% of all infections related to surgery (Smyth *et al.* 2008). Nowadays, up to 5% of surgical patients may develop an SSI (Leaper 2010), leading to pain and discomfort and thereby contributing to high risks of the patient developing morbidity or mortality. The Health Protection Agency (HPA 2011) also detected SSI rates of around 10% for patients undergoing bowel surgery. SSI rates are therefore continuing but sometimes are not monitored due to early discharge of the patient and lack of follow-up by medical staff once they have returned home.

Surgical site infections

During surgery, microorganisms from exposed tissues, such as skin, bowel or stomach, can spread throughout the wound site and infiltrate tissues that are being operated on (Aziz 2014). Once the microorganisms access the tissues, they then begin to multiply, leading to infections. Normally SSIs arise within 30 days of surgery, but if an implant is placed within the body, SSIs can arise within 12 months as any infection may take time to affect the incision or the deep tissues. Once the body is infected, the patient may suffer from fever, inflammation, swelling and pain; and in some cases organisms are released into the bloodstream, causing sepsis (Leaper 2010).

However, patients may remain in hospital for a short time, and SSIs often do not appear for up to 30 days. Therefore, monitoring these patients is a vital part of their care pathway following their return home. There must be monitoring of postoperative patients at home in order to ensure prevention of developing SSIs; furthermore, in the event SSIs do develop, immediate action needs to be implemented to treat the infection. Patients may not develop SSIs, but if they do then actions need to be taken to prevent or cure the infections (Tanner *et al.* 2009).

Risks associated with SSIs

Patients run varying risks of developing SSIs depending on the surgical procedure they receive. Further risks include high body mass index (BMI; e.g. morbid obesity) and pre-existing conditions in patients. The status of the patient can cover these areas:

- Minor surgery where no microbes are encountered and body spaces are not entered. For example, gastrointestinal, respiratory or urinary tracts may be entered under controlled conditions and without contamination occurring.
- Major surgery or trauma surgery where parts of the body including the gastrointestinal or urinary tracts are incised, leading to contamination by microbes.
- Patients who have an existing infection already present prior to surgery can inadvertently contribute to infection of tissues that have been incised or opened.

Rapid Perioperative Care, First Edition. Paul Wicker and Sara Dalby.

Surgery may be carried out with no incisions into organs which contain microbes. However, the patient may be given antibiotics prior to surgery, reducing the risk of acquiring an infection. Similarly, small and superficial wounds which become infected can be treated by oral antibiotics and are generally not serious infections. However, infections deep within the body, including in the organs or bowels, can result in serious side effects leading to readmission to hospital, intravenous antibiotics, wound debridement and possibly further surgery (Leaper 2010).

Causes of SSIs

Although SSIs often occur because of infections during surgery, it is also possible for the patient to increase the risk of SSIs because of their wellbeing. For example, smoking, diabetes and old age can all contribute to SSIs developing because of the impact that these conditions have on the health of the patient (Leaper 2010). Following accidents or trauma, the patient will not be able to improve their health before surgery as urgent surgery is likely to be needed. However, if the patient is undergoing normal surgery and has several weeks to plan for their own care, then it is advisable for patients to stop smoking, improve their diet, control diabetes and so on. GPs and surgeons, as well as practitioners, should encourage the patient to develop a healthy lifestyle in preparation for surgery to reduce the likelihood of developing an SSI (Aziz 2014).

The National Institute for Health and Clinical Excellence (NICE 2008) produced guidelines on preventing surgical wound infections which provide a comprehensive list of recommendations for best practice. Some of the priorities identified include:

- Ensure the patient is clean and healthy before anaesthesia and surgery.
- Remove hair using electric clippers.
- Give antibiotics before surgery.
- Prepare the skin for surgery using an antiseptic prep (Darouiche *et al.* 2010).
- Maintain sterility during surgery and anaesthesia.
- Use suitable dressings to adequately and effectively protect the wound following surgery (NICE 2008).

Perioperative care

On entry to the operating room, the patient must be prepared and cared for effectively to reduce the chances of developing SSIs. Various actions need to be taken at each stage of perioperative care, including the following.

Preoperative phase

- Advise patient to have a shower or bath before surgery.
- Remove hair using electric clippers – which should ideally be carried out before the patient has a shower before surgery to prevent stray hairs going into the incision site.
- Provide suitable theatre wear to the patient.
- Keep the patient warm.
- Ensure the patient has visited the toilet before surgery.
- Remove jewellery, artificial nails, nail polish and so on.
- Ensure patient receives antibiotics if prescribed by doctors (NICE 2008).

Intraoperative phase

- The surgical team will scrub hands and don theatre scrubs and gloves before starting surgery.

- The surgical team must all wear face masks.
- Prepare the patient's skin using antiseptic solutions, for example povidone–iodine or chlorhexidine.
- Place drapes carefully on the patient, ensuring sterility is maintained.
- Ensure antiseptic skin preparations are dry before using diathermy.
- Ensure the patient's temperature is above 36.5 °C as a minimum.
- Maintain respirations, breathing and oxygen saturation throughout the surgery.
- Consider using wound irrigation, but only if required.
- Cover the wound with a dressing post surgery.

Postoperative phase

- Change dressing if needed using an aseptic non-touch technique.
- Use sterile saline for cleaning the wound soon after surgery.
- Advise patients not to shower up to 48 h after surgery.
- Although infected wounds are unlikely to happen during the recovery period, ask the doctor for prescription of antibiotics if the wound shows signs of infection, possibly due to trauma or an accident prior to surgery.
- Monitor the patient regularly to identify any issues that may be developing, for example pain, vomiting, pressure sores and so on (NICE 2008).

On return to the ward, following assessment and discharge from the Recovery Room, ward nurses will provide instructions to the patient regarding how to care for their wounds appropriately. The ward staff will also ensure the patient has contact details of relevant support in the community on their return home for any concerns or issues they may have. They will also let them know who to contact if any issues arise once they return home.

Conclusion

Perioperative practitioners working effectively and efficiently can aim to reduce the risk of harm to patients in the development of surgical site infections. It is also essential that recovery room practitioners are aware of the need to protect the patient against infection by assessing and managing postoperative wounds and detecting postoperative wound infection if it occurs (Aziz 2014). All perioperative practitioners therefore need to have a good understanding of preventative measures and the importance of avoiding SSIs in perioperative care.

13 Skin Preparation for Surgery

Ward nurses must ensure that the patient's skin for surgery is safe and aseptic in order to prevent the risk of infection to the wound site, so that infection of the skin does not arise or spread into the wound site. This may include bathing, showering, removing hair and so on. It is also important that the patient's dignity is maintained as much as possible while skin preparation occurs to prevent the patient from becoming anxious or undergoing stress.

Surgical site infections (SSIs) can occur when surgical wounds become infected from causes such as bacterial contamination (because of unclean skin or lack of preparation), the presence of viruses, and any allergies which the patient is suffering from (WHO 2009). SSIs can occur because of bacterial contamination on the patient's skin or mucous membranes, or in areas where bacteria or viruses occur such as within the bowel or vagina (NICE 2013). Organisms that cause harm to the patient may include aerobic Gram-positive staphylococci, or faecal flora in areas such as the perineum, groin, vagina or anus.

The reason for disinfecting skin is to prevent SSIs by removing and destroying any skin flora close to the surgical incision. Skin disinfectant should therefore be fast acting, be persistent and contain antiseptics to ensure skin is cleaned well and remains free from bacteria or viruses. Hair is also often removed if it is close to the surgical site, using a surgical hair clipper before prepping and draping the patient.

It is advisable that patients should undertake a shower or bath using soap or skin-cleansing fluids before surgery (Webster *et al.* 2012). Undertaking showers or baths before surgery helps to remove dirt, soil or any other debris in order to reduce the presence of bacteria or viruses. Antiseptic solutions (e.g. chlorhexidine), used for washing skin before surgery, are not normally undertaken. However, NICE do recommend skin cleansing with soap in order to ensure that the skin is clean and has a reduction in the amount of bacteria or viruses (NICE 2013).

Surgical skin preparation

Practitioners or surgeons should use a painting technique with the antiseptic solution, starting at the centre of the surgical site and moving to the periphery. The swab should not be returned to the centre of the surgical site after moving to the periphery in case of bacteria or viruses being taken back to the main incision site. The solution should be dry before applying the drapes; this can be achieved either by waiting for it to dry, or by using a dry swab to effectively dry the area.

Actions to take involving skin preparation may include:

- The surgical site and positioning of the patient must be confirmed using the WHO checklist, and confirmed with the surgeon, before commencing skin prepping.
- Skin prep lotions must be checked to ensure they are the correct solution and are in date before use.
- Marking of the surgical site using a pen should not be removed during skin prepping, to allow the pen marks to remain visible after draping has occurred.

Rapid Perioperative Care, First Edition. Paul Wicker and Sara Dalby.

- Surgical preparation will only start once nonsterile practitioners move away from the surgical site.
- Scrub practitioners can only prep the area after they have received specific training on the methods for skin prepping. Otherwise, surgeons will prep the area themselves.
- Swabs or sponges are used at the tip of an instrument holder to prevent the skin from being damaged.
- Aqueous-based skin prep solutions must be used if the patient has sensitive areas, such as mucous membranes or open wounds. In other cases, alcoholic skin prep solutions will be used.
- Alcohol-based prep solutions which pool underneath patients or under drapes may result in fire following the use of diathermy, and may also burn the patient's skin.
- Prep solutions should be applied carefully to prevent solutions from pooling beneath the patient or underneath drapes.

Skin prep solutions

Alcoholic prep solutions provide good service as an antiseptic agent because they act rapidly and also evaporate quickly, compared to aqueous solutions (Maiwald *et al.* 2012). Alcohol solutions also support the skin and do not produce stains on the skin. The best alcohol concentrations are usually around 60–90% which help to destroy bacteria and viruses (Maiwald *et al.* 2012). Chlorhexidine gluconate (CHG) is a very useful solution which has high antibacterial activity (Larson *et al.* 1990). CHG also protects the skin and does not tend to irritate the skin or normally produce allergic reactions; however, it should not be used for eyes or inside the patient's ear, especially if the patient is being treated for head or neck surgery.

However, using alcoholic-based skin prep solutions can lead to operating room fires originating from them. This occurs because electrosurgery may be used to stop bleeding or to seal blood vessels; electrosurgery creates sparks that may ignite the alcohol vapour. The patient may suffer from burns, and the drapes may catch fire. Fire can be prevented by ensuring the skin is dry before applying the drapes and also ensuring that there is no alcoholic solution pooling underneath the patient or soaking into the operating table cover. It is also essential that alcoholic solutions are not used in areas with excessive hair (e.g. the groin) as this can prevent the alcohol from vaporising (Hemani *et al.* 2009).

Povidone–iodine is an iodophor which reduces the effects of tissue irritation, staining of skin or absorption within the skin (WHO 2009). Aqueous iodine, however, may lead to a rise in serum iodine in the patient's bloodstream. This can lead to severe allergic reactions, which in some cases have been seen to happen in some patients. Iodophors, however, have little effect on the patient and are usually inactivated by blood or serum proteins.

Summary

Preparation of patients for surgery is important and essential to ensure that they are kept safe and healthy and do not develop SSIs. In summary:

1. Patients should have a shower or bath before surgery.
2. Skin prep should be applied from the centre of the surgical site to the periphery and allowed to dry completely before applying drapes.
3. Alcohol-based prep solutions (in particular, 2% chlorhexidine gluconate) should be used whenever possible.
4. Patients requiring cervical surgery must use low levels of alcohol prep or aqueous prep solutions.
5. Prep solutions should be kept away from eyes, ears and mouths to prevent harm to the patient.

References and Further Reading

1. The Role of the Anaesthetic Practitioner

References

Association of Anaesthetists of Great Britain and Ireland (AAGBI) (2012) *Checking Anaesthetic Equipment*. Available at http://www.aagbi.org/sites/default/files/checking_anaesthetic_equipment_2012.pdf (accessed 15 November 2014)

Copley S, Ottley E, Rigby J (2006) Anaesthesia Practitioner Role Development. *The Clinical Services Journal*. Available at http://www.clinicalservicesjournal.com/Print.aspx?Story=982 (accessed 19 November 2014)

Fynes E, Martin DSE, Hoy L, Cousley A (2014) Anaesthetic nurse specialist role: leading and facilitation in clinical practice. *Journal of Perioperative Practice* **24** (5): 97–102.

Goodman T & Spry C (2014) *Essentials of Perioperative Nursing*, 5th ed. Burlington MA, Jones & Bartlett Learning.

NHS Modernisation Agency (2005) *Anaesthesia Practitioner Curriculum Framework*. London, NHS Modernisation Agency.

O'Neill J (2010) Patient Care During Anaesthesia. In Wicker P & O'Neill J, *Caring for the Perioperative Patient*. Chichester, Wiley-Blackwell.

Royal College of Anaesthetists (RCA) (2006) *The Workforce Consequences of Anaesthesia Practitioners*. London, RCA.

Smith B, Rawling P, Wicker P, Jones C (eds.) (2007) *Core Topics in Operating Department Practice: Anaesthesia and Critical Care*. Cambridge, Cambridge University Press.

Valdez-Lowe C, Ghareeb S, Artinian N (2009) Pulse Oximetry in Adults. *American Journal of Nursing* **109** (6): 52–59.

Wicker P & Smith B (2008) Checking the Anaesthetic Machine. *Journal of Perioperative Practice* **18** (8) 354–359.

Further Reading

Francis C (2006) *Respiratory Care*. Oxford, Blackwell Publishing.

McConachie I (2014) *Anesthesia and Perioperative Care of the High Risk Patient*. Cambridge, Cambridge University Press.

Websites

The Anaesthesia Team: http://www.aagbi.org/sites/default/files/anaesthesia_team_2010_0.pdf (accessed 15 November 2014)

The Anaesthetic Practitioner: http://www.docnet.org.uk/anaesthetic-practitioner.html (accessed 15 November 2014)

Videos

The Anaesthetic Machine Check: https://www.youtube.com/watch?v=DojLuUsoEBg (accessed 15 November 2014)

Checking Anaesthetic Equipment: https://www.youtube.com/watch?v=-JnMRrVdsJw (accessed 15 November 2014)

ODP Anaesthetic Machine Check: https://www.youtube.com/watch?v=bu5nXPe6w_U (accessed 15 November 2014)

Rapid Perioperative Care, First Edition. Paul Wicker and Sara Dalby.

2. The Role of the Surgical Practitioner

References

Conway N, Ong P, Bowers M, Grimmett N (2014) *Clinical Pocket Reference: Operating Department Practice*, 2nd ed. Oxford. www.clinicalpocketreference.com

D'Lima D, Sacks M, Blackman W, Benn J (2014) Surgical Swab Counting: A Qualitative Analysis from the Perspective of the Scrub Nurse. *Journal of Perioperative Practice* **24** (5): 103–111.

Goodman T & Spry C (2014) *Essentials of Perioperative Nursing*, 5th ed. Burlington MA, Jones & Bartlett Learning.

Smith C (2005) Care of the Patient Undergoing Surgery. In Woodhead K & Wicker PA (eds.) *Textbook of Perioperative Care*. Elsevier, Edinburgh, pp. 161–180.

Wicker P & Nightingale A (2010) Patient Care during Surgery. In: Wicker P & O'Neill J (eds.) *Caring for the Perioperative Patient*, 2nd ed. Chichester, Wiley-Blackwell, pp. 339–378.

Further Reading

Gruendemann BJ & Fernsebner B (1995) *Comprehensive Perioperative Nursing*. London, Jones & Bartlett.

Manley K & Bellman L (2000) *Surgical Nursing: Advancing Practice*. Edinburgh, Churchill Livingstone.

Woodhead K & Fudge L (2012) *Manual of Perioperative Care: An Essential Guide*. Chichester, Wiley-Blackwell.

Websites

Duties of the Scrub Practitioner: http://www.meht.nhs.uk/EasysiteWeb/getresource.axd?AssetID=2674&type=full&servicetype=Attachment (accessed 18 November 2014)

Nontechnical Skills of the Scrub Practitioner: http://chfg.org/wp-content/uploads/2013/09/JPP-December-2012-NonTechSkillsScrubPract-McClelland.pdf (accessed 18 November 2014)

Role of the Circulating Nurse: http://nursingcrib.com/nursing-notes-reviewer/role-of-circulating-nurse/ (accessed 18 November 2014)

Videos

A Comprehensive Guide to the Surgical Scrub: https://www.youtube.com/watch?v=L8OLnyJ3mAc (accessed 18 November 2014)

Surgery Instruments: https://www.youtube.com/watch?v=COjJxfbmdWY (accessed 18 November 2014)

What Is an Operating Department Practitioner (ODP)?: https://www.youtube.com/watch?v=lPbP7rToi7c (accessed 18 November 2014)

3. The Role of the Recovery Practitioner

References

Alfaro NI (2013) *Roles of the Postanesthesia Care Unit Nurse*. Available at http://www.slideshare.net/najr2006/roles-of-the-postanesthesia-care-unit-nurse (accessed 11 December 2014)

Association of Anaesthetists of Great Britain and Ireland (AAGBI) (2013) *Immediate Post-anaesthesia Recovery*. London, AAGBI. Available at http://www.aagbi.org/sites/default/files/immediate_post-anaesthesia_recovery_2013.pdf (accessed 18 December 2014)

Hatfield A & Tronson M (2009) *The Complete Recovery Book*, 4th ed. Oxford, Oxford University Press.

Further Reading

Association of Anaesthetists of Great Britain and Ireland (AAGBI) (2002) *Immediate Postanaesthesia Recovery*. Available at http://www.aagbi.org/sites/default/files/postanaes02.pdf (accessed 18 December 2014)

Rawlinson A, Kitchingham N, Hart C, *et al.* (2012) Mechanisms of Reducing Postoperative Pain, Nausea and Vomiting: A Systematic Review of Current Techniques. *Journal of Evidence Based Medicine* **17**: 75–80.

Stephens DS & Boaler J (2007) The Nurse's Role in Immediate Postoperative Care. *British Journal of Medicine* **1** (6070): 1119–1202. Available at http://www.ncbi.nlm.nih.gov/pmc/articles/PMC1606846/ (accessed 18 December 2014)

Websites

Postoperative Care: http://www.surgeryencyclopedia.com/Pa-St/Postoperative-Care.html (accessed 18 December 2014)

Phillips J (2013) *Post-operative Care*. Available at https://www.rcoa.ac.uk/system/files/CSQ-ARB2012-SEC3.pdf (accessed 16 December 2014)

Videos

Enhanced Recovery after Surgery: http://www.youtube.com/watch?v=9Ec_CsdjbP4 (accessed 18 December 2014)

Postoperative Initial Assessment: https://www.youtube.com/watch?v=sdnM5ZuPfl0 (accessed 18 December 2014)

Postoperative Nursing Care: https://www.youtube.com/watch?v=0wSkUPiOQoA (accessed 18 December 2014)

4. Preoperative Assessment of Perioperative Patients

References

Berger R (2005) Bacteria of Preoperative Urinary Tract Infections Contaminate the Surgical Fields and Develop Surgical Site Infections in Urological Operations. *The Journal of Urology* **174** (6): 2244–2244.

Goodman T & Spry C (2014) *Essentials of Perioperative Nursing*, 5th ed. Burlington MA, Jones & Bartlett Learning.

Holmes J (2005) Preoperative Visiting: Landmarks of the Journey. *British Journal of Perioperative Nursing* **15** (10): 434–443.

Mood G & Tang W (2009) Perioperative DVT Prophylaxis. Available at http://emedicine.medscape.com/article/284371-overview (accessed 10 August 2014)

Nelson EA, Mani R, Vowden K (2008) Intermittent Pneumatic Compression for Treating Venous Leg Ulcers. *Cochrane Database of Systematic Reviews* (**2**): CD001899. doi:10.1002/14651858.CD001899.pub2

Schultz A (2005) Predicting and Preventing Pressure Ulcers in Surgical Patients. *AORN Journal* **81** (5): 986–1006.

Sweitzer B (2008) *Handbook of Preoperative Assessment and Management*. Philadelphia, Lippincott Williams & Wilkins

Waterlow J (1985) A Risk Assessment Card. *Nursing Times* **81** (48): 49–55.

Wicker P (2010) Preoperative Preparation of Perioperative Patients. In Wicker P & O'Neill J (eds.) *Caring for the Perioperative Patient*. Chichester, Wiley-Blackwell.

Wicker P (2015) Caring for Perioperative Patients. *Journal of Operating Department Practitioners* **3** (1): 27–32.

Wicker P, Cox F (2010) Patient Care during Recovery. In Wicker P & O'Neill J. (eds.) *Caring for the Perioperative Patient*. Oxford, Wiley-Blackwell.

Further Reading

Aitkenhead A, Moppott I, Thompson J (2013) *Textbook of Anaesthesia*, 6th ed. Edinburgh, Elsevier Health Sciences.

Current Nursing (2013) Application of Roy's Adaptation Model in Nursing Practice. Available at http://currentnursing.com/nursing_theory/application_Roy's_adaptation_model.htm (accessed 10 August 2014)

Holdcroft A & Jagger S (2005) *Core Topics in Pain*. Cambridge, Cambridge University Press.

Websites

Preoperative Assessment and Planning: http://www.institute.nhs.uk/quality_and_service_improvement_tools/quality_and_service_improvement_tools/pre-operative_assessment_and_planning.html (accessed 12 May 2014)

Preoperative Assessments: http://www.nhs.uk/Video/Pages/Pre-operativeassessments.aspx (accessed 20 December 2014)

Videos

Head to Toe Nursing Assessment: https://www.youtube.com/watch?v=9Fxb8icOTOA (accessed 12 May 2014)

Pre-operative Assessments: https://www.youtube.com/watch?v=wl7Td5ehgl4 (accessed 12 May 2014)

5. Perioperative Patient Care

References

Goodman T & Spry C (2014) *Essentials of Perioperative Nursing*. Burlington MA, Jones & Bartlett.

Griffiths R (2000) *Anaesthetic Drugs*. NATN Back to Basics Perioperative Practice Principles. Harrogate, National Association of Theatre Nurses.

Harris P (2015) The Soothing Patients' Anxiety 'SPA' Experience. *Journal of Perioperative Practice* **25** (6): 97–100.

Phillips N (2004) *Berry & Kohn's Operating Room Technique*, 10th ed. St. Louis, Mosby.

Reed H (2003) Criteria for the Safe Discharge of Patients from the Recovery Room. *Nursing Times* **99** (38): 22–24.

Rothrock J (2007) *Alexander's Care of the Patient in Surgery*, 14th ed. St Louis, Elsevier.

Wicker P, O'Neill J (2010) *Caring for the Perioperative Patient*. Oxford, Wiley-Blackwell.

World Health Organization (WHO) (2009) Safe Surgery Checklist. Available at http://www.nrls.npsa.nhs.uk/resources/?Entryld45=59860 (accessed 12 May 2014)

Further Reading

Woodhead K & Fudge L (2012) *Manual of Perioperative Care: An Essential Guide*. Chichester, Wiley-Blackwell.

Pudner R (2005) *Nursing the Surgical Patient*. Edinburgh, Elsevier.

Websites

Perioperative Patient Care: http://www.patientsafetyfirst.nhs.uk/ashx/Asset.ashx?path=/How-to-guides-2008-09-19/periopcareLATEST%206%20Oct.pdf (accessed 12 July 2014)

Perioperative Care: http://www.surgical-tutor.org.uk/default-home.htm?principles/perioperative.htm~right (accessed 12 July 2014)

Videos

Patient Care Plans and Pathways: http://www.youtube.com/watch?v=2lPZJQJvja4 (accessed 12 July 2014)

Perioperative Care Part 1: https://www.youtube.com/watch?v=vliJiVonig0 (accessed 12 July 2014)

Pre and Post-operative Care: https://www.youtube.com/watch?v=XZq1gExGh8k (accessed 12 July 2014)

6. Operating Theatre Attire and Personal Protective Equipment

References

Department of Health (2010) *Uniforms and Workwear: Guidance on Uniform and Workwear Policies for NHS Employers*. Available at http://webarchive.nationalarchives.gov.uk/20130107105354/http://www.dh.gov.uk/en/Publicationsandstatistics/Publications/PublicationsPolicyAndGuidance/DH_114751 (accessed 18 November 2014)

Goodman T, Spry C (2014) *Essentials of Perioperative Nursing*. Burlington MA, Jones and Bartlett Learning.

National Institute for Health and Clinical Excellence (NICE) (2008) *Clinical Guideline 74 – Surgical Site Infection: Prevention and Treatment of Surgical Site Infection*. London, NICE.

National Institute for Health and Clinical Excellence (NICE) (2013) *Surgical Site Infection*. Available at https://www.nice.org.uk/guidance/qs49/chapter/quality-statement-4-intraoperative-staff-practices (accessed 22 August 2015)

Wicker P & O'Neill J (2010) *Caring for the Perioperative Patient*. Oxford, Wiley Blackwell.

Further Reading

Davey A & Ince CS (2005) *Fundamentals of Operating Department Practice*. London, Greenwich Medical Media.

Websites

Operating Theatre Dress Policy (Royal United Hospital Bath): http://www.ruh.nhs.uk/about/policies/documents/clinical_policies/blue_clinical/Blue_741_Operating_Theatre_Dress.pdf (accessed 27 November 2014)

Personal Protective Equipment: http://www.hse.gov.uk/toolbox/ppe.htm (accessed 27 November 2014)

Theatre Attire: http://www.afpp.org.uk/filegrab/theatre-attire-a2-poster-v5-final.pdf?ref=1458 (accessed 27 November 2014)

Videos

Hospital PPE – Standard Precautions: Donning and Doffing: https://www.youtube.com/watch?v=oxdaSeq4EVU (accessed 27 November 2014)

Personal Protective Equipment Training Video: https://www.youtube.com/watch?v=9NCV6-qGE8c (accessed 27 November 2014)

Theatre Attire and Hygiene: https://www.youtube.com/watch?v=qjyQv-g5XZs (accessed 27 November 2014)

7. Surgical Safety Checklist

References

Cvetic E (2011) Communication in the Perioperative Setting. *AORN Journal* **94** (3): 261–270.

Haynes AB, Weiser TG, Berry WR, Lipsitz SR (2009) A Surgical Safety Checklist to Reduce Morbidity and Mortality in a Global Population. *New England Journal of Medicine* **360** (5): 491–499.

Hunter DN & Finney SJ (2011) Follow Surgical Checklists and Take Time Out, Especially in a Crisis. *British Medical Journal* **334**: d8194.

National Patient Safety Agency (NPSA) (2009) *WHO Surgical Safety Checklist*. Available at http://www.nrls.npsa.nhs.uk/resources/?EntryId45=59860 (accessed 21 November 2014)

Patient Safety First (2015) *Supporting the WHO Surgical Safety Checklist*. Available at http://www.patientsafetyfirst.nhs.uk/Content.aspx?path=/Campaign-news/current/Supporting-Surgical-Safety-Checklist/ (accessed 22 August 2015)

World Health Organization (WHO) (2013) *Pilot Evaluation of the "WHO Surgical Safety Checklist"*. Available at http://www.who.int/patientsafety/safesurgery/pilot_sites/en/index.html (accessed 21 November 2014)

Further Reading

Kao LS & Thomas EJ (2008) Research Review: Navigating towards Improved Surgical Safety Using Aviation Strategies. *Journal of Surgical Research* **145**: 327–335.

Patient Safety First (2014) *Implementing the Surgical Safety Checklist: The Journey So Far. …* Available at http://www.patientsafetyfirst.nhs.uk/ashx/Asset.ashx?path=/Implementing+the+Surgical+Safety+Checklist+-+the+journey+so+far+2010.06.21+FINAL.pdf (accessed 19 December 2014)

Websites

Using Checklists to Ensure Patient Safety: http://www.aaos.org/news/aaosnow/nov13/research4.asp (accessed 19 December 2014)

WHO SSCL and Getting Started Kit (2014): http://www.ihi.org/resources/Pages/Tools/WHOSurgicalSafetyChecklistGettingStartedKit.aspx (accessed 19 December 2014)

WHO Surgical Safety Checklist: http://www.gloshospitals.nhs.uk/SharePoint1/Clinical%20Policies/A2089.pdf (accessed 19 December 2014)

Videos

5 Steps to Safer Surgery: http://www.nrls.npsa.nhs.uk/patient-safety-videos/five-steps-to-safer-surgery/ (accessed 19 December 2014)
How to Do the WHO Surgical Safety Checklist: http://www.youtube.com/watch?v=CsNpfMldtyk (accessed 19 December 2014)
How NOT to Do the WHO Surgical Safety Checklist: http://www.youtube.com/watch?v=REyers2AAel (accessed 19 December 2014)
How to Implement the Surgical Safety Checklist: http://www.youtube.com/watch?v=pFG9ihbPT-A (accessed 19 December 2014)

8. Teaching Students How to Use Operating Theatre Equipment

Further Reading

British Journal of Anaesthesia (2012) *Improving Patient Safety in the Operating Theatre and Perioperative Care: Obstacles, Interventions, and Priorities for Accelerating Progress*. Available at http://bja.oxfordjournals.org/content/109/suppl_1/i3.full (accessed 2 June 2016)
Eredie A (2016) *Operating Room Technique*. Available at http://www.cartercenter.org/resources/pdfs/health/ephti/library/lecture_notes/nursing_students/LN_OperatingRoomTechnique.pdf (accessed 2 June 2016)
Mangold T (2016) *Supplies and Equipment for the Laboratory*. Available at http://www.ast.org/uploadedFiles/Main_Site/Content/Educators/Supplies_Equipment_Laboratory.pdf (accessed 2 June 2016)
Reid WMN (2016) *Teaching and Learning in Operating Theatres*. Available at http://www.faculty.londondeanery.ac.uk/e-learning/explore-further/teaching_and_learning_in_operating_theatres.pdf (accessed 2 June 2016)
Royal Cornwall Hospitals (2016) *Clinical Guideline for Theatre Practice Standards*. Available at http://www.rcht.nhs.uk/DocumentsLibrary/RoyalCornwallHospitalsTrust/Clinical/Theatres/TheatrePracticeStandardsGeneric.pdf (accessed 2 June 2016)

Videos

Common Surgical Instruments used in Operation Theatre: https://www.youtube.com/watch?v=yUMnUrl-HkE (accessed 12 January 2016)
Inside Jobs Surgical Technology: https://www.youtube.com/watch?v=kClAxlXFQrY (accessed 12 January 2016)
Operating Theatre Equipment and Table Disinfection: https://www.youtube.com/watch?v=8r05jzQdAlQ (accessed 12 January 2016)
Operating Theatre Etiquette for Medical Students: https://www.youtube.com/watch?v=E3VX-Ij6ch8 (accessed 12 January 2016)
Surgery Instruments: https://www.youtube.com/watch?v=COjJxfbmdWY (accessed 12 January 2016)

9. Perioperative Equipment

References

Association for Perioperative Practice (AFPP) (2011) *Standards and Recommendations for Safe Perioperative Practice*, 3rd ed. Harrogate, AFPP.
Association of Anaesthetists of Great Britain and Northern Ireland (AAGBI) (2012) *Checking Anaesthetic Equipment*. London, AAGBI.
Cunnington J (2006) Facilitating Benefit, Minimising Risk: Responsibilities of the Surgical Practitioner during Electrosurgery. *Journal of Perioperative Practice* **6** (4): 195–202.

Department of Health (DH) (2013) *Management and Decontamination of Surgical Instruments Used in Acute Care.* London, DH. Available at https://www.gov.uk/government/publications/management-and-decontamination-of-surgical-instruments-used-in-acute-care (accessed 5 December 2014)

Goodman T & Spry C (2014) *Essentials of Perioperative Nursing*, 5th ed. Burlington MA, Jones & Bartlett Learning.

Health and Safety Executive (HSE) (1999) *Management of Health and Safety at Work*. Richmond, HSE.

Wicker P, O'Neill J (2010) *Caring for the Perioperative Patient.* Oxford, Wiley-Blackwell.

Further Reading

Association for Perioperative Practice (AFPP) (2011) *Standards and Recommendations for Safe Perioperative Practice*, 3rd ed. Harrogate, AFPP.

Davey A & Ince CS (2005) *Fundamentals of Operating Department Practice*. London, Greenwich Medical Media.

Klenerman L (2003) *The Tourniquet Manual: Principles and Practice*. London, Springer Verlag.

Medicines and Healthcare Products Regulatory Agency (MHRA) (2006) *Guidelines for the Perioperative Management of Patients with Implantable Pacemakers or Implantable Cardioverter Defibrillators, Where the Use of Surgical Diathermy/Electrocautery Is Anticipated.* Available at http://www.mhra.gov.uk/home/groups/dts-bi/documents/websiteresources/con2023451.pdf (accessed 19 December 2014)

Websites

Managing Medical Devices: http://www.mhra.gov.uk/Publications/Safetyguidance/DeviceBulletins/CON2025142 (accessed 21 December 2014)

The Operating Room: http://www.surgeryencyclopedia.com/La-Pa/Operating-Room.html (accessed 21 December 2014)

Videos

Dedicated Robotic Assisted Surgery Operating Room: https://www.youtube.com/watch?v=aE9Bare2NzE (accessed 21 December 2014)

Diathermy Generator: https://www.youtube.com/watch?v=vBOxbqt8AnE (accessed 21 December 2014)

Operating Theatre Equipment and Table Disinfection: https://www.youtube.com/watch?v=8r05jzQdAIQ (accessed 21 December 2014)

Surgical Instrument Tracking and Management: http://www.youtube.com/watch?v=85ZjZFbBbUs (accessed 21 December 2014)

10. Managing Perioperative Medication

References

Hollevoet I, Herregods S, Vereecke H, Vandermeulen E, Herregods L (2011) Medication in the Perioperative Period: Stop or Continue? A Review. *Acta Anaesthesiologica Belgica Journal* **62**: 193–201. Available at http://www.sarb.be/fr/journal/artikels_acta_2011/acta_62_4/2011_4-03-Hollevoet%20et%20al.pdf (accessed 11 December 2014)

Kennedy JM, van Rij AM, Spears GF, *et al.* (2000) Polypharmacy in a General Surgical Unit and Consequences of Drug Withdrawal. *British Journal of Clinical Pharmacology* **49**: 353.

Kroenke K, Gooby-Toedt D, Jackson JL (1998) Chronic Medications in the Perioperative Period. *Southern Medical Journal* **91**: 358.

Reiss TF, Chervinsky P, Dockhorn RJ (1998) Montelukast, a Once-Daily Leukotriene Receptor Antagonist, in the Treatment of Chronic Asthma: A Multicenter, Randomized, Double-Blind Trial. Montelukast Clinical Research Study Group. *Archives of Internal Medicine Journal* **158**: 1213.

Saber WS (2006) Perioperative Medication Management: A Case Based Review of General Principles. *Cleveland Clinic Journal of Medicine* **73** (Suppl. 1): P82–87.

Shammash JB, Trost JC, Gold JM (2001) Perioperative Beta-Blocker Withdrawal and Mortality in Vascular Surgical Patients. *American Heart Journal* **141**: 148.

Spell NO (2001) Stopping and Restarting Medications in the Perioperative Period. *Medical Clinics of North America Journal* **85**: 1117.

University of Michigan (2015) *Perioperative Management of Chronic Medications*. Available at http://med.umich.edu/preopclinic/guidelines/meds_to_stop1.pdf (accessed 2 June 2015)

Visala M, Macpherson DS (2012) *Perioperative Medication Management*. Available at http://clinicaldepartments.musc.edu/medicine/education/residency/perioperative%20medication%20management%20up%20to%20date.pdf (accessed 10 December 2014)

Further Reading

Whinney C (2009) Perioperative Medication Management: General Principles and Practical Applications. *Cleveland Clinical Journal of Medicine* **76** (Suppl. 4): S126–S132.

Websites

Perioperative Medication Management: http://emedicine.medscape.com/article/284801-overview (accessed 10 December 2014)

Perioperative Medication Management:
http://www.unmc.edu/media/catt/medicationrecommendationspriortosurgery1.pdf (accessed 10 December 2014)

Videos

Medication Safety in Perioperative Care: https://www.youtube.com/watch?v=enMSkLAmRwQ (accessed 10 December 2014)

The Importance of Warfarin after Joint Replacement Surgery:
https://www.youtube.com/watch?v=CGXKNA0NDNc (accessed 10 December 2014)

11. Interprofessional Learning and Collaboration

References

Centre for the Advancement of Interprofessional Education (2011) *Principles of Interprofessional Education*. Available at http://caipe.org.uk/resources/principles-of-interprofessional-education/ (accessed 14 December 2014)

Health Education England (2014) *Better Training Better Care*. Available at http://hee.nhs.uk/work-programmes/btbc/ (accessed 14 December 2014)

Quick J (2011) *Modern Perioperative Teamwork: An Opportunity for Interprofessional Learning. Journal of Perioperative Practice* **21** (11): 387–390.

Wicker P (2011) Interprofessional Learning. *Journal of Perioperative Practice* **21** (3): 83.

Wooding A (2013) Interprofessional Learning: A Student's Perspective. *Journal of Operating Department Practitioners* **1** (2): 95–99.

World Health Organisation 2010 *Framework for Action on Interprofessional Education and Collaborative Practice*. Geneva, WHO. Available at http://www.who.int/hrh/resources/framework_action/en/ (accessed 14 December 2014)

Further Reading

Chan AK, Pharma B, Wood V (2010) Preparing Tomorrow's Healthcare Providers for Interprofessional Collaborative Patient-Centred Practice Today.

University of British Columbia Medical Journal **1**(2). Available at http://www.ubcmj.com/pdf/ubcmj_1_2_2010_22-24.pdf (accessed 13 December 2014)

Körner M (2010) Interprofessional Teamwork in Medical Rehabilitation: A Comparison of Multidisciplinary and Interdisciplinary Team Approach. *Clinical Rehabilitation* **24** (8): 745–755.

Websites

Framework for Action on Interprofessional Education & Collaborative Practice:
http://www.uea.ac.uk/documents/4006821/4007300/FMH+-+CIPP+-+Framework+for+Action.pdf/6e15515c-0744-45cd-97b4-15fcc344113d (accessed 14 December 2014)

Interprofessional Teamwork:
http://www.ttuhsc.edu/qep/images/Miller_Poster.pdf (accessed 14 December 2014)

Videos

Inter-professional Learning: https://www.youtube.com/watch?v=RHV9Omb2RgA (accessed 14 December 2014)

Interprofessional Teamwork: https://www.youtube.com/watch?v=IqpT95TKumY (accessed 14 December 2014)

12. Preventing Surgical Site Infection

References

Aziz AM (2014) Preventing Infection after an Invasive Surgical Procedure. *Journal of Operating Department Practitioners* **2** (6): 266–268.

Darouiche RO, Wall MJ Jr, Itani KM, Otterson MF, Webb AL, Carrick MM, *et al.* (2010) Chlorhexidine-Alcohol versus Povidone-Iodine for Surgical-Site Antisepsis. *New England Journal of Medicine* **362**: 1, 18–26.

Health Protection Agency (HPA) (2011) *Surveillance of Surgical Site Infections in NHS Hospitals in England 2010/2011*. London, HPA.

Leaper DJ (2010) Surgical Site Infection. *British Journal of Surgery* **97**: 1601–1602.

National Institute for Health and Clinical Excellence (NICE) (2008) *Surgical Site Infection: Prevention and Treatment of Surgical Site Infection*. London, NICE. Available at https://www.nice.org.uk/guidance/cg74 (accessed 17 December 2014)

Smyth ET *et al.* (2008) Four Country Healthcare Associated Infection Prevalence Survey 2006: Overview of the Results. *Journal of Hospital Infection* **69** (3): 230–248.

Tanner J *et al.* (2009) Post-discharge Surveillance to Identify Colorectal Surgical Site Infection Rates and Related Costs. *Journal of Hospital Infection* **72**: 3, 243–250.

Further Reading

Aziz AM (2014) Supporting Infection Prevention in the Operating Room. *Journal of Operating Department Practitioners* **2** (3): 121–129.

Barnes GB & Sheikh A (2013) Preventing Surgical Site Infection in the Operating Theatre. *Journal of Operating Department Practitioners* **1** (2): 101–102.

Johns Hopkins Medicine (2014). Surgical Site Infections. Available at http://www.hopkinsmedicine.org/healthlibrary/conditions/surgical_care/surgical_site_infections_134,144/ (accessed 19 December 2014)

Rutala W & Weber D (2010) Guidelines for Disinfection and Sterilisation of Prion-Contaminated Medical Instruments. *Infection Control & Hospital Epidemiology* **21** (2): 107–117.

UK Government (2014). Surgical Site Infection (SSI): Guidance, Data and Analysis. Available at https://www.gov.uk/government/collections/surgical-site-infection-ssi-guidance-data-and-analysis (accessed 19 December 2014)

Websites

Surgical Site Infection (SSI): Guidance, Data and Analysis: https://www.gov.uk/government/collections/surgical-site-infection-ssi-guidance-data-and-analysis (accessed 19 December 2014)

Surgical Site Infections: http://www.cdc.gov/HAI/pdfs/ssi/SSI_tagged.pdf (accessed 19 December 2014)

Videos

Definitions of Surgical Site Infections (SSI): https://www.youtube.com/watch?v=nsBTVFyu0IY (accessed 19 December 2014)

Preventing Surgical Site Infections (SSI): https://www.youtube.com/watch?v=ylghY0dRk2M (accessed 19 December 2014)

Surgical Site Infections: http://www.cdc.gov/HAI/pdfs/ssi/SSI_tagged.pdf (accessed 2 June 2016)

Tackling Surgical Site Infections: https://www.youtube.com/watch?v=s_MiT-HwOz4 (accessed 19 December 2014)

13. Skin Preparation for Surgery

References

Hemani ML, Lepor H (2009) Skin Preparation for the Prevention of Surgical Site Infection: Which Agent Is Best? *Reviews in Urology Journal* **11** (4): 190–195.

Larson EL, Butz AM, Gullette DL, Laughon BA (1990) Alcohol for Surgical Scrubbing? *Infection Control and Hospital Epidemiology Journal* **11** (3): 139–143.

Maiwald M, Chan ESY (2012) The Forgotten Role of Alcohol: A Systematic Review and Meta-Analysis of the Clinical Efficacy and Perceived Role of Chlorhexidine in Skin Antisepsis. *PLoS One* **7** (9): e44277. doi:10.1371/journal.pone.0044277

National Institute for Health and Clinical Excellence (NICE) (2013) *Surgical Site Infection*. London, NICE.

Webster J & Osborne S (2012) Preoperative Bathing or Showering with Skin Antiseptics to Prevent Surgical Site Infection. *Cochrane Database of Systematic Reviews* (9): CD004985. DOI: 10.1002/14651858.CD004985.pub4

World Health Organization (WHO) (2009) *Guidelines for Safer Surgery*. London, WHO.

Further Reading

Kac G, Podglajen !, Gueneret M, Vaupre S, Bissery A, Meyer G (2005). Microbiological Evaluation of Two Hand Hygiene Procedures Achieved by Healthcare Workers during Routine Patient Care: A Randomized Study. *Journal of Hospital Infection* **60** (1): 32–39.

Vernon MO, Hayden MK, Trick WE, Hayes RA, Blom DW, Weinstein RA (2006) Chlorhexidine Gluconate to Cleanse Patients in a Medical Intensive Care Unit: The Effectiveness of Source Control to Reduce the Bioburden of Vancomycin-Resistant Enterococci. *Archives of Internal Medicine* **166** (3): 306–312.

Websites

Preoperative Skin Antiseptic Preparations for Preventing Surgical Site Infections: http://www.medscape.com/viewarticle/763958 (accessed 13 September 2015)

Skin Preparation for the Prevention of Surgical Site Infection: Which Agent Is Best?: http://www.ncbi.nlm.nih.gov/pmc/articles/PMC2809986/ (accessed 13 September 2015)

Standards of Practice for Skin Prep of the Surgical Patient: http://www.ast.org/uploadedFiles/Main_Site/Content/About_Us/Standard_Skin_Prep.pdf (accessed 13 September 2015)

Videos

Aseptic Nursing Technique in the OR: Gowning, Gloving, and Surgical Skin Preparation: https://www.youtube.com/watch?v=su8R-wNIKcg (accessed 13 September 2015)

Betadine Scrub and Paint: https://www.youtube.com/watch?v=2GAoHDDScC8 (accessed 13 September 2015)

Demonstration and Observation of ChloraPrep Antiseptic Surgical Agent: https://www.youtube.com/watch?v=Pmsgl7scl2o (accessed 13 September 2015)

Surgical Site Infection Improvement Programme – Surgical Skin Preparation: https://www.youtube.com/watch?v=aR73lk_GthM (accessed 13 September 2015)

SECTION 2

Anaesthesia

Paul Wicker

14 Preoperative Evaluation of the Anaesthetic Patient

As the population ages, combined with much more complex anaesthesia and surgery, patients find themselves under more and more stress. It is therefore essential that patients are prepared before anaesthesia and given information which may help them to feel more at ease and relax a little (Mitchell 2013). Preoperative evaluation of the patient is therefore to assess any risks and prevent harm to the patient during anaesthesia (Wicker 2010). Two essential elements that need investigating before anaesthesia or surgery are the presence of heart or respiratory diseases and the patient's well-being. A fall in their physiological reserves, usually in elderly people, could lead to dementia following anaesthesia. It is also essential for the surgeon and anaesthetist to work together in order for the surgeon and anaesthetist to understand the risks associated with each individual patient. Surgery, for example, can lead to problems related to anaesthesia, and vice versa.

Identification of high-risk patients

Patients who are likely to die postoperatively may be elderly or may have serious medical disorders. To assess the patient before anaesthesia, the anaesthetist assesses the patient using the ASA (American Society of Anaesthetists) grade which is an assessment of a patient's health based on five classes:

ASA I	A healthy and fit person
ASA II	Mild systemic disease which can be treated
ASA III	Severe systemic disease, such as angina or renal failure
ASA IV	Severe systemic disease that may lead to morbidity
ASA V	A moribund person who is likely to die with or without surgery (Woodhead & Fudge 2012).

However, patients often have other issues which can affect both their anaesthesia and their surgery, for example:

- Cardiorespiratory problems
- Severe trauma incident
- Blood loss >8 units
- Age over 70 years old
- Low blood pressure
- Septicaemia
- Renal failure
- Obesity
- Vascular problems.

Rapid Perioperative Care, First Edition. Paul Wicker and Sara Dalby.

Patients therefore need to undergo physiological assessment to ensure they are healthy enough for anaesthesia and surgery (Wicker 2010). For example, patients with any cardiovascular problems may experience low blood pressure, low pulse rate and severe respiration problems, possibly leading to death. It is possible, therefore, that surgeons and anaesthetists may treat the patient earlier to optimise their health before anaesthesia and surgery (Goodman & Spry 2014).

Preoperative visits

Theatre practitioners sometimes visit patients preoperatively the day before surgery or the day of surgery, the latter especially if it is a day case patient. Patient care plans are essential to assess the patient and to outline actions that need to be undertaken (Goodman & Spry 2014). Pre-assessment clinics are also becoming more common, and often they contain practitioners as well as doctors. There are many general aspects that need assessment by the practitioner, and questions which the patient may have about their surgery and anaesthesia (Woodhead & Fudge 2012). Practitioners therefore take time to go through the care plan, discuss the patient's issues and prepare for any problems which may occur during anaesthesia and surgery (Goodman & Spry 2014).

Previous problems

Patients may have had issues during previous anaesthetics, for example postoperative nausea and vomiting, or inadvertent hypothermia, caused by anaesthetic drugs (Wicker 2010). Patents may also have had malignant hyperthermia previously, caused because of inherent problems acquired from parents or family. Once these are identified, then the issues require a detailed discussion within the team to ensure the best care possible for the patient during surgery (Woodhead & Fudge 2012).

Smoking

Patients who smoke can have cardiovascular and respiratory problems, including postoperative pulmonary complications and high levels of carbon monoxide in their blood leading to lower levels of oxygen (Woodhead & Fudge 2012). Given the seriousness of these issues, it is advisable for the patient to stop smoking at least three months before surgery. In some cases, patients will continue smoking up to the day before surgery, although this does help to reduce carbon monoxide levels before anaesthesia. If a patient is smoking on the day of surgery, then their surgery may be cancelled because of the high risk of associated problems before, during and after anaesthesia.

Alcohol and medications

Alcohol intake by patients leads to the induction of hepatic enzymes which alter the actions of anaesthetic drugs. Patients undergoing major surgery should avoid alcohol for at least a month before anaesthesia. Certain medications can also affect anaesthesia, for example the regular use of sedatives or analgesics increases the need for anaesthetic drugs, potentially leading to further problems. Drugs which need to be stopped before anaesthesia include antidiabetic agents (e.g. chlorpropamide and tolbutamide), antidepressants, anticoagulants (e.g. warfarin or heparin) and corticosteroids. (See Chapter 9 for more information.)

Obesity

Obesity in patients can cause serious problems for both anaesthesia and surgery (Goodman & Spry 2014). This includes:

- Difficulty in venous access, airway management, moving the patient, local anaesthesia and so on
- Increased demand on the heart leading to hypertension or cardiac failure
- Risk of hypoxia and other respiratory problems
- Increased risk of pressure sores
- Chance of deep vein thrombosis (DVT) or pulmonary embolus
- Increased risk of diabetes and the like.

Preparation of the obese patient is therefore essential before the start of anaesthesia or surgery to prevent or reduce the chance of incidents such as these from occurring.

Bleeding problems

Several possible bleeding problems may occur, although most are usually associated with surgery (Wicker 2010). Long-term anaemia is normally well tolerated if erythropoietin is given to patients. Erythropoietin is a hormone developed in the kidneys which increases red blood cells when oxygen is reduced in the tissues. However, acute anaemia can lead to low haemoglobin (Hb) levels which can cause oxygen and circulatory problems. If the patient has pallor or shortness of breath, then treatment is usually given with iron, erythropoietin or folate, or in severe cases packed red cells will be transfused. The normal Hb level should be around 9–10 g/dl, and following surgery the patient would be monitored for their cardiovascular and respiratory status. If the patient remains low on Hb throughout their surgery, then a higher fraction of oxygen (FiO_2) will need to be delivered (i.e. greater than 0.4). Any bleeding problems that occur need to be treated quickly and efficiently to prevent harm to the patient (Goodman & Spry 2014).

Conclusion

Many more problems can occur during anaesthesia and surgery, including:

- Cardiovascular problems: myocardial infarction, dysrhythmias, hypertension, angina pectoris and so on
- Respiratory problems: respiratory tract infection, asthma, chronic obstructive pulmonary disease, bronchospasm and so on
- Neuromuscular problems: myopathies and myasthenia gravis
- Renal disease
- Liver disease
- Epilepsy.

It is possible for the patient to receive preoperative medications, including analgesics, atropine, antacids, anti-emetics and the like, to provide support for their health. Whatever the situation, it is important that the anaesthetist communicates with the theatre team in regards to the health status of the patient in the preoperative briefing, so all members of the team are aware of issues which may develop (Wicker 2010).

15 Preparing Anaesthetic Equipment

The anaesthetic machine is the most important machine to check before anaesthesia. However, there are many other types of equipment which must also be checked to ensure they are working correctly. This chapter will provide an outline of how items of equipment need to be checked prior to the patient's arrival in theatre, to ensure their safety.

Anaesthetic machine

As part of their daily duties, it is the anaesthetic practitioner's responsibility to always check that the anaesthetic machine is working before the anaesthetist arrives. The practitioner will then confirm and verify it is working correctly with the anaesthetist on their arrival before the patient arrives. The stability of the equipment is important during induction of anaesthesia because faulty equipment can put the patient at high risk of harm because of lack of oxygen, high levels of anaesthetic gases and so on (Shaikh & Stacey 2013). Anaesthetic practitioners need to use the Association of Anaesthetists of Great Britain and Northern Ireland (AAGBI) checklist (AAGBI 2012) as well as the manufacturer's manual to ensure the correct checking of the anaesthetic machine.

Basic Steps for Checking an Anaesthetic Machine Using the AAGBI (2012) Guidelines

Step 1 – Carry out the manufacturer's automatic machine check.
Step 2 – Plug in the machine, and ensure the backup battery is charged.
Step 3 – Check flowmeters, hypoxic guard, cylinders, gas and suction pipelines to ensure the gas supplies and suction are working.
Step 4 – Use the 'two-bag' test to identify any leaks in the breathing system, check that vaporisers are not leaking, soda lime should be pink, and check the availability of alternative breathing systems, for example the Bains Circuit (Hughes & Mardell 2012).
Step 5 – Check that the ventilator and scavenging systems are working properly.
Step 6 – Check the monitors are working, and set alarm parameters.
Step 6 – Check airway equipment availability, for example laryngoscope, endotracheal tube (ETT), oral airways and so on. And check where emergency equipment is located in the department.

These steps show basic steps needed by the practitioner for checking the anaesthetic machine prior to the arrival of the anaesthetist. The anaesthetist will also check the machine before the patient arrives, and normally after each case (AAGBI 2012). The checks carried out after the patient has left the operating room include checking (as a minimum) the breathing system, ventilator, airway equipment and suction (Shaikh & Stacey 2013). All pieces of equipment should be clean, and airway equipment (e.g. ETTs) should be sterile.

Other checks required include consumable items such as facemasks, oxygen masks, oral and nasal airways, laryngeal mask airways, ETTs, laryngoscopes and bougies, anaesthetic

Rapid Perioperative Care, First Edition. Paul Wicker and Sara Dalby.

medications, syringes, needles, giving sets, IV cannulae, alcoholic wipes and Band-Aids, amongst others (Hughes & Mardell 2012). Anaesthetic assistants normally check and sign the anaesthetic checklist to provide the best and safest patient care.

Anaesthetic equipment

Monitors

Anaesthetic practitioners usually attach monitors to the patient before anaesthesia so that physiological parameters are recorded (Green *et al.* 2003). There are many monitoring devices used during anaesthesia; therefore, they need to be known and understood to monitor the patients' physiological parameters correctly (AAGBI 2012). Examples of anaesthetic monitors include:

- Oxygen analyser
- Pulse oximeter
- Capnograph
- Non-invasive blood pressure monitor
- Electrocardiography
- Airway monitor
- Airway pressure monitor
- Nerve stimulator
- Invasive arterial pressure
- Temperature probe.

The anaesthetist and practitioner work together to ensure the monitors are available and working properly. The oxygen analyser, pulse oximeter and capnograph are the most important monitoring devices, and they need to function correctly to preserve the health of the patient (Hughes & Mardell 2012). It is also important that the parameters and alarms for all monitors have been set appropriately before using the anaesthetic machine (Green *et al.* 2003).

Airway equipment

Airway equipment is essential for anaesthesia to maintain the patient's oxygen supply and circulation, because any problems with airway equipment can lead to major problems. Checking airway equipment will include (Shaikh & Stacey 2013, Higginson & Parry 2015):

- Ensuring that laryngoscopes must be working correctly and available in a suitable size for the patient (Higginson & Parry 2015).
- Checking availability of various sizes of tracheal tubes, laryngeal mask airways, Guedel airways and facemasks; and ensuring that these are working correctly.
- Checking availability of the bacterial filter and angle piece/catheter mount; they must be checked and working correctly before use. These devices are used singly for each patient.
- Checking gas flow through the airway system and the breathing circuit.
- Patients with airway problems (e.g. stiff necks or small mouths) will need specialised equipment that must also be checked to ensure it is available and working.

Ancillary and resuscitation equipment

Patients sometimes need resuscitation before, during or after surgery. Resuscitation equipment must be available within the operating rooms and working correctly (Hughes

& Mardell 2012). All other equipment within the operating room must also be checked. Checks include:

- Ensuring the operating table is functioning and fully charged.
- Ensuring the operating table can be tilted head-down rapidly, in case of vomiting. The patient's bed or patient trolley also needs to be functioning correctly.
- Identify the location of the difficult-airway trolley, resuscitation equipment and defibrillator.
- Ensure equipment and drugs for management of emergencies, such as malignant hyperthermia or local anaesthetic toxicity, are available and working.

Central venous pressure

Central venous pressure (CVP) lines measure fluid balance, filling pressure of the right atrium and circulating volume (Shaikh & Stacey 2013). The process used to insert CVP lines involves:

- Inserting a needle into the patient via the internal jugular or the subclavian route
- Inserting the guide wire inside the needle
- Removing the needle
- Inserting the catheter over the guide wire.

Correct placement of the CVP is confirmed by x-ray, and risks to the patient include pneumothorax, air embolus, haematomas and infection. Once the CVP is installed correctly, an electronic transducer is connected to a monitor which then records the patient's CVP (Green *et al.* 2003).

Arterial blood gases

A syringe of patient blood containing heparin monitors arterial blood gases, and it is then analysed in a laboratory to indicate the level of carbon dioxide and oxygen in the blood. These results identify the patient's respiration, ability to breathe and acid–base balance within the blood. The normal ranges for arterial blood results are:

PAO_2	12–15 KPa (90–110 mmHg)
$PaCO_2$	4.5–6 KPa (34–46 mmHg)
HCO_3	21–27.5 mmol/L
H+ ions	36–44 nmol/L (pH 7.35–7.45) (Hughes & Mardell 2012).

Fluid warmers

Patients sometimes become hypothermic in operating rooms because of low room temperature, inadequate coverings, cold fluid infusions and the like. Therefore, using fluid warmers to inject warm fluids into patients helps to warm them up. Heated plates are used which allow the fluid to warm up as it passes through the fluid warmer. There are many different types of fluid warmers which are effective in warming blood and fluids. For example, heating water to 40 °C then heats the fluids as it passes through the machine (Shaikh & Stacey 2013). In all fluid warmers, the infusion never makes direct contact with the warming fluid as this may lead to problems for the patient (AAGBI 2012).

Total intravenous anaesthesia

Total intravenous anaesthesia (TIVA) is used for some patients, especially if there are medical problems. TIVA involves the use of intravenous medications which are used in place of anaesthetic gases (Shaikh & Stacey 2013). TIVA equipment needs to be checked and made available if this process is carried out:

- IV pumps must be available, configured correctly and either fully charged or plugged into a wall socket.
- Appropriate IV administration sets must be available and checked to be appropriate for the patient. This includes giving sets, tubes, valves, pumps and so on.

There are many more items of equipment used to support anaesthesia, and anaesthetic practitioners need to be fully aware of the need to understand how they work and ensure they are clean and ready to use before anaesthesia.

16 Checking the Anaesthetic Machine

The anaesthetic machine is one of the most important pieces of equipment and therefore has to be checked before patients receive anaesthesia. The anaesthetic practitioner will check the machine, and then the anaesthetist will also confirm that it is working properly before starting anaesthesia (Al-Shaik & Stacey 2002, Chilton & Thomson 2012). Airway obstruction, circulatory problems, reduced blood oxygenation or even death due to errors such as flow reversal though the back bar on the anaesthetic machine can occur during induction of the patient. This leaves patients in a vulnerable position (Cheng & Bailey 2002) if the anaesthetic machine is not carefully checked.

The AAGBI checklist (AAGBI 2012) and the manufacturer's manual are essential guides for practitioners while checking the anaesthetic machine. Following these guidelines will help to ensure the anaesthetic machine is safe and effective. Before the anaesthetist arriving, the anaesthetic practitioner assembles and checks the equipment in preparation for the anaesthetic (Hughes & Mardell 2012). When the anaesthetist arrives, he or she will then ensure the correct equipment is available for the anaesthetic procedure. The anaesthetic practitioner and the anaesthetist work together to ensure that the equipment is checked and working normally, and the patient is safe (Wicker & Smith 2008).

Errors can occur during anaesthesia because of lack of equipment checks. Kumar (1998) suggested many years ago that using a checklist when checking an anaesthetic machine may lead to a decrease of problems for the patient. New anaesthetic machines, or machines that have been returned from servicing, need to be thoroughly checked to ensure they are assembled correctly, working properly and ready for use.

Using the AAGBI (2012) anaesthetic checklist will help to reduce risks to the patient from faulty equipment, and ensure the best patient care during anaesthesia (Wicker & Smith 2008).

Checking the anaesthetic machine

The rest of this chapter highlights some of the checks that are needed on first entry to the operating room, and before and during the use of the anaesthetic machine. The checks can be taken by the anaesthetic practitioner and then confirmed by the anaesthetist, or if possible, both will work together to confirm that all the equipment is working correctly (Chilton & Thomson 2012).

Checks before the patient's arrival

Gases

- Check the monitoring panel for the **gas line supply**.
- Identify **who to contact** if there is a problem with the gas supply.
- Locate the **gas isolation valves**, and ensure they are working correctly.

Rapid Perioperative Care, First Edition. Paul Wicker and Sara Dalby.

- Check the **gas line pressure indicators**.
- Discover where the spare **oxygen cylinders** are stored.
- Understand how to manage failure of the gas supply.

Electricity

- Check the **electrical safety system**.
- **Know which mains power outlets are 'always on'.**
- Identify an action to take if there is a **mains power failure**.
- Assess the status of the **battery backup devices** such as the monitors, anaesthetic machine, ventilator and so on (Hughes & Mardell 2012).
- Carry out an action plan if the **mains power failure** does not resume.

Facilities

- Confirm the availability of the **anaesthetic machine, equipment, monitors** and so on. Ensure they are working effectively, and that they comply with hospital guidelines and recommendations for patient safety, safe administration of anaesthetic gases and monitoring.
- Ensure the **equipment has been serviced** – check the label dates.
- **Ensure essential drugs are available** and you know how to obtain others as needed.
- Check for spare **self-inflating airway bags**.
- Check for **difficult intubation equipment**.
- Check the way to **start a cardiac arrest call** – in your own theatre or a different one.
- Locate a **defibrillator** close to your area of work.
- Find the actions to take if there is a fire: the fire drill, fire extinguisher and meeting points (AAGBI 2012, Chilton & Thomson 2012, Hughes & Mardell 2012).

Checking the anaesthetic machine

Delivering anaesthesia requires an anaesthetic machine, equipment or apparatus which supplies gases, vapours, local anaesthesia and intravenous anaesthetic agents.

Safely maintaining anaesthetic equipment includes ensuring that equipment is working effectively, monitors have appropriate alarms, backup equipment for ventilation and oxygenation is available, the checklist for checking the anaesthetic machine has been completed and appropriate anaesthetic equipment is available (Wicker & Smith 2008).

The anaesthetic machine must be checked thoroughly by using the checklist and the manufacturer's guidelines, although different anaesthetic machines may have different checking systems.

Level 1 check

The Level 1 check is very detailed and includes:

- Checking anaesthetic machines after servicing
- Electrical safety testing
- Testing for gas leaks
- Calibration of monitors and equipment
- Checking of alarms (Wicker & Smith 2008).

The Operating Department Manager will inform staff of the Level 1 check and ensure that all test results are documented and retained on a file.

Level 2 Check

Before the start of anaesthesia, the anaesthetic team will check all aspects of the anaesthetic machine (Chilton & Thomson 2012), including:

- Ensure the service label for the anaesthetic machine is current and not out of date.
- Check pipeline and cylinder pressures to ensure they are adequate. Cylinders will be switched off after checking.
- Ensure the oxygen failure alarm is working.
- Ensure oxygen supply is working correctly – check O_2 rotameters and oxygen level in the circuit.
- Check that the airway bag is not leaking and that it fills correctly.
- Check additional equipment attached to the anaesthetic machine, for example the oxygen monitor.
- Ensure that vaporisers are full, sealed and attached correctly to the anaesthetic machine.
- Confirm the secure fixing of the back bar on the vaporiser.
- Check that the airway circuit is assembled properly, there are no leaks, valves are working correctly and manual ventilation is possible using a second airway bag.
- Check that the ventilating system is working correctly, including alarms and bellows.
- Check other devices attached to the anaesthetic machine, such as the scavenging system, suction devices, airway and intubation equipment, monitors and so on.
- Check the availability of anaesthetic medicines, IV infusions, syringe pumps and so on. (Wicker & Smith 2008, AAGBI 2012, Hughes & Mardell 2012)

Level 3 Check

The anaesthetist will normally check the anaesthetic machine and associated equipment before starting the first anaesthetic, and subsequent anaesthetic equipment for the next patient (Wicker & Smith 2008). This will include:

- Complete check of the anaesthetic machine, and ensuring that airway circuits and vaporisers have been filled or changed according to requirements.
- Update drugs, suction, IVs, pumps, monitoring, airway and intubation equipment and so on.

Manual Ventilation

The anaesthetic practitioner may check that manual ventilation is possible before each case by undertaking the following tests.

1. *The Bag Test*
    - Keep the fresh gas flow to zero, and set the adjustable pressure-limiting (APL) valve to 30.
    - Close off the Y-piece.
    - Switch on the oxygen flush.
    - Squeeze the airway bag, and check that it remains tight for at least 10 sec.
    - Check that the valves work by going up and down with intermittent squeezing. (AAGBI 2012, Chilton & Thomson 2012)
2. *Airway circuit*
    - Check that the patient can breathe easily through the circuit before induction.
    - Keep the fresh gas flow to zero, with the APL valve open, and attach a suitable mask to the patient.
    - Check that the mask is comfortable and gently sealed.
    - Confirm that the bag inflates and deflates as the patient breathes (Hughes & Mardell 2012).

If the bag test fails, then check and feel for leaks. This may need another airway bag or tubing, or testing of the back bar; and then test the airway bag again to confirm it is working correctly and leaks have been repaired.

3. *Non-electronic machines*
   - Check gas levels in cylinders, line pressures and mains power.
   - Test for delivery of gases:
     - Turn on the nitrous oxide or oxygen rotameters.
     - Check that the bag starts to fill.
     - Check for leaks at the Y-piece.
     - Turn off the nitrous or oxygen, and hit the oxygen flush button until the bag is nearly full.
     - Check the level of O_2 at the Y-piece.
   - Turn on vaporiser No. 1 and check that it is working efficiently, for example via its back bar, contents and filler cap:
     - At the same time, check other equipment such as suction, monitors, airway tubing and so on.
     - Confirm that the circuit pressure has increased to 30 cm H_2O or more.
     - Turn the vaporiser off (AAGBI 2012).
   - Repeat the tests for vaporiser No. 2 if it is going to be used by the anaesthetist for the patient.

Conclusion

There are often many other checks that need to take place within the anaesthetic room; for example, equipment for drugs needs to be available, including syringes, needles, giving sets, alcoholic wipes, Band-Aids and so on. Problems with intubation can occur, so specific intubation equipment should also be accessible in case of ongoing problems. A primary concern for the anaesthetist is that the anaesthetic practitioner must be qualified and experienced in the relevant speciality (AAGBI 2012).

The above checks do not necessarily follow all the AAGBI (2012) guidelines; however, the AAGBI (2012) checklist is one of the most effective and useful checklists which enable the practitioner to carry out a thorough check of the anaesthetic equipment. If this checklist is used, the anaesthetic practitioner should ensure they check and sign the checklist so a record is kept in case of future problems or issues. This checklist will help to provide the best and safest patient care by checking the anaesthetic machine at a high standard.

17 Anatomy and Physiology: The Cardiovascular System

The cardiovascular system is responsible for transporting oxygen, carbon dioxide, nutrients, hormones and cellular waste throughout the organs and tissues of the body via the heart and blood vessels (Figure 17.1). This chapter will consider the heart, blood, circulation, blood pressure regulation and haemostasis.

The heart

The heart is a muscular organ which pumps blood throughout the body. The bottom of the heart is the apex; the top of the heart is the base that connects to the aorta, vena cava, pulmonary arteries and veins. The heart has four chambers, and the left and right sides work separately as they pump the blood around the body. The septum of the heart, a muscular wall, separates the left and right sides. The heart functions efficiently by simultaneously pumping both sides of the heart (Marieb 2006).

The pulmonary and systemic circulation form circulatory loops which allow blood to leave the heart and then return to it. The heart uses the right atrium and right ventricle to create the pulmonary circulation. The pulmonary circulation carries deoxygenated blood from the right side of the heart to the lungs, where it deposits the carbon dioxide in the lungs, and then the blood collects oxygen from the lungs and returns to the left side of the heart. The left atrium and left ventricle provide pumps for the systemic circulation which send oxygenated blood from the left side of the heart to the rest of the body, and they collect wastes from the body to send to organs and return deoxygenated blood to the right side of the heart for reoxygenation via the lungs (Clancy & McVicar 2009, Tortorra & Derrickson 2011).

The left and right coronary arteries of the heart stem from the aorta and provide oxygenated blood and nutrients to the left and right sides of the heart, enabling the heart to continue pumping blood throughout the body. The heart also contains veins, such as the coronary sinus, on the reverse side of the heart which returns the blood to the vena cava. If the arteries of the heart get blocked because of thrombosis, then the heart may stop working, leading to angina or heart attack (Marieb 2006).

Blood vessels

Blood vessels, including arteries, veins and capillaries, provide blood flow from the heart, to the body and then back to the heart, ensuring that tissue cells receive blood and nutrients and can also offload waste materials which can be directed to the organs of the body (Tortorra & Derrickson 2011). The blood vessels are like tubes with a lumen, allowing blood to flow quickly and efficiently.

The blood vessels contain tissues in the walls of the blood vessels which hold the lumen open. The inner layer is the endothelium which secures the blood within the vessels and helps to prevent clots from forming. Blood vessels are named according to the direction

Rapid Perioperative Care, First Edition. Paul Wicker and Sara Dalby.

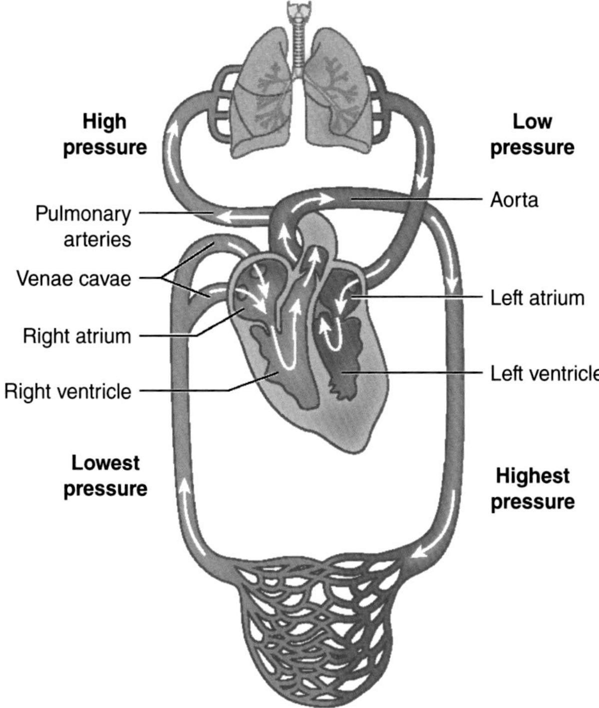

Figure 17.1 The cardiovascular system

of their blood flow or their proximity to nearby structures. For example, the femoral artery carries blood though the upper leg, the axillary artery carries blood into the axilla and the carotid artery carries blood to the brain.

Arteries and arterioles

Blood carried by arteries is oxygenated and is sent around the body to ensure all tissues are oxygenated. Arteries contain high pressure because the blood is being strongly pushed out of the heart. Arteries therefore need strong and thick walls, which contain muscles and elastic tissues, to prevent swelling or bursting of the arteries. This is especially the case with vessels such as the aorta which contain elastic tissues, allowing them to stretch because of the high pressure of the heart as it contracts and ejects the blood (Marieb 2006).

Smaller arteries have more muscular tissues in their walls which can contract or expand to regulate blood flow to the areas of the body where they are sending the blood. These arteries may also affect blood pressure, depending on the amount of blood they allow to pass through the area. Arterioles have thinner walls and are narrower than small arteries; they have very low blood pressure because of their high number and less pressure from the heart. The smooth muscles of the arteriole walls can also regulate the blood flow through their vessels.

Capillaries

Capillaries are small and thin and are found in almost every tissue of the body. They normally connect to arterioles on the proximal end and then to venules on the distal end. Capillaries exist because they are able to exchange gases, nutrients and waste products between their lumens and the tissues that surround them. The capillaries are thin and have a thin layer of endothelium, allowing liquids, gases and chemicals to diffuse into or out of the tissues (Clancy & McVicar 2009). At the end of capillaries are precapillary sphincters which are composed of smooth muscle which regulate the blood flow into active or inactive tissues.

Veins and venules

Veins return blood to the heart and then via the pulmonary arteries to the lungs so the blood can be reoxygenated. Venules are small blood vessels, similar to capillaries, which return blood to the veins. As there is little pressure on veins and venules from the heart, the walls are much thinner and less elastic than arteries. Veins also have little or no muscular layers, so they need gravity or skeletal muscle contraction to help them return blood to the heart (Marieb 2006). Some veins, such as leg and arm veins, contain one-way valves which help to force blood back to the heart. The valves also stop the blood from moving backwards or forwards in the veins if the skeletal muscles fail to contract. When the muscles do contract again, they push the blood towards the heart via the main veins, for example the vena cava or the femoral veins (Tortorra & Derrickson 2011).

Blood

The human body normally contains around 4.5 to 5.5 L of blood which consists of red blood cells, white blood cells, platelets and plasma. Red blood cells are called erythrocytes, which are produced in red bone marrow from stem cells. Erythrocytes carry oxygen in the blood by using haemoglobin which contains iron and proteins. Because erythrocytes have a large surface area, they allow oxygen to be transferred easily between lungs and tissues.

White blood cells are called leukocytes, and they play an important part in the body's immune system. The two types of leukocytes are granular and agranular. Granular leukocytes are neutrophils, eosinophils and basophils, which can neutralise bacteria and viruses, and protect the body against parasites. Agranular leukocytes are called lymphocytes and monocytes; they produce antibodies and can also engulf and ingest dead cells from infected wounds (Clancy & McVicar 2009).

Platelets are also called thrombocytes, which help to clot blood and form scabs on surface wounds. Platelets are also made in bone marrow from pieces of membrane from internal cells. Platelets survive in the body for up to a week, and then they are destroyed by the macrophages (Tortorra & Derrickson 2011).

Plasma makes up about 50% of the blood volume and is a mix of water, proteins (containing antibodies and albumins) and other substances such as glucose, oxygen, carbon dioxide, electrolytes and nutrients. The antibodies prevent pathogens from infecting the body. The albumins provide an isotonic solution for the body cells to maintain osmotic balance. The plasma therefore helps to move the substances found in blood throughout the body.

Cardiovascular system physiology

The cardiovascular system is one of the most important systems of the human body. It delivers and removes essential materials to and from the body, protects the body from pathogens and regulates homeostasis.

The cardiovascular system provides blood to all the body's tissues, and by doing so it delivers essential nutrients and oxygen and removes wastes and carbon dioxide which are processed by organs and removed from the body. Plasma in the blood holds onto hormones which are transported throughout the body and delivered to their destinations (Marieb 2006).

Leukocytes collect debris from cells and attack pathogens in the bloodstream, thereby protecting the body. Wounds are sealed by platelets and red blood cells which form scabs that prevent pathogens from entering the body, leading to infection, and also stop liquids from leaking out and prevent blood loss. Antibodies prevent diseases from developing and are present in the blood if the patient has been vaccinated or has developed immunity from previous illnesses or diseases (Clancy & McVicar 2009).

Homeostasis of the body is controlled and regulated by various systems, but the cardiovascular system is one of the main systems that helps to control homeostasis (Wicker 2010). The patient's temperature is maintained at ±37 °C by blood vessels which circulate the blood flow from the core of the body to the skin surface. If the patient has a high temperature, then the surface blood vessels allow the heat to be dissipated throughout the tissues and then possibly leave the body. If the patient is hypothermic, blood vessels tend to constrict the blood flow to the body's core, in particular the essential organs. Other activities by the blood flow include balancing the body's pH by using bicarbonate ions and using albumins in blood plasma to help maintain an isotonic environment (Wicker 2010).

Blood pressure

High heart rate and strong contractions can lead to high blood pressure, whereas low heart rate and weak contractions can reduce blood pressure. Hormones within the blood supply and nerve signals from the brain can also alter the rate and strength of the heart contractions, which in turn can affect blood pressure. Vasoconstriction of blood vessels reduces blood flow through the vessels and can also increase blood pressure as the blood flow is restricted (Marieb 2006). Vasodilation of blood vessels by particular hormones, chemicals or anaesthetic drugs can reduce blood pressure because of the expansion of blood vessels.

Haemostasis

Platelets in blood create haemostasis, clotting of blood and formation of scabs on wounds, when they approach damaged tissues or wounds. When platelets become active, they develop into a ball with spines that attach onto damaged tissues. The platelets then start to form blood clots by releasing clotting factors and producing a structure by using fibrin (Marieb 2006). The platelets also attach to each other to form a 'plug' which is a temporary seal to stop the loss of blood and also prevents external materials from entering the blood vessels. The plug remains in place until the tissues or vessels heal.

18 Anatomy and Physiology: The Lungs

People may survive for a long period of time without food and water; however, they can only survive for a few minutes without oxygen. Body cells need to grow, repair or replace themselves, and maintain vital functions in order to accomplish this, and to do that they need a constant supply of oxygen to produce energy to stay healthy. Oxygen must be inhaled into the lungs safely and effectively, and delivered in the required amounts (Clancy & McVicar 2009).

The lungs are in the chest and are located on the left and right sides (Figure 18.1). The right lung consists of the upper lobe, middle lobe and lower lobe. The left lung only has two lobes which are the upper and lower lobes. Between the lungs is the heart which is located in the centre of the chest, although it extends further into the left side. The heart and lungs interact with each other to provide oxygenation to the entire body.

Inhalation initiates from the mouth and nose, and the air travels down the trachea, then the bronchus, and dissipates into the separate bronchi which distribute the air to both of the lungs. The bronchi themselves become smaller and smaller and extend throughout the lungs similar to tree branches. Finally, the bronchi turn into alveoli, which are grape-like objects which exchange oxygen and carbon dioxide between the air contents and the blood supply (Clancy & McVicar 2009).

Cilia line the bronchi; they are tiny hairs which move backwards and forwards constantly. This enables mucus to be collected by the cilia, and the mucus moves upwards towards the throat (Marieb 2006). Cilia also transport objects, materials, bacteria and viruses out of the lungs and bronchi, protecting the lungs from infection.

Breathing occurs mainly by the diaphragm which is a large dome-shaped muscle that contracts and relaxes, and also prevents the abdominal cavity from interacting with the chest. Muscles associated with the ribs also help to expand and contract the chest to assist with breathing (Wicker 2010).

The lungs expand because of the pleural membranes, intercostal muscles between the ribs and the diaphragm which help to expand the lungs and the alveoli within the lungs. Pleurae are membranes lining the thoracic cavity (parietal pleura), and they cover the lungs (visceral pleura). In between the two pleurae is the pleural cavity which aids the expansion and constriction of the lungs to aid breathing. The pleural cavity contains pleural fluid which lubricates the pleural membranes, allowing them to slide against each other easily during breathing. The fluid in the pleural space originates from the lymphatic system and moves from inside the lungs into the pleural space (Clancy & McVicar 2009).

The tissue network surrounding the alveoli is called the 'pulmonary interstitium'. The interstitium has strong fibres that support the alveoli and prevent them from being overstretched, preventing rupture. The pulmonary interstitium also supports and strengthens other areas of the lungs including the pulmonary capillary endothelium, basement membrane and perivascular and perilymphatic tissues.

Rapid Perioperative Care, First Edition. Paul Wicker and Sara Dalby.

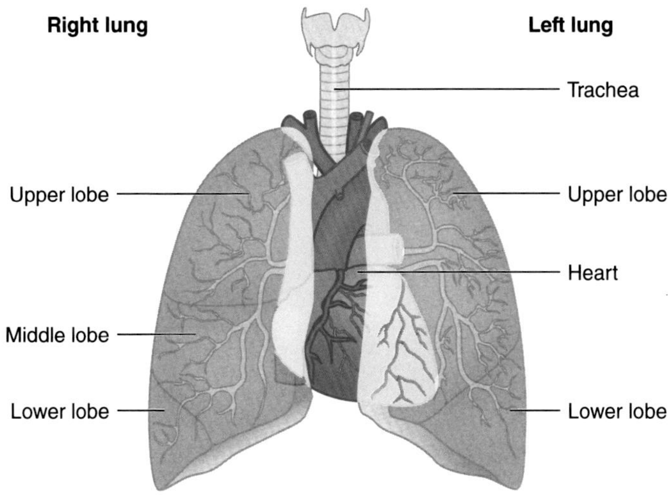

Figure 18.1 Anatomy of the lungs

Oxygen exchange

Once the air enters the alveoli, which have thin walls, the oxygen can transfer from the alveoli to the surrounding capillaries. The capillaries then carry the oxygenated blood from the lungs to the rest of the body via arteries and blood vessels which supply oxygen to all parts of the body (Marieb 2006). Carbon dioxide is also released from the blood via the capillaries and enters the alveoli, which is then released from the lungs by breathing out. Hypoventilation, or low breathing, can happen if there are high levels of carbon dioxide in the blood. Alternatively, too little carbon dioxide in the bloodstream can result in hyperventilation or rapid breathing.

A spirometry/diffusion capacity (DLCO) test is used to evaluate and diagnose any breathing difficulties. The purpose of this test can include identifying shortness of breath, assessing the effectiveness of respiratory drugs, identifying obstruction in the air passages or limited volume within the lungs and evaluating the presence of a respiratory disease. The DLCO test also measures the amount of oxygen diffusing from the lungs to the bloodstream.

Lung problems

Lung parenchyma is a medical term which is used to describe the functioning systems and tissues of a human lung. It includes the alveolar walls as well as the blood vessels and the bronchi. If any part of the parenchyma becomes damaged or diseased, a person's life may be at risk due to poor oxygen and carbon dioxide exchange (Clancy & McVicar 2009). Lung parenchyma is involved in O_2 and CO_2 gas transfer via the alveoli, alveolar ducts and respiratory bronchioles and blood vessels which are located inside the lungs.

Pleurisy

Pleurisy occurs because inflamed pleural layers rub against each other when the lungs expand during breathing or inhalation. This can result in severe and sharp pain caused by the presence of pain sensors and nerve fibres which are in the lining of the pleura. This can also result in the pleura sticking to the chest wall, reducing the patient's ability to breathe easily. High levels of fluid can also collect in the pleural space, resulting in pleural effusion. If there are high levels of fluid, then the pleura is pushed against the lung, resulting in the lung collapsing (Clancy & McVicar 2009).

The symptoms of pleural effusion include sharp chest pain, coughing, fever, hiccups, rapid breathing and shortness of breath. Treatment can be carried out using thoracentesis which is a procedure used to remove fluid from the space between the lining of the outside of the lungs (pleura) and the wall of the chest. Removing the fluid will allow the lung to expand more and make breathing easier. Complications from pleurisy include damage to the lungs and infected pleural fluids that may need a chest tube to drain the fluids (Pudner 2010).

Asbestosis

Asbestos fibres can damage lungs as they can be inhaled deeply into the lungs and become embedded in the lung tissues. Some of the asbestos fibres may become embedded in the pleura surrounding the lung. The fluid in the pleural space, however, may also remove the fibres out of the lung and deposit them throughout the body. White blood cells attempt to remove these fibres, but sometimes the asbestos fibres can destroy the macrophages, and the fibres will remain within the body.

Asbestosis results in the scarring of the lung tissues caused by asbestos fibres, resulting in inflammation in the lung tissue. This inflammation may also lead to scarring in the interstitium, resulting in the alveoli not exchanging oxygen with the blood, and reducing the oxygen supply to the body. Scarring can also damage capillaries, reducing the exchange of oxygen and carbon dioxide in the bloodstream.

When macrophages are destroyed, their contents exit their cells and lead to inflammation of the pleura, leading to scarring which hardens and thickens the pleura. The hardened pleura will make it hard for the lungs to expand during inhalation and may also cause the lungs to contract in size, leading to poor breathing and reduced oxygenation of the blood (Marieb 2006).

Mesothelioma

When the pleural lining of the chest or abdomen becomes cancerous, it is called a mesothelioma. Lung cancer normally occurs in the lung tissue, and it is often caused by smoking or by exposure to asbestos. Cigarette smoking also greatly increases the likelihood of a person developing lung cancer as the result of tar and tobacco contents collecting in the lung.

Conclusion

The lungs are one of the most important organs of the body, as they supply oxygen to the body cells which keep the body alive. However, lungs are susceptible to damage because of inhaling toxic materials and irritants (e.g. smoking, pollution and smog). If this happens, then the body is at risk because the body's need for oxygen is essential (Pudner 2010). The effective functioning of the respiratory system therefore greatly affects the health of the body since any damage or disease in the lungs can result in further harm to the rest of the body's organs and tissues. And because the heart and lung are connected closely, any lung disease can also result in heart problems.

19 General Anaesthesia

General anaesthesia (GA) has developed over time and changed in many ways, to work in association with even more complex surgical procedures. As a result, GA has improved vastly and become safer than ever before. However, there are still risks associated with GA because of faulty equipment or patient problems, including airway complications, allergic reactions and so on, during induction and recovery. In the early 1960s and 1970s, young patients often undertook GA by dentists; however, as GA has become safer, anaesthetic gases are rarely used outside of hospitals these days.

Preoperative assessment of patients is essential to ensure safe anaesthesia (O'Neill 2010). This is usually carried out mainly by the anaesthetist, but also by practitioners. Preoperative assessment involves assessing the patient's health, informing the patient of the anaesthetic drugs and gases which are going to be used and letting them know of the need for monitoring and observations (Young & Griffiths 2006, AAGBI 2007). Often, the anaesthetist will visit the patient alongside the surgeon or someone from the surgical team in order to ensure the patient has a full understanding of the actions that are going to be carried out.

The type of operation being undertaken by the patient will also affect the type of anaesthetic being delivered. For example, a patient who has a full stomach may inhale some of the food contents, in which case a rapid sequence induction (RSI) will be required. In other situations, such as a circumcision, local anaesthetics can also be used alongside GA, reducing the level of general anaesthetic drugs needed. Other actions needed during anaesthesia can include difficult intubation, muscle relaxation, venous access, monitoring, intravenous fluids, circulatory problems and so on (O'Neill 2010).

Given the health status of the patient, there are many reasons which may affect anaesthesia. Assessment of the patient helps to identify the requirements for anaesthesia and any risks which the patient may develop. Assessment needs investigation of the patient's history, examination and further investigation if problems are identified.

Investigation of the patient's history includes pre-existing conditions such as heart disease, liver disease, blood disorders, diabetes mellitus and respiratory disease (O'Neill 2010). Medication, such as antidepressants and barbiturates that the patient takes because of these conditions, can also have an effect on the impact of anaesthetic drugs. The patient should also be asked about any previous anaesthesia and whether any adverse events occurred.

Examination of the patient can identify areas such as cardiovascular and respiratory system problems. The patient should be checked for heart rate, blood pressure, cardiovascular problems and respiratory disease. The patient also needs to be assessed for neck problems, loose teeth or crowns, opening of the mouth and so on. It is also important to check that veins are available for intravenous access for drugs or fluids.

Further investigations can include:

- Checking blood for anaemia, and cross matching if needed
- Use of diuretics or renal impairment
- Sickle cell disease
- Patients with existing heart disease will need electrocardiograph (ECG) monitoring (Young & Griffiths 2006).
- Spirometry to investigate lung diseases.

Rapid Perioperative Care, First Edition. Paul Wicker and Sara Dalby.

Premedication

Premedication may be given up to 2 h before surgery in most patients, but especially for those who are anxious. Anxiety is a major issue for the patient which needs actions taken by anaesthetists and practitioners in order to help the patient relax (Mitchell 2013). Anxiolytic drugs are sometimes used in the anaesthetic room and include temazepam and midazolam, both to reduce anxiety and to reduce the level of the induction agent. Patients with gastric acidity may also be given ranitidine or sodium citrate pre-induction, to reduce the risk of gastric content aspiration. Postoperative nausea and vomiting (PONV) can be common when surgical procedures are carried out in areas such as the middle ear, female reproductive organs, bowel, gallbladder or eyes. One of the best drugs to administer to patients is Ondansetron which can prevent PONV from occurring in patients (Gan 2006).

Anaesthetic induction

Induction is usually carried out with the use of IV drugs. Sodium thiopentone has been used for many years, but new drugs, such as propofol, fentanyl or alfentanil, have emerged which work faster and are safer. Once the induction drug is given to the patient, the patient becomes unconscious, and a face mask is connected to oxygen and attached to the patient to enable them to breathe (Photo 3). When muscle relaxants are given to the patient, laryngeal mask airways (LMAs) or endotracheal tubes (ETTs) will be attached, as the patient will need the use of the respirator attached to the anaesthetic machine to be able to breathe. When ETTs are used, the patient will normally require propofol, muscle relaxants and intubation via a laryngoscope. Sevoflurane has a rapid onset of action and has now superseded isoflurane, halothane and other agents during induction and maintenance of anaesthesia.

Suxamethonium remains a popular depolarising muscle relaxant because it can cause rapid paralysis in about 10–20 sec and last for about 5–10 min (Conway *et al.* 2014). It is often used during a rapid sequence induction because of its fast action. Rocuronium is a

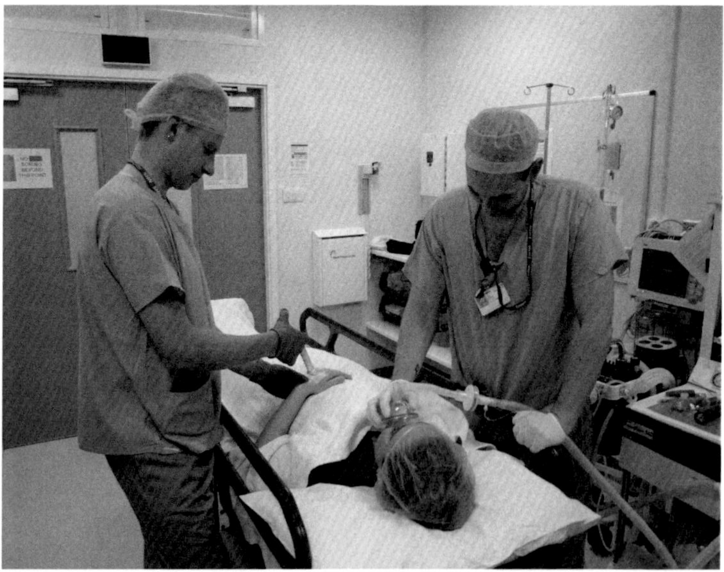

Photo 3 Preoperative anaesthetic induction. Courtesy of Aintree Hospital, Liverpool

modern non-depolarising drug, but it has a slower onset of action than suxamethonium. Rocuronium relaxes muscles after 1–3 min and lasts for around 45 min. Suxamethonium is rapidly metabolised in the body, resulting in the reverse of muscle paralysis; however, rocuronium lasts longer and keeps the patient's muscles paralysed. Suxamethonium does have some problems and can result in scoline apnoea and malignant hyperthermia in some patients if they are not able to metabolise the drug. Suxamethonium can also cause muscle aching postoperatively because of the fasciculation during induction.

Airway management

ETTs and LMAs are used to maintain respiration and enable ventilation (O'Neill 2010). ETTs in particular can prevent gastric reflux if the patient has undergone trauma and needs a rapid sequence induction, has a hiatus hernia or is undergoing abdominal surgery. However, the LMA is useful for minor procedures such as plastic surgery or carpal tunnel surgery if the patient undergoes GA. The LMA is an alternative to bag ventilation which allows the anaesthetist or assistant to free their hands, but it does not eliminate the risk of gastric aspiration. The LMA does not enter the trachea as it sits in the patient's hypopharynx and covers the supraglottic structures.

Maintenance of anaesthetic

The main aims for maintaining GA in patients include:

- Controlling unconsciousness
- Maintaining pain relief
- Providing muscle relaxation
- Reducing signals from the autonomic nervous system (ANS) (O'Neill 2010).

The ANS has two branches, the sympathetic nervous system and the parasympathetic nervous system, and is regulated within the brain by the hypothalamus. The ANS connects with the peripheral nervous system which influences the function of internal organs, for example regulating the heart rate, digestion, respiratory rate, pupillary response and urination. Anaesthetic drugs help to reduce signals from the ANS and allow the anaesthetist to regulate the function of the body's organs.

Maintenance of anaesthesia is achieved by combining anaesthetic drugs, opioids and muscle relaxants. Volatile anaesthetic gases may be combined with nitrous oxide and oxygen to reduce the amount of volatile gases needed for anaesthesia. However, nitrous oxide can result in PONV, and therefore it is used less now, especially in cases where patients may be susceptible to PONV (Gan 2006).

Monitoring

Monitoring occurs before, during and after anaesthesia, and it is important to ensure the patient is safe and is not receiving high or low dosages of anaesthetic drugs or inhalation gases (AAGBI 2007). Examples of the equipment used during anaesthesia include a pulse oximeter, non-invasive blood pressure monitor, temperature monitor, capnograph, nerve stimulator and electrocardiograph. Airway gases, such as oxygen, carbon dioxide and anaesthetic vapours, also need to be monitored, usually by monitors on the anaesthetic machine (Conway *et al.* 2014). Airway pressure is also monitored by ventilators to prevent damage to the lungs and to ensure the volume of oxygen received is suitable (AAGBI 2007).

Complications

There are many potential complications during GA, because of the health of the patient, faulty equipment, inappropriate drugs, low oxygen levels, gastric reflux and so on. However, given the learned knowledge and skills of both the anaesthetist and the anaesthetic practitioner, complications tend to be rare and don't occur often. Examples of risks associated with anaesthesia (Conway *et al.* 2014) can include:

- Damage to the mouth, teeth or crowns during intubation.
- Minor allergic reactions to anaesthetic drugs leading to PONV.
- Major allergic reactions to anaesthetic drugs, leading to cardiovascular problems, respiratory depression or jaundice.
- Slow recovery from the anaesthetic because of drug interactions, incorrect drug dosage or inadequate reversal of drugs, leading to poor cardiac, hepatic or renal functions.
- Malignant hyperpyrexia caused by a reaction to anaesthetic gases or suxamethonium.
- Prolonged apnoea caused by inability of the patient to inactivate suxamethonium.

'Anaesthetic awareness' can also occur during surgery when anaesthetic dosages are too low and the patient is awake but still paralysed by the muscle relaxant. This can result in the patient being aware of the surgery being performed and also hearing the conversations happening within the operating room by the surgical team. A patient who is paralysed but undergoing low levels of anaesthetic drugs must be monitored carefully in case of any signs of intraoperative awareness or pain. Midazolam may be given if this occurs, leading to induction of amnesia. Normally, however, the extensive range of monitoring during anaesthesia will inform the anaesthetist of any problems the patient is experiencing (Young & Griffiths 2006).

20 Local Anaesthesia

Local anaesthetics (LAs) are used to remove pain during surgery, which can then be continued or stopped after surgery. There are various techniques used for local anaesthesia, including topical anaesthesia, infiltrative anaesthesia, ring blocks and peripheral nerve blocks (Wicker & Bocos 2010). LAs are safer than general anaesthetics as they have a lesser impact on the physiology of the body; they are also easy to administer and readily available. LAs have been undergoing development since 1884, when Sigmund Freud and Karl Koller (Reis 2009) were the first to use a LA agent during surgery on a patient's eye. LAs have now become safe and effective during surgical procedures.

Pathophysiology

Electrical impulses in nerves will transmit sensations to all parts of the body. The electrical impulses occur because the ion gradient on the cell wall alternates depending on the membrane potential.

When the nerve is not active, it has a negative membrane potential of –70 mV, developed by two major ions, Na^+ and K^+ (Torpy & Lynm 2011). The concentration of ions is adjusted by the sodium–potassium pump which moves sodium ions out of the cell and potassium ions into the cell. However, the nerve has a negative resting potential when it is not active because K^+ ions move out of the cell, giving the cell a negative status.

When a nerve becomes stimulated by the electrical impulses, the nerve depolarises and the nerve transmits sensations. Sodium ions pass through sodium channels in the nerve cell membrane and enter the cell body, increasing the electric potential. As the number of sodium ions increase, the nerve membrane becomes depolarised and reaches a level of +35 mV or higher. When the electrical impulse stops and the nerve relaxes, the membrane starts to absorb sodium and potassium ions which re-establishes the negative resting membrane potential (Torpy & Lynm 2011).

Action of local anaesthetics

The nerve membrane is stopped from depolarising by LAs which interfere with the influx of Na^+ and K^+ ions. This stops the threshold level of the ions and stops the action potential from propagating.

LAs of all types have three components – an aromatic portion, an intermediate chain and an amine group. The aromatic portion is made from benzene and is lipophilic (combines or dissolves in lipids), and the amine group provides hydrophilic properties (absorbing or dissolving in water). The level of lipid solubility in the LA enables its diffusion through the nerve membrane. The length of action of the LA is established by its ability to bind to anaesthetic receptors on the outside of the nerve cell membrane, which are proteins. The aromatic and amine portions are connected to a chain which is composed of either an ester or an amide linkage, which in turn classifies LAs as either aminoamide or aminoester (Torpy & Lynm 2011).

Rapid Perioperative Care, First Edition. Paul Wicker and Sara Dalby.

Local anaesthetics

The two groups of anaesthetic drugs are the ester and amide groups. The difference between the two groups can affect the metabolism of the LA and also lead to an allergic reaction.

Ester anaesthetics metabolise by a plasma enzyme called pseudocholinesterase. If patients cannot metabolise ester-type anaesthetics because of a genetic defect, this may result in toxic reactions, allergy and raised levels of LA in their bloodstream. Patients therefore need to be assessed before the use of the ester anaesthetic to ensure safety (Becker & Reed 2006).

The liver uses enzymes to metabolise amide-type LAs. However, patients with liver disease, or who are taking medications, may not be able to metabolise the LA and should be monitored closely for any signs of toxicity or adverse reactions such as increased levels of LA in blood. Medications that can affect LAs include antiarrhythmic agents (Quinidine), antibiotics (Erythromycin, Tetracycline), benzodiazepines (Midazolam) and calcium channel blockers (Nifedipine) (Tables 20.1 and 20.2) (Becker & Reed 2006).

Examples of ester group LAs include procaine, chloroprocaine and tetracaine. Amide groups include lidocaine, bupivicaine, etidocaine and prilocaine (Becker & Reed 2006).

Table 20.1 Amides for infiltrative injection

Common local anaesthetics	Concentration(s)	Maximum total adult dose per procedure*	Volume of maximum total adult dose	pH	Onset, duration
Lidocaine (or xylocaine)	1–2%	4.5–5 mg/kg, not to exceed 300 mg	30 mL of 1%; 15 mL of 2%	pH: 5–7	Onset: < 2 min Duration: 0.5–1 h
Lidocaine with epinephrine	1–2% lidocaine with epinephrine 1:100,000 or 1:200,000	7 mg/kg, not to exceed 500 mg	50 mL of 1%; 25 mL of 2%	pH: 3.3–5.5	Onset: < 2 min Duration: 2–6 h
Bupivacaine	0.25%	2.5 mg/kg, not to exceed 175 mg	70 mL	pH: 4–6.5	Onset: 5 min Duration: 2–4 h
Bupivacaine with epinephrine	0.25% bupivacaine with epinephrine 1:200,000	Not to exceed 225 mg	90 mL	pH: 3.3–5.5	Onset: 5 min Duration: 3–7 h
Mepivacaine	1%	Not to exceed 400 mg	40 mL of 1%	pH: 4.5–6.8	Onset: 3–5 min Duration: 0.75–1.5 h (with epinephrine: 2–6 h)

Table 20.2 Esters for infiltrative injection

Common local anaesthetics	Concentration(s)	Maximum total adult dose per procedure*	Volume of maximum total adult dose	pH	Onset, duration
Procaine	0.25–0.5% (via dilution)	350–600 mg	140–240 mL of 0.25%; 70–120 mL of 0.5%	pH: 3.5–5	Onset: 2–5 min Duration: 0.25–1 h
Chloroprocaine	1–2%	Not to exceed 800 mg	80 mL of 1%; 40 mL of 2%	pH: 4.5	Onset: 6–12 min Duration: 0.5 h

Local anaesthetic drugs are given to patients to ensure they remain pain free during surgery, and stay healthy during the surgical procedures.

Administration of LAs

Mechanism of action

LAs provide a loss of sensation in a limited area by blocking nerve conduction. Nerve conduction is blocked by inhibiting sodium channels along the axon of the nerve. The reduction in sodium ions decreases depolarisation which prevents the formation of the nerve action potential.

Infiltrative local anaesthetic agents

LAs can be used for infiltration and nerve block anaesthesia, depending on the surgical procedure. Infiltration anaesthesia is used for minor surgical procedures, whereas nerve block anaesthesia is used for major surgical procedures and for pain management (Wicker & Bocos 2010). Infiltrative anaesthetics are used for several procedures, including subcutaneous (suturing, IV infusions), submucosal (laceration repairs), wound infiltration (to control pain at the incision), intra-articular injections (to reduce arthritic joint pain) and nerve blocks (e.g. ankle block) (Torpy & Lynm 2011).

Dosage and administration

LAs are normally given in low concentrations when used for infiltration, depending on the procedure and the patient's individual needs or situation. Patients with problems such as being young or old, suffering from liver disease or arterial diseases or being acutely ill normally have a much reduced dosage to preserve their safety during delivery of the LA (Wicker & Bocos 2010).

Administrative techniques

It is important to ensure the patient's comfort during the administration of LAs, since the administration can be painful or disturbing for the patient. Infiltration anaesthesia is administered via intradermal, subcutaneous or submucosal layers, above or across the nerve pathway in the area where the surgical procedure takes place. The most common technique for injecting the LA is by using a field block technique, subcutaneously, in a circular pattern around the surgical procedure area (Becker & Reed 2006).

Adverse effects

LAs often create adverse effects when the LA enters the bloodstream, resulting in high plasma concentrations of the LA. Other issues include high dosages, delay in clearing the LA and infiltration into vascular tissue. Systemic effects can occur when LA drugs enter the blood and increase to toxic levels (Torpy & Lynm 2011). This can happen if the LA is injected by accident into an artery or vein, or if an excessive dose of the anaesthetic is delivered. Systemic toxicity by LAs can also result in damage to the central nervous system and the cardiovascular system. Other possible systemic effects on the patient may include:

- Seizures
- Respiratory arrest
- Cardiovascular effects such as bradycardia, arrhythmias or cardiac arrest
- Hypotension or hypertension
- Skin discoloration
- Swelling (Wicker & Bocos 2010).

There may also be other adverse reactions depending on the health and physiology of the patient. For example, infection may happen when a sterile technique is not carried out effectively. Using alcohol swabs to clean the skin before injection can help to reduce the chances of infection. If infection develops, then antibiotics will be given and drainage of an abscess may be required (Wicker & Bocos 2010).

Allergic reaction to LAs

LA agents are in the amide group or the ester group. Because of the different structure of the LAs, each may result in an allergy depending on the state of the patient. The liver metabolises the amide groups, whereas plasma cholinesterases metabolise the ester groups. When broken down, the ester group of LAs develops para-aminobenzoic acid (PABA), which is a well-known allergen, and they are more likely to produce allergy compared to the amide group (Torpy & Lynm 2011). Allergy caused by the amide local anaesthetics therefore rarely occurs.

Allergic reactions can also be caused by acute toxicity, patient anxiety and actions of other anaesthetic drugs such as epinephrine. Examples of allergic reactions include facial swelling, wheezing, dyspnoea, cyanosis, nausea, vomiting, oedema and abdominal cramping. However, there are few allergies developed by LAs in most patients.

21 Regional Anaesthesia

Regional anaesthesia involves injecting a local anaesthetic (LA) into an area of the body where there are multiple nerves; the LA then numbs that part of the body where surgery is going to take place. Patients usually remain awake, or they may be given a sedative to calm them down if they are anxious. Injecting LA into the spinal canal can create spinal and epidural blocks which will block feeling in the legs and abdomen. Other areas that can be blocked include extremities, arms and legs. The most commonly used regional anaesthetics are a femoral nerve block for leg surgery and a brachial plexus block in the arm or shoulder (Hadzic 2007).

In general anaesthesia, the patient is unconscious and has no awareness of the surgery or of pain. However, in regional anaesthesia, the patient may be awake, be aware of the surgery being undertaken, be able to speak and occasionally feel pain over time. If the patient is anxious, they are often given a sedative to reduce pain and allow them to drop into a semiconscious state, allowing the patient to remain comfortable during the surgical procedure (Burkard *et al.* 2005). If minimal sedation is given to the patient, then the patient may be able to answer questions from the surgeon or anaesthetist, and may be fully aware of the procedures being undertaken. If the patient does receive sedation during surgery, their vital signs, such as heart rate, blood pressure and oxygen level, are monitored to avoid any problems.

Examples of surgical procedures

Anaesthetists provide regional anaesthesia after consulting with the surgeon over the type of surgery being performed. Although a wide variety of surgical procedures can use regional anaesthesia, it is important for the patient's safety and comfort that the best method of anaesthesia is used, which may also include sedation or general anaesthesia (Burkard *et al.* 2005). Regional techniques may be used with the following procedures (Hadzic 2007):

Surgery	Techniques
Gastrointestinal or liver surgery	Epidural, spinal or paravertebral nerve blocks, with catheters to provide ongoing local anaesthetics
Gynaecology, including hysterectomy, pelvic procedures and caesarean sections	Epidural, spinal or paravertebral nerve blocks can provide effective regional anaesthesia and analgesia.
Ophthalmology, involving eye surgery	Injection of local anaesthetics will provide pain relief.
Orthopaedics, including fingers, toes and joints	Epidural, spinal, and peripheral nerve blocks, depending on the area requiring surgical intervention
Thoracic surgery, including surgery in the chest or oesophagus	Epidural, paravertebral or intercostal nerve blocks and catheters will control pain effectively.
Urology, including surgery on the kidney, prostate and bladder such as prostatectomy or nephrectomy	Epidural, spinal or paravertebral nerve blocks and catheters
Vascular surgery, including carotid artery, aortic artery and femoral arteries	Cervical blocks (for carotid surgery), and epidural or paravertebral nerve blocks for other areas

Rapid Perioperative Care, First Edition. Paul Wicker and Sara Dalby.

To maintain patient safety, the anaesthetist will assess the patient before deciding on the type of anaesthesia to undertake and also discuss with the surgeon the type of surgical procedure being undertaken.

Regional blocks

Epidural and spinal anaesthesia

Spinal and epidural anaesthetics involve injecting an LA into the vertebral canal which prevents nerve sensations in the chest, abdomen and legs. The spinal cord has a dural sac containing spinal fluid which surrounds the spinal nerves (Hadzic 2007).

Patients will be connected to monitors before spinal anaesthesia to monitor vital signs. The patient will then be placed on their side, with their knees close to their chest, or alternatively the patient may be asked to sit upright with their arms resting on a table in front of them (McConachie 2014). This positioning allows the anaesthetist to gain access to the patient's spine.

The anaesthetist marks the patient's back in the area required, cleans the skin with an antiseptic solution wipe and then places a sterile drape around the area needed for injection (Burkard *et al.* 2005). LA is often injected around the area to reduce pain for the patient. The anaesthetist inserts the needle through the skin into the space between the vertebrae. Patients sometimes feel tingling feelings because of irritation of the nerves during injection (Wedel & Horlocker 2005).

To provide spinal anaesthesia, the anaesthetist will push the needle into the patient's back until it perforates the dural sac, and then inject the LA into the spinal fluid. Spinal injections are normally undertaken once, and the duration of the spinal anaesthesia will depend on the amount of LA injected (Wedel & Horlocker 2005).

Providing epidural anaesthesia requires the anaesthetist to use a sterile technique and push the needle into the epidural space, on the outside of the dural sac. The anaesthetist will then insert a small flexible plastic catheter and remove the needle, which will allow for continuous injections of LA. Epidural analgesia is often used during childbirth or after painful surgical procedures to reduce pain in the patient (Hadzic 2007).

Once the anaesthetist has completed the spinal or epidural block, the patient will start to feel numbness, and eventually they will not be able to move their legs. Once the pain relief has become established, the surgical procedure will start. Patients may be given a sedative to help relax them during the surgery, or alternatively the patient may stay wide awake depending on their condition.

Following surgery, the patient is escorted to the recovery room to be closely monitored and cared for by the recovery practitioner until the spinal or epidural block wears off. A spinal block will normally last for 2–6 h, depending on the amount of LA injected. An epidural block can last longer if the catheter remains in place, allowing a continuous infusion of LA (Wedel & Horlocker 2005).

Brachial plexus block

The brachial plexus is a network of nerves which starts at the spine and then continues through the neck, to the axilla (armpit region) and then into the arm. Depending on the surgical procedure, the anaesthetist will inject LA into specific parts of the brachial plexus (McConachie 2014). Surgery on the shoulder would require a nerve block in the brachial plexus above the clavicle. Surgery in the axilla, in the shoulder joint or down the arm would need a nerve block below the clavicle or under the axilla. An ultrasound device or nerve stimulator is used to locate the brachial plexus and the correct area for injecting the LA. Before the block is started, the patient will be asked to inform the anaesthetist of any pain or any nerve injuries or problems experienced before surgery. Blocking the brachial plexus may also interfere with breathing; therefore, any breathing problems may also need to be discussed with the anaesthetist prior to anaesthesia, and general or local anaesthetic may be administered as an alternative instead (McConachie 2014).

Paravertebral block

Paravertebral blocks can occur in several different parts of the body and numb the specific areas where the block is performed (Hadzic 2007). Paravertebral blocks can include blocks in the chest or abdomen to allow breast, thoracic and abdominal surgery, or in the neck to allow surgery on the thyroid gland or carotid artery. They can also be used at the hip to enable surgery on the hip, knee or thigh.

Most paravertebral blocks use similar techniques. The anaesthetist will check the patient's area where the surgery is going to be conducted, cleans the skin and then injects LA firstly into the skin and then deeper into the tissues. The anaesthetist then inserts a needle and injects LA which numbs the nerves. The anaesthetist may also insert a small flexible catheter, and then remove the needle, to allow for continuous injections of LA to prolong the pain relief. A nerve stimulator is often used to locate the nerves, resulting in twitching of the local muscles. If the patient experiences any pain when injecting the LA, the anaesthetist needs to be made aware of this as it may be causing damage to the nerves. The anaesthetic practitioner also needs to be aware of any issues the patient may be experiencing during the paravertebral block and inform the anaesthetist of any problems experienced by the patient (McConachie 2014).

Femoral nerve block

The femoral nerve block provides anaesthesia for the entire anterior thigh, the knee and the femur (McConachie 2014). The patient is normally positioned in the supine position. The anaesthetist cleans the groin and numbs the skin area by injecting a minor dose of LA. A nerve stimulator is set up, and the anaesthetist then inserts a needle deeper into the tissues and injects an LA to numb the femoral nerves. A flexible plastic catheter may replace the needle to allow continuous infusion of LA if the surgical procedure is likely to progress for a long time, to ensure the patient does not feel pain. The patient will let the anaesthetist know if he or she suffers any sharp or radiating pain during injection. Postoperatively, the patient may also not be able to walk well due to weakness of the leg, so assistance will be needed (e.g. a wheelchair may be used).

Sciatic and popliteal nerve block

This sciatic nerve is located in the back of the thigh, and the popliteal nerve is located around the knee and lower leg. Therefore, sciatic and popliteal blocks are used for surgery on the knee and lower leg, including the calf, Achilles tendon, ankle and foot. The patient will normally be placed in a prone position or on their side to receive the sciatic nerve block. The process is the same as the femoral nerve block and may include adding a catheter for long surgical procedures (McConachie 2014). Again, the patient may have difficulty standing, and care must be provided to support the patient postoperatively.

22 Rapid Sequence Induction

Introduction

Rapid sequence intubation (RSI) is carried out on patients who have severe airway problems, suffered a serious accident or require surgery after having eaten a full meal which can result in gastric reflux leading to airway problems. RSI provides anaesthesia which induces immediate unconsciousness and muscular relaxation by using anaesthetic induction agents and muscle relaxants. RSI offers an effective and efficient method to ensure the patient's emergency airway is managed.

Airway protection

During RSI, the anaesthetist and anaesthetic practitioner need to work quickly to ensure the patient's safety. This includes:

- Maintaining airway protection and patency
- Checking for respiratory failure, and airway secretion management
- Relaxing the patient to minimise oxygen consumption, and ensuring oxygen delivery is appropriate
- Ensuring patient is unresponsive to pain, terminating seizures occurring in the patient and preventing secondary brain injury if there are head injuries
- Maintaining temperature control (McConachie 2014).

On occasion, it may be necessary to carry out RSI outside the hospital because of the condition of the patient. However, it is important that a correct decision is made, because RSI can also lead to harm to the patient if there is little equipment available or the patient needs to be transported from a demolished house or car accident. Reasons to carry out RSI outside the hospital can include lack of airway protection, hypoventilation, prolonged transfer to the hospital or spinal injuries. Reasons to avoid RSI outside the hospital can include lack of close proximity to an operating room, paediatric cases, a hostile environment or lack of skills within the team.

There are also many factors which can make emergency intubation difficult to carry out, especially when the patient is seriously ill. In this situation, RSI needs to be carried out quickly, safely and efficiently (McConachie 2014). Issues with patients can include (Nolan & Soar 2012):

- A seriously ill patient with a potential to die quickly
- An argumentative or non-cooperative patient
- Major airway and breathing problems, or patient apnoea, caused by phlegm, secretions, blocked airway or the like
- Low levels of oxygen delivered to the patient
- Patient's full stomach leading to increased risk of gastric reflux and aspiration into the lungs
- Damaged anatomy of the airway, for example damaged vocal chords or crushed trachea.

Rapid Perioperative Care, First Edition. Paul Wicker and Sara Dalby.

Steps taken for rapid sequence induction

There are many ways that anaesthetists start RSI, but the most common is to follow the '10 Ps' (Nolan & Soar 2012). This involves addressing RSI step by step:

- Compose a plan before starting the RSI.
- Prepare drugs, equipment, practitioners, anaesthetic machine and so on.
- Protect the neck from too much stretching or turning.
- Position the patient correctly, normally in the supine position.
- Pre-oxygenate the patient to provide high levels of oxygen before intubation.
- Give drugs before starting RSI, including atropine, fentanyl and/or lignocaine.
- Apply cricoid pressure to reduce the chance of gastric reflux.
- Deliver sedatives and muscle relaxants to produce paralysis and induction.
- Placement of the endotracheal tube (ETT), and checking of the patient's O_2 and CO_2 levels using monitors.
- Manage the patient post intubation by checking that the ETT is attached correctly; a chest x-ray may be taken to confirm correct placement and continuous sedation and paralysis during anaesthesia until surgery is complete.

Under normal circumstances, there would be a minimum of three people involved in proceeding with RSI (Simpson 2013). This will include the anaesthetist, who is responsible for managing the airway, and an anaesthetic practitioner, who will be responsible for applying cricoid pressure and providing the anaesthetist with the necessary equipment. An assistant anaesthetist may also help with administering drugs and assisting the anaesthetist for airway management, monitoring of blood pressure and pulse and so on (McConachie 2014).

Preparing for RSI

Preparation of the anaesthetic room is essential to ensure the safety of the patient, especially in an emergency situation. Normally, the anaesthetic practitioner would prepare the anaesthetic room with equipment and then discuss anything further with the anaesthetist. A sterile environment is also essential, especially in regards to oral airways, ETTs and so on.

The main items of equipment needed include:

- *Suction*: The suction machine must be checked to ensure it is working, and at least one suction catheter and tubing should be easily available for the anaesthetist.
- *Oxygen*: A mask that does not allow re-breathing or a bag valve mask may be used with an oxygen flow of 15 litres per minute (L/PM) (Simpson 2013).
- *Airways*: Normally, a 7.5 ETT fits most adults; however, a size 7.0 may be used for smaller females and a size 8.0 for larger males. The balloon is tested before intubation and filled with a syringe, with approximately 10 cc of air (Simpson 2013).
- *Stylet*: A stylet is a smooth, malleable metal or plastic rod that is placed inside an ETT to adjust the curvature and enhance its rigidity. It is normally bent at around 30°.
- *Laryngoscopes*: There are various types of blade that will be attached to laryngoscopes depending on the patient's age, size and condition (McConachie 2014). These include:
  - Curved Macintosh blade size 3 or 4 for adults
  - Straight Miller blade size 3 or 4 for adults
  - Blade is attached to the laryngoscope handle and checked to ensure the light source works correctly.
- An emergency cricothyrotomy kit enables a surgical procedure which is used to gain prompt access to an inaccessible airway (Yentis *et al.* 2009).

- Extra equipment may include a video laryngoscope, laryngeal mask airway or bougie or the like.
- Monitoring equipment includes electrocardiograph monitor, pulse oximeter, blood pressure monitor, capnography monitor (measures CO_2) and so on.
- Medications need to be available, drawn up into syringes and available for immediate use, for example sedatives, muscle relaxants, resuscitation drugs and so on (Nolan & Soar 2012).

Drugs used for RSI

The drugs used for RSI render the patient unconscious and unresponsive quickly via intravenous injection, usually into the arm. The drugs also provide analgesia, maintain cardiovascular status and have few side effects. Drugs are given according to body weight and the physiological health of the patient (Yentis *et al.* 2009). These drugs can usually be reversible if required. Examples of drugs used for RSI include induction agents and neuromuscular agents.

Induction Agents

- Propofol 1.5–2.5 mg/kg
- Fentanyl 2–10 mcg/kg
- Midazolam 0.1–0.3 mg/kg
- Thiopental 3–5 mg/kg
- Etomidate 0.3–0.4 mg/kg
- Ketamine 1.5–2 mg/kg IV (rarely used) (Nolan & Soar 2012, Simpson 2013).

See also Table 22.1.

Neuromuscular Agents

- Suxamethonium 1–2 mg/kg
- Rocuronium 0.6–1.2 mg/kg
- Vecuronium 0.15–0.25 mg/kg (Nolan & Soar 2012, Simpson 2013).

See also Table 22.2.

Undertaking RSI in different settings

While RSIs may be undertaken within a hospital setting, which can guarantee patient safety, it is also possible that RSIs may need to be undertaken outside the hospital because of the urgency of the need to intubate the patient to maintain oxygen levels (Nolan & Soar 2012).

Following assessment of the patient, it may be possible to take the patient quickly to a local hospital. However, if the patient is miles away from any hospital, then RSI may be needed immediately. The patient will need to be positioned correctly, and the anaesthetist and team need full access to the patient. Airway equipment and the necessary drugs will be needed and are usually placed beside the patient (Yentis *et al.* 2009).

RSIs may happen in ambulances due to airway problems suffered by the patient. Normally, the patient will be placed in the ambulance on a trolley in a supine position. If the patient needs urgent help with airway obstruction, it is possible to intubate the patient on the ground, although this can be challenging to the team because of the hard ground and possible lumps and bumps under the patient.

Initiating RSI in an aircraft is challenging because of the lack of space, possible turbulence and lack of equipment. There may be some intubation equipment and drugs available, but if not then the patient will need to be pre-oxygenated using an oxygen mask and have a clear airway with visible signs of breathing. RSI may occur once the plane has landed and health professionals become available to assist and help the patient.

Table 22.1 Induction agents

Ketamine
Dose: 1.5 mg/kg IV (4 mg/kg IM)
Onset: 60–90 sec
Duration: 10–20 min
Use: Used occasionally for RSI, especially if the patient is haemodynamically unstable or if the patient has a constrictive airway. Ketamine will lead to bronchodilation but can also increase saliva.
Problems: Ketamine may lead to increased secretions, hypertension, tachycardia, laryngospasm and raised intraocular pressure.

Thiopentone
Dose: 3–5 mg/kg IV (via a vein, not an artery)
Onset: 30–45 sec
Duration: 5–10 min
Use: Often used for RSI if the patient is haemodynamically stable.
Problems: Thiopentone can result in histamine release, myocardial depression, vasodilation and hypotension.

Propofol
Propofol 1.5–2.5 mg/kg IV
Onset: 15–45 sec
Duration: 5–10 min
Use: Haemodynamically stable patients, reactive airways disease and status epilepticus.
Drawbacks: Hypotension, myocardial depression, reduced cerebral perfusion, pain on injection, variable response and very short acting.

Fentanyl
Dose 2–10 mcg/kg IV
Onset: <60 sec
Duration: Depending on the dosage given, approximately 30 min for 1–2 mcg/kg, and up to 6 h for 100 mcg/kg
Use: Fentanyl may be used as a premedication or may be used at low doses along with other drugs (such as propofol) when a patient is haemodynamically unstable.
Problems: Fentanyl may result in respiratory depression, apnoea, hypotension, nausea and vomiting, bradycardia and so on.

Midazolam
Dose: 0.3 mg/kg IV
Onset: 60–90 sec
Duration: 15–30 min
Use: Midazolam is usually not used directly for RSI, but low doses can be used if patients are in shock or in a state of anxiety.
Problems: Respiratory depression, hypotension, slow onset and so on.

Etomidate
Dose: 0.3 mg/kg IV
Onset: 10–15 sec
Use: Etomidate can be used for RSI, especially if the patient is haemodynamically unstable.
Problems: Adrenal suppression, myoclonus, and pain on injection.
From McConachie (2014).

RSI in a ward environment can also be difficult because of the number of patients and visitors close to the area where the patient is located. Transfer to a recovery room or intensive care unit would be ideal if possible; otherwise, the RSI may need to be carried out in the ward itself. Crowd control would need to be managed, and also moving beds and equipment may be necessary. There should also be full access to the patient. Anaesthetists and anaesthetic practitioners would need to be called urgently to provide the skills necessary to intubate the patient.

Table 22.2 Muscle relaxants

Suxamethonium
Dose: 1.5 mg/kg IV
Onset: 45–60 sec
Duration: 6–10 min
Use: Suxamethonium is widely used for RSI due to its quick onset of action.
Problems: There are many problems associated with suxamethonium in certain patients, including hyperkalaemia, malignant hyperthermia, bradycardia, fasciculations and elevated intraocular pressure. Anaesthetists must ensure patients are safe to use this drug.

Rocuronium
Dose: 1.2 mg/kg IV
Onset: 60 sec
Duration: 50 min or longer, depending on dosage
Use: Rocuronium is now often used for RSI unless rapid recovery is needed following intubation. Rocuronium can be reversed by Sugammadex.
Problems: There are few problems with rocuronium, although allergy may happen in some patients.

Vecuronium
Dose: 0.15 mg/kg IV
Onset: 120–180 sec
Duration: 45–60 min
Use: Vecuronium can be reversed by sugammadex, but it is not usually used for RSI, unless suxamethonium and rocuronium are not able to be used for the patient.
Problems: Allergy, slow onset and long duration.
From McConachie (2014).

Following intubation of the patient, various steps need to be taken which include securing the ETT, monitoring pulse oximetry, assessing vital signs frequently and potentially considering long-term sedation. It is also important to restrain the patient to prevent him or her from falling off the table or bed.

23 Total Intravenous Anaesthesia (TIVA)

Total intravenous anaesthesia (TIVA) is a technique which uses intravenous drugs to anaesthetise the patient without the use of any inhalational agents (Aitkenhead *et al.* 2014). Propofol was developed in 1986 and became one of the most popular induction agents for TIVA. The pharmacokinetic and pharmacodynamics properties of propofol and certain opioids have been found to be useful for TIVA due to their short-acting properties, and they are also more effective at times than general anaesthetics (Nimmo & Cook 2014). TIVA has become safer over time since machines now provide drug administration and monitor the level of drugs being delivered, leading to safe and effective use of the intravenous anaesthetic agents (Table 23.1).

TIVA is an alternative to general anaesthesia, and it involves the use of intravenous drugs for induction and ongoing maintenance of anaesthesia. Propofol is normally the preferred induction agent because of its rapid onset and minimal side effects; however, alfentanil and remifentanil may also be used (Aitkenhead *et al.* 2014). Postoperatively, the patient will recover quickly and also be 'clear-headed' on waking up. TIVA is also effective when surgery on the airway is carried out and use of an inhaled anaesthetic agent is not possible. In emergency situations where the correct equipment is not available, for example anaesthetic machines or anaesthetic gases, then TIVA is also more likely to be used (Aitkenhead *et al.* 2014).

Propofol can affect the brains of older people, and therefore they require reduced levels of propofol in comparison to younger patients (Reves et al., 2007). Remifentanil may also be given to reduce the concentration of propofol to be administered. Major surgical procedures may require an increased amount of propofol due to the extended length of surgery and the potential of pain, but if regional anaesthesia is used then the amount of drugs used in TIVA can be reduced (Reves *et al.* 2007). Target controlled infusion devices (TCIs) are normally used to control the drugs being administered and to ensure they are at safe levels.

TIVA actions

TIVA is commenced by administering a bolus of an induction agent and then providing a continuous infusion at an approved rate. The average blood propofol concentration is normally about 3.67 μg/ml; this is achieved within two min and then maintained at that level for the remainder of the surgical procedure (Aitkenhead *et al.* 2014). If an increase in the blood propofol concentration is needed, then another injection may be given, followed by a higher rate of infusion. If the blood propofol concentration rises beyond appropriate levels, then the infusion may be paused for a few seconds or minutes and then resumed at a reduced rate of infusion. TIVA has now become a more expensive option due to the high cost of the drugs and the use of the equipment (Aitkenhead *et al.* 2014).

TIVA uses a TCI to calculate the drug concentration and any delays in the transfer of drugs through the blood–brain barrier. Propofol needs to be monitored effectively as high levels can lead to a decrease in cardiac output and also hepatic blood flow, which can have

Rapid Perioperative Care, First Edition. Paul Wicker and Sara Dalby.

Table 23.1 Advantages of TIVA

1. Enhanced emergence from anaesthesia, compared to use of inhalational agents
2. Used for patients undergoing airway procedures
3. Reduction of contamination in theatre environment (e.g. caused by gases)
4. Reduction of risk of malignant hyperthermia
5. Reduction of chance of postoperative nausea and vomiting
6. Rapid induction and recovery using propofol
7. Can be used more easily than intubation and general anaesthesia outside of the operating theatre environment.

significant impact on the physiology of the patient. The TCI uses an infusion pump which injects the drugs into the intravenous circulation.

The infusion pump needs to be watched carefully as it is responsible for the delivery of the drugs. The first bolus of an induction agent rapidly increases the plasma concentration of the drug administered, which leads to the patient relaxing and becoming sedated. The infusion pump is normally able to function effectively even if the anaesthetist lowers the flow rates. Alarms on the TCI can identify any issues such as improper positioning of the syringe in the pump, high dosages of drugs, faulty rates of flow and so on. Normally, the syringe is fixed into place in the TCI to ensure that it remains firmly in place when the pump is in use. There is also a battery indicator on the TCI which informs practitioners if the battery level has fallen below normal levels.

There are several precautions which need to be considered and taken during the use of the syringe pump. These include (Yentis *et al.* 2009):

1. High concentrations of drugs that have a long onset and are long lasting should be avoided.
2. The patient needs to have the syringe pump connected close to the area of intravenous injection.
3. Vasoactive drugs (which cause vasodilation or vasoconstriction) should not be added to the main drug in the syringe pump.
4. The syringe pump should be placed equal to the level of the patient (Nimmo & Cook 2014).

A major problem of TIVA is the difficulty in measuring the level of the intravenous drugs in the plasma, which may affect the patient's physiological well-being (Smith *et al.* 2007). However, the advantages of TIVA include:

- Lack of problems caused by inhalational gases, for example hypoxia
- Prevents malignant hyperthermia in patients susceptible during general anaesthesia
- Reduction of postoperative nausea and vomiting.
- Remifentanil, which is an ultra-short-acting opioid, can be added to reduce the level of anaesthetic agents needed (Smith *et al.* 2007).

Main aims of TIVA

The main aims of TIVA are to provide a safe and effective method of sedation and pain relief for the patient. The patient will have a catheter inserted intravenously before drug dosage. Normally, the patient will lie in a supine position or a sideways position once the drugs have been injected. Inhalational gases are not administered; however, oxygen is usually given via an oxygen mask or a laryngeal mask (LMA) (Wicker & O'Neill 2010). The patient will be monitored closely in case of any issues arising.

Actions to be taken for TIVA include:

1. Smooth induction – intubation is not required, and induction is rapid if propofol is used.
2. Maintenance of TIVA by monitoring drug levels and monitoring the condition of the patient.
3. Rapid recovery following surgery because of the fast reduction in drug levels.
4. Drug combinations used in TIVA include:
   a. Propofol with remifentanil
   b. Propofol with sufentanil
   c. Midazolam with sufentanil (often used for patients with potential for developing malignant hyperthermia) (Nimmo & Cook 2014).

Conclusion

Patients undergoing TIVA using propofol may require a mixture of air or oxygen via a face-mask or LMA to maintain SpO_2 within normal limits, due to the low levels of breathing (Wicker & O'Neill 2010). TIVA also reduces the risk of hypoxia, compared to general anaesthesia (GA) when patients may be maintained on a combination of N_2O and O_2.

Postoperative recovery is also improved in terms of the patient's shorter duration of stay, because of the short action time of propofol and other intravenous agents, compared to GA because of the inhalation of anaesthetic gases and other drugs. Patients undergoing TIVA wake up quickly, opening their eyes and lifting their limbs, whereas under GA it can take some time for the patient to recover. TIVA is therefore associated with a much improved recovery on entering the recovery room (Wicker & O'Neill 2010).

Few patients who undergo TIVA experience postoperative nausea and vomiting (PONV) during recovery, whereas almost half the patients undergoing GA may suffer from PONV. This makes TIVA much more useful for minor cases, such as day case surgery (Nimmo & Cook 2014).

TIVA therefore provides better stability hemodynamically, rapid recovery and less chance of postoperative nausea and vomiting. Day case surgery also uses TIVA often because of the improved recovery profile of patients and earlier discharge, helping patients to be fully orientated, alert and healthy on exit from the hospital.

24 Airway Management

Evaluation and management of a patient's airway are essential for both routine and difficult cases. The actions that an anaesthetist or an anaesthetic practitioner should take, following issues with airway problems, could include:

1. Evaluate the patient's airway to support intubation or mask ventilation.
2. Identify the need for tracheal intubation due to blockage of the airway.
3. Provide adequate bag-mask ventilation, and/or intubation and insertion of a laryngeal mask airway (LMA) or endotracheal tube (ETT) into the patient.
4. Decide on actions following failed intubation, to ensure support of the patient's airway.
5. Consider awake intubation under local anaesthesia, if intubation fails.
6. A patient who cannot be intubated or ventilated will need an emergency airway to be established.
7. Assess an obstructed airway, and take actions on poor ventilation, low oxygenation and failed intubation (Quasim 2010, Yentis *et al.* 2013).

Anaesthetists and anaesthetic practitioners are airway experts and need to manage a patient's airway to provide suitable levels of oxygen for the patient. Normally, the anaesthetist understands best the difficulties that might be encountered and usually prepares equipment and drugs for a difficult or failed intubation. Practicing airway management techniques is also essential so patients can be treated effectively under emergency situations (Smith *et al.* 2007).

Assessing the airway

Difficult intubation may be caused by known or unexpected difficult airways. Patients with difficult airways can therefore have problems with intubating because of difficulties with viewing the airway using the laryngoscope. Deaths related to anaesthesia can be caused by hypoxia, often because of the inability to manage the airway (Cook & MacDougall-Davis 2012).

Airway assessment is therefore essential to predict possible complications and create techniques for ensuring alternative airway management. Preoperative assessment may not always predict airway problems; however, patients still need airway assessment to ensure their safety (Smith *et al.* 2007).

The anaesthetist will evaluate the patient's history of previous anaesthesia and evaluate the airway through examination. A previous history of difficult intubation will assist the anaesthetist to understand airway difficulties in the past and give vital information on how this was managed previously, especially if the airway is clear when evaluated (Cook & MacDougall-Davis 2012). The patient should also tell the anaesthetist about any problems such as breathing problems, difficulty sleeping, and abnormal voice quality. If the patient experiences stridor while at rest, this also highlights airway obstruction caused by narrowing of the airway, vocal chords or other areas of the airway (Yentis *et al.* 2013). Any future problems about airways can be assessed through various tests before anaesthesia. These include tests such as the ability of the patient to open their mouth more than 3.5 cm,

Rapid Perioperative Care, First Edition. Paul Wicker and Sara Dalby.

problems with jaw movement and the Mallampati score which identifies the ability to see the oropharyngeal structures (Yentis *et al.* 2013). Ventilation using a mask can also lead to problems, for example if the patient has a large beard, missing teeth, old age (>55 years) or a history of snoring while sleeping.

Physical conditions may also increase problems with difficult airway management, for example obesity, pregnancy, rheumatoid arthritis, airway infection and trauma of the head and neck (Smith *et al.* 2007).

During airway assessment, the anaesthetist will consider various issues and probably also inform the anaesthetic assistant. These include:

1. Is airway control needed? If so, is general anaesthesia appropriate?
2. Does the patient have the physiological reserve to be able to tolerate apnoea?
3. Is an awake intubation technique required and possible?
4. Has the patient eaten recently? Is there a risk of aspiration?
5. Is difficult laryngoscopy likely to happen?
6. Can the patient be ventilated using a mask, without intubating? (Cook & MacDougall-Davis 2012).

Airway management techniques

When airway management is successful, it helps to ensure satisfactory oxygenation in the body tissue. If patients suffer from poor ventilation and receive low levels of oxygen, then they are more likely to suffer or die, even if their intubation fails. Therefore, it is important that anaesthetists and their assistants are skilled in airway management.

Facemask ventilation

Facemasks, which have various sizes, are designed for use during anaesthesia; they form a seal on the patient's face, apply minimum pressure and prevent the leakage of gases. However, when patients are in the supine position and undergo anaesthesia, breathing can be blocked because of the tongue and epiglottis falling backwards and blocking the airway (Smith *et al.* 2007). The patient's head can be tilted backwards by performing a chin lift and jaw thrust, which then opens the airway and allows breathing. The anaesthetist or anaesthetic practitioner will hold the face mask using the thumb at the bridge of the nose, the fifth finger behind the mandible and the rest of the fingers pulling the mandible into the mask. This will allow breathing and seal the gases from escaping the mask (Yentis *et al.* 2013).

Oropharyngeal airways

When a patient becomes unconscious, the jaw muscles relax and the tongue falls backwards, covers the epiglottis and obstructs the airway. When intubation is not possible or develops problems, or the patient has an airway problem, an oral airway, which is also known as an oropharyngeal airway or Guedel airway, is used to help maintain the patient's airway. The oral airway does this by preventing the tongue from falling backwards and covering the epiglottis, allowing the patient to be able to breathe. However, oral airways can only be used for sedated or unconscious patients, otherwise the patient may start coughing or choking, resulting in vomiting leading to an obstructed airway or inhalation of stomach contents (Cook & MacDougall-Davis 2012).

Oral airways come in several sizes which are suitable for children and adults. The anaesthetist, anaesthetic assistant or recovery practitioner will measure the distance from the corner of the patient's mouth to the angle of the jaw to identify the correct size needed. The oral airway is inserted into the patient's mouth upside down. When the airway touches the back of the throat, the oral airway is then turned around (rotated 180°) and pushed a little further down the throat. The patient's mouth is closed to allow grip on the 'bite block', at the proximal end of the oral airway, to prevent the airway from falling further down the throat. When the patient recovers from anaesthesia or regains a swallow reflex, the oral airway can be removed by gently pulling it out of the mouth, as the patient will be able to protect his or her own airway (Yentis *et al.* 2013).

Using an oral airway still requires patients to adopt a recovery position, and further consistent assessment of the airway will remain essential as it does not prevent obstruction of the airway by gastric reflux (e.g. fluid or food). However, the oral airway will support ventilation well if the patient has a heart attack and needs cardiopulmonary resuscitation (CPR).

The main risks associated with oral airways include gag reflex leading to vomiting, closure of the glottis (vocal chords and the split between them) leading to blockage of the airway, and damage to the airway leading to bleeding.

Laryngeal mask airway

The LMA allows the patient to breathe spontaneously under anaesthesia. However, the LMA does not prevent aspiration of regurgitated contents and does not support positive pressure ventilation (Yentis *et al.* 2013).

The LMA is a tube with an elliptical bowl-shaped mask that is surrounded by a cuffed rim and is connected to a breathing circuit. The LMA comes in several sizes suitable for adults and children. There are different types of LMA, including ProSeal which reduces the risk of regurgitation by blocking the upper oesophagus, and a reinforced version with metal hoops to prevent it bending.

Inserting the LMA requires the following actions:

1. The patient will be sedated before insertion of the LMA to avoid coughing and laryngospasm.
2. The cuff is fully deflated, and the tip of the LMA is lubricated using lubricating jelly.
3. The patient's head is tilted backwards.
4. The mask is inserted into the mouth, is curved downwards towards the throat and finally resides in the upper oesophagus.
5. The cuff is inflated to stabilise the LMA.
6. The LMA is taped to the sides of the face.

The LMA has a similar effect as anaesthesia using a face mask. However, there may be difficulties with LMAs, including improper positioning, gas leaks caused by the cuff deflating or not being fully inflated, no protection against gastric aspiration and the possibility of laryngeal spasm occurring (Nolan & Kelly 2011).

Endotracheal intubation

Insertion of an endotracheal tube (ETT) is followed by connection to the anaesthetic machine and a ventilator which supports control of the airway and ventilation. ETTs are inserted when there is a risk of gastric aspiration and when the patient has major surgery requiring muscle relaxants (Nolan & Kelly 2011). Following intubation, the patient can lie in any position as the ETT supports the passage of gases in and out of the airway.

Preparation for intubation

The anaesthetist and anaesthetic practitioner work together to prepare for intubation of the patient. The anaesthetic assistant will hand over equipment (e.g. the ETT and laryngoscope) and apply cricoid pressure when needed. If there is an airway emergency, the anaesthetic assistant will work hard with the anaesthetist to solve the problems (Smith *et al.* 2007, Quasim 2010).

Equipment that is required for intubation will include:

- A source of positive pressure oxygen via the wall unit
- Anaesthesia machine
- Monitoring equipment (e.g. electrocardiograph (ECG), capnograph, pulse oximeter and blood pressure cuff)
- Suction
- Equipment for facemask ventilation
- Self-inflating bag
- Laryngoscopes – with intubation stylets or bougies
- Oropharyngeal or nasopharyngeal airways
- Magill forceps (to guide tracheal tubes into the larynx)
- Any other equipment which may be needed following difficult intubation.

Patient preparation would include information about anaesthesia, the need for intravenous access, monitoring vital signs, determining best positioning of the head and neck using a pillow and optimising the view at laryngoscopy. Monitoring of the patient's vital signs is also important during anaesthesia and would include oxygen monitoring, oxygen saturation, blood pressure, circulation, ECG and end-tidal carbon dioxide (Nolan & Kelly 2011).

Complications of intubation can include:

- Hypoxia caused by lack of oxygen or faulty insertion of ETT
- Oesophageal intubation instead of tracheal intubation
- Failed intubation – caused by narrow airways, blockages and so on
- Failed ventilation – caused by faulty equipment
- Aspiration – caused by gastric regurgitation
- Trauma to trachea leading to damage or blockages (Nolan & Kelly 2011).

During airway manipulation or the presence of airway secretions, laryngeal spasm and bronchospasm may also occur. Patients who smoke or have a respiratory tract infection or asthma are more susceptible to laryngeal spasm. Treatment of laryngeal spasm commences by placing a face mask on the patient and administering 100% oxygen. A small dose of suxamethonium (0.25 mg/kg) may also be given to try to stop the laryngeal spasm (Yentis *et al.* 2013).

Airway emergencies

During an airway emergency, it is important that a planned approach is used to clear the airway as quickly as possible to prevent severe hypoxia in the patient. A review of the techniques used include:

1. Recognise early airway problems.
2. Call for help – anaesthetist or practitioner.
3. Start immediate treatment – give the patient oxygen, use suction and so on.
4. Re-evaluate the patient's airway.
5. Diagnose underlying causes for airway blockage.
6. Initiate definitive treatment – for example, intubation or tracheostomy.

Following treatment of the patient, it is worthwhile to find out the reasons for airway difficulties to prevent future 'never events' from occurring (Nolan & Kelly 2011).

Upper airway obstruction can occur for many reasons, and it should be recognised if the patient has a reduction in expiration, extended expiration, cyanosis or stridor and the like. Anatomical causes can include infection, oedema, tumours, trauma, foreign bodies and so on. Management of the airway in these situations can be difficult, but certain actions need to be taken, including:

- Provide suitable care for the patient to avoid complete airway obstruction.
- Consider other investigations if required, for example chest x-ray, computed tomography (CT), lateral neck x-ray or arterial blood gas (ABG).
- Call for essential personnel such as theatre staff, surgeons and anaesthetists.
- Prepare equipment to be ready for emergency intubation, including laryngoscopes, ETTs, oral airways, LMAs, suction catheters, intubating stylets, intravenous equipment and local anaesthetics.
- Monitor oxygen and carbon dioxide using pulse oximeters and capnography (Quasim 2010, Nolan & Kelly 2011).

Other issues can include:

- Infection in the airway – provide local anaesthetics, incise and drain the abscess, provide antibiotics and intubate if possible.
- Foreign body aspiration – remove foreign body if possible, using a bronchoscope or laryngoscope.
- Trauma – give local or topical anaesthetic before intubation, offer sedation or perform a tracheostomy if essential.
- Oedema – provide oxygen, adrenaline, early intubation or tracheostomy if required (Yentis *et al.* 2013).

Conclusion

Successful airway management will maintain patient safety and keep the patient secure. Sometimes this may not happen, but knowledge and understanding about managing airways will help support both the anaesthetist and practitioner when problems arise with patients.

25 General Anaesthetic Pharmacology

General anaesthetics (GAs) provide drugs which produce unconsciousness and loss of sensation; anaesthesia also depresses the central nervous system (CNS), allowing surgery to be carried out with minimum nerve stimulation. The *triad of anaesthesia* describes three areas of anaesthesia – unconsciousness, analgesia and muscle relaxation.

Premedication

Anaesthetists often prescribe premedication before administration of a general anaesthetic, depending on the state of the patient. Anaesthetic premedication also improves the quality of the anaesthetic by combining drugs to give an overall anaesthetic effect on the patient. For example, clonidine, which is an alpha-2 adrenergic agonist, reduces the need for anaesthetic induction agents, volatile anaesthetic agents and postoperative analgesics. Premedication of clonidine also reduces the following problems:

- Postoperative shivering
- Postoperative nausea and vomiting (PONV)
- Emergence delirium associated with sevoflurane.

Clonidine is therefore a popular premedication drug, but it can lead to problems such as hypotension and bradycardia (Bergendahl *et al.* 2006).

Midazolam is a benzodiazepine which has a rapid onset and short duration, and it is effective in reducing preoperative anxiety (Cox *et al.* 2006). Other antipsychotic agents may be used in patients who are uncooperative or particularly anxious (Bozkurt 2007).

Melatonin is also an effective drug used in adults and children, providing hypnotic, anxiolytic, sedative and anticonvulsant actions. Melatonin provides faster recovery compared to other drugs, and it also helps reduce postoperative agitation and delirium, improving recovery of patients postoperatively (Naguib *et al.* 2007). Using melatonin as a premedication also helps to reduce the levels of propofol or thiopentone during induction (Naguib *et al.* 2007).

Other examples of premedication drugs include:

- Beta adrenergic antagonists which reduce the incidence of postoperative hypertension, cardiac dysrhythmia or myocardial infarction
- Antiemetic agents, for example droperidol or dexamethasone, to reduce the incidence of PONV
- Subcutaneous heparin to reduce the incidence of deep vein thrombosis
- Opioids such as fentanyl or sufentanil
- Metoclopramide to reduce gastric reflux.

Rapid Perioperative Care, First Edition. Paul Wicker and Sara Dalby.

Anaesthetic induction

Anaesthetic induction agents are often administered intravenously, or sometimes via inhalation, to exert their pharmacologic effects, and once they are in the circulatory system they affect the central and autonomic nervous systems.

Onset of anaesthesia via intravenous injection is rapid and can take around 10–20 sec to induce total unconsciousness, depending on the drug being used. This prevents patients from becoming anxious if they are inhaling volatile gases instead. Propofol, sodium thiopental, etomidate and (sometimes) ketamine are the most commonly used intravenous induction agents. Sevoflurane is one of the most popular inhalational gases used for induction as it is effective, is quick acting and also provides less irritation inside the airways, compared to other volatile anaesthetic agents.

Neuromuscular blocking agents

A neuromuscular blocking agent provides total paralysis or temporary muscle relaxation to enable anaesthesia and surgery to continue. Curare was the first muscle relaxant to be used in the 1940s; however, it had several side effects and also took a long time to relax the muscles. This drug has now been replaced by more recent and improved modern drugs with fewer side effects and a shorter duration of action. Examples of skeletal muscle relaxants in use today are pancuronium, rocuronium, vecuronium, atracurium, mivacurium and suxamethonium. Muscle relaxation supports surgery within, for example, the abdomen or thorax, and it reduces the need for deep anaesthesia and supports endotracheal intubation.

Acetylcholine is a neurotransmitter which causes muscles to contract when it is released from nerve endings at the neuromuscular junction. Muscle relaxant drugs prevent acetylcholine from attaching to its receptor at the neuromuscular junction, preventing muscle contraction. This can prevent breathing, and therefore ventilators will be required along with the anaesthetic machine to support the patient's breathing. The muscles of the larynx also become paralysed, hence the need for an ETT to maintain the airway. A peripheral nerve stimulator will monitor muscle paralysis by sending electrical pulses through the skin over a peripheral nerve to observe the contraction, or no contraction, of the muscle which is covered by the nerve. Using anticholinesterase drugs helps to reverse the actions of muscle relaxants following the end of the anaesthetic and surgical procedures.

Maintenance of anaesthesia

Following the short duration of intravenous induction agents, volatile anaesthetic gases are delivered to the patient via the anaesthetic machine and into the endotracheal tube or laryngeal mask airway. The patient will normally breathe a mixture of oxygen and a volatile anaesthetic agent, with or without nitrous oxide or, alternatively, by infusing a medication such as propofol through an intravenous catheter. Inhalation agents move to the brain via the lungs and bloodstream which enables the patient to remain unconscious. Inhaled gases are often used with intravenous anaesthetics, such as fentanyl or midazolam, to augment the anaesthetic and also reduce the need for inhalational gases. Following the completion of surgery, the anaesthetist will discontinue the anaesthetic agents. The patient will recover following the drop of concentration of the anaesthetic agents in the brain, usually within 30 min after the anaesthetic drugs have stopped being used.

Various other drugs may be given to the patient during anaesthesia to treat side effects or prevent complications. These include antihypertensives, ephedrine or phenylephrine to raise blood pressure, salbutamol to treat laryngospasm or bronchospasm, and epinephrine to treat allergic reactions. Antibiotics may also be given to prevent infection, for example if the bowel is opened and the patient has faeces within the abdomen.

Emergence from anaesthesia

Following surgery, anaesthetic agents will be stopped, and the patient will emerge from anaesthesia and return to normal physiologic function of the organs and body systems. During emergence from anaesthesia, the patient may suffer side effects such as agitation, mental confusion, inability to speak or lack of sensory or motor function. The patient is also likely to shiver because of exposure during surgery, which can lead to issues such as a rise in oxygen consumption, high levels of carbon dioxide, raised cardiac output and heart rate and high levels of blood pressure. Cardiovascular and respiratory events may also happen on emergence from anaesthesia, including dyspnoea, changes in blood pressure, rapid heart rate and cardiac dysrhythmias.

Postoperative care

The anaesthetist will discuss with recovery staff the various needs for the postoperative care of the patient; one of the main aims is to ensure they are pain free on awakening. Analgesics may include regional analgesia, oral drugs, transdermal injections or parenteral medication. Oral medications for minor surgery may include paracetamol and ibuprofen or other nonsteroidal anti-inflammatory drugs (NSAIDS). If the patient has a moderate level of pain, they are likely to need mild opiates, such as tramadol. Following major surgery, the patient may need a stronger dose of drugs such as patient-controlled analgesia (PCA) involving powerful opiates such as morphine or fentanyl. The patient is able to activate the syringe device by pressing a button and receiving a small dose of the drug. To allow the drug to take effect and to prevent overdose with the drug, the PCA device will then be inoperative for about 5 min.

Postanaesthetic shivering also happens frequently on awakening, sometimes because of the low temperature within the operating room. This can lead to discomfort, increased pain, and breathing and cardiovascular problems. When this occurs, recovery staff will provide warm blankets, heated intravenous fluids, Bair Huggers (which provide warm air under the blanket) and other ways of warming the patient (English 2002).

26 Intraoperative Fluid Management

Almost all patients who undergo general anaesthesia (GA) and intermediate or major surgery are provided with IV fluids. The correct and suitable delivery of fluid therapy is common practice during anaesthesia, and it is essential that the anaesthetist and anaesthetic practitioner know the type of fluids needed, the amount needed and the timing of its administration. Ensuring that patients receive appropriate levels of fluid therapy during surgery may help to increase postoperative outcomes. Patients who undergo major surgical procedures may be given large amounts of crystalloid fluids; however, high amounts of fluid can lead to fluid-based weight gain, leading to the risk of morbidity or mortality (Kuper *et al.* 2011). Preoperative dehydration has now been reduced by allowing patients to drink fluids, and eat small amounts of food, up to two h before anaesthesia and surgery. Low-risk patients who undergo major surgery may be given high amounts of crystalloids (20–30 ml kg^{-1}) via an IV infusion, which helps to reduce postoperative nausea and vomiting (PONV), dizziness and pain (Bamboat & Bordeianou 2009). This chapter reviews the distribution of water in the body, highlights the need for fluid balance and discusses the use of managing fluid therapy by the use of an oesophageal Doppler monitoring device.

The main issues to consider include maintaining fluid therapy at an appropriate level, ensuring it is distributed throughout the body, monitoring fluid therapy using haemodynamic monitors and discussing the use of crystalloid and colloid fluids during surgery.

Body water distribution

Water in the body provides around 60% of the body mass, equivalent to around 42 L in a 70 kg patient: 28 L are intracellular volume (ICV), and 14 L are extracellular volume (ECV) (Lobo *et al.* 2006). Body fluid compartments contain ions in intracellular fluid (ICF) and extracellular fluid (ECF).

Soluble substances such as water, anions, cations and glucose can pass in and out of capillaries; however, larger molecules such as protein cannot do that and remain in the blood. Sodium (cation) and chloride (anion) are in the ECF, whereas in the ICF, potassium is the major cation and PO_4^{2-} (phosphate ion) is the most common anion which has a high protein content. Osmotic equilibrium is maintained since the membrane of the cell is permeable to water but not to ions. The basal fluid requirement in a normothermic adult with a normal metabolic rate is 1.5 ml kg^{-1} h^{-1} (Bamboat & Bordeianou 2009).

Capillary fluid shifts

Fluid shifts occur at the endothelial layer of the capillaries, allowing fluids to shift between the intravascular and extracellular spaces. Most fluid contained within the blood stays within the vessels, because of the inward pull of osmotic pressure caused by the high level of protein content in the plasma. This helps to push plasma out of the vessels and into the interstitium, which is the space between cells in tissues. This results in a leak of fluid and

Rapid Perioperative Care, First Edition. Paul Wicker and Sara Dalby.

protein from the blood vessel to the interstitium, which is then returned to the blood vessels by the lymphatic system. Fluid movement across the capillary endothelium happens in both directions: moving inwards reduces interstitial oedema, and moving outwards can lead to excessive oedema interstitially (Bamboat & Bordeianou 2009).

The endothelium of blood vessels is a barrier between the blood and tissues, and also provides haemostasis, coagulation, fibrinolysis, inflammation and regulation of vasomotor tone (Ait-Oufella *et al.* 2010). However, the endothelial covering can be damaged and then leads to problems such as clumping of platelets, adhesion of leucocytes and permeability of the blood vessel leading to higher levels of interstitial oedema. Therefore, during surgery, it is important that the endothelial glycocalyx (glycocalyx is a glycoprotein–polysaccharide covering that surrounds the cell membranes) is protected and not damaged to prevent interstitial oedema (Chappell *et al.* 2010). Sevoflurane (Chappell *et al.* 2011), hydrocortisone and anti-thrombins can preserve the integrity of the endothelium by reducing shedding of the glycocalyx and reducing adhesion of leucocytes following ischaemia or injury to the endothelium (Chappell *et al.* 2010).

Distribution of crystalloid fluids

Crystalloid solutions, such as normal saline and lactated Ringer's solution, are the most common fluids used. When IV fluids are infused into the patient, the composition of the fluids determines the way the fluid spreads throughout the body. For example, when IV glucose 5% is given, it is only water which collects in the extracellular and intracellular areas because the glucose is metabolised by the liver (Bamboat & Bordeianou 2009). When isotonic sodium solution is administered, the fluid is confined to the extracellular space because sodium is stopped by the cell membrane from being transported into the intracellular space within cells.

Plasma expansion is supported more by normal saline 0.9% than by Hartmann's solution. Normal saline retains around 56% volume for as long as 6 h, whereas Hartmann's solution retains around 30% (Kuper *et al.* 2011). However, normal saline can lead to hyperchloraemia which can lead to adverse physiological changes to the body, which may affect organ functions and also affect surgery.

Distribution of colloid fluids

Examples of colloids include hydroxyethyl starch 6% (HES, aka Voluven), albumin 5% and succinylated gelatine 0.4% (gelofusine).

Colloid fluids expand plasma because they contain macromolecules, for example polysaccharides or polypeptides, which cannot pass through the endothelium and therefore help to expand plasma. Normally, 0.9% sodium chloride and Hartmann's solution (crystalloids) are used to suspend the macromolecules and prevent haemolysis. However, colloids may cause anaphylaxis, coagulation or pruritus (skin itching) because of the large molecules which may become embedded within tissues (Bamboat & Bordeianou 2009). However, there are also benefits from the effects of colloids, including reduction of inflammation, improved microcirculation and activation of the endothelial tissues.

When patients lose fluids, such as blood or plasma, crystalloids provide a much higher volume replacement than colloids, because of the ability of crystalloids to permeate the blood vessels. However, infusing colloids improves other factors, such as increasing cardiac volume and cardiac output (Kuper *et al.* 2011).

Administering intravenous fluids is essential during surgery to prevent loss of fluids leading to poor circulation. Colloids are of course an alternative to crystalloids, depending on the need for colloids and their actions. Therefore, the choice between crystalloids and colloids has been a very controversial subject in perioperative care over the past 50 years. It is therefore essential that consideration is given regarding the use of either a crystalloid solution or a colloid solution, to confirm the safety and efficacy of these intravenous fluids.

Administration of intraoperative fluids

The main aim of intraoperative fluid therapy is to provide an acceptable amount of fluid in the circulation to provide satisfactory organ perfusion and to improve oxygen delivery around the tissues of the body. In the past, patients were hypovolaemic because of long fasting times before anaesthesia and surgery, expulsion of bowel contents, perspiration and urinary output. Normally, in the old days, large volumes of crystalloid solutions would be given to the patient to restore their fluid volume. Nowadays, however, loading IV fluids does not help hypotension caused by anaesthetic drugs; therefore, vasopressors are more likely to be used.

Prolonged preoperative fasting no longer happens since research has shown that solid-food fasting for 6 h and drinking fluids up to 2 h before anaesthesia is safe and improves patient outcomes (Lobo *et al.* 2006). Bowel preparations have also reduced substantially as it has been found that there is little effect on the patient or body during surgical procedures (Contant *et al.* 2007).

During major abdominal surgery, the patient needs IV fluids infused using balanced crystalloid fluids. Evaporation of fluids from the skin, airway and abdomen during surgery showed a loss of 0.5–1.0 ml kg^{-1} h^{-1} (Lamke *et al.* 1977). Also, when major haemorrhage does not occur, excessive doses of IV infusions should not be given, as it may cause hypervolemia causing ANP (atrial natriuretic peptide) release, leading to damage of the endothelial glycocalyx and interstitial oedema. ANP is released by muscle cells in the atria of the heart in response to high blood volume, reducing the water, sodium and adipose levels and leading to reduced blood pressure (Bamboat & Bordeianou 2009).

An important factor when giving IV fluids preoperatively is that patients should not be given high levels of fluid or, alternatively, low levels of fluids. The reason behind this is that high-risk patients can suffer physiological problems as a result of excess or reduction in fluid levels (Bundgaard-Neilson 2009).

Oesophageal doppler monitoring

The oesophageal Doppler monitor (ODM) can be used in the perioperative setting to measure cardiovascular performance (Kuper *et al.* 2011) by analysing the blood flow in the descending aorta. To measure blood flow, the oesophagus has a probe inserted which can then detect the stroke volume during each heartbeat. The stroke volume is the amount of blood leaving the left ventricle of the heart and is used to indicate the volume of blood leaving the heart. The ODM is therefore recommended for use in major colorectal surgery patients to ensure the blood flow is at the recommended level.

Conclusion

Low-risk adult patients undergoing minor or intermediate surgery may be given around 2 L of crystalloid infusions over a period of 30 min, as this will stabilise anaesthesia and reduce problems such as pain, nausea and dizziness. Adult patients undergoing major surgery need to be monitored to ensure their fluids are restricted to an appropriate level, to ensure urine output remains at a normal level and fluid levels do not rise above normal. Under normal circumstances, colloid and/or crystalloid fluids may be used, depending on the health of the patient and the surgery being performed.

27 Monitoring Perioperative Patients

The anaesthetic practitioner must understand and be familiar with monitors and how they work. This may involve the anaesthetic practitioner undertaking training, being aware of their own competence and technical ability and understanding the results shown on the monitors and any risks the patient may undergo. This may also include infection control if a probe has to be inserted into the patient (Milton 2009). The anaesthetic practitioner will also work alongside the anaesthetist, who should be able to give them good advice on the issues involved with monitoring patients.

Monitoring patients by using monitoring devices and equipment helps to reduce risks, by detecting physiological problems and informing the perioperative team of the status of the patient (AAGBI 2007). Monitoring the patient's physiological status is therefore a very important task during anaesthesia and surgery to maintain the patient's health. Clinical observation of the patient is also essential, for example if the equipment provides wrong results or the patient is not being monitored because the equipment is not available. The lack of monitors attached to patients may result in major problems during anaesthesia and surgery (ANZCA 2013). The anaesthetic team has the responsibility of recording the results of monitoring on the patient's notes and in the care plan to provide a record of the patient's physiological status, which may be useful postoperatively as the patient is recovering. The anaesthetic practitioners often attach the monitors and leads to the patient following entry to the anaesthetic room, to identify the physiological parameters, for example pulse, blood pressure and oxygen saturation. Monitors are used throughout anaesthesia to provide continuous assessment of the patient's physiological status and the depth of anaesthesia (O'Neill 2010).

Setting up monitors before anaesthesia

The anaesthetist and anaesthetic practitioner will check that all equipment is available and working correctly before use to ensure it is in working order and the various parts attached to it (e.g. wires or probes) are working. Sometimes, the anaesthetic practitioner will check the equipment and then inform the anaesthetist that it is working correctly. However, the anaesthetist, being responsible for the patient's health, may also double check the equipment to ensure it is working and effective (AAGBI 2007). The anaesthetic team must understand the purpose of the monitors and how the equipment works, and also ensure they check the equipment following the manufacturer's guidelines. If equipment is complex and detailed, then training may be required.

Examples of equipment used to monitor patients include:

Oxygen analyser: This positioning of this device on the anaesthetic machine is essential to ensure that the mixture of oxygen and volatile gases is appropriate and is continuously monitored. An audible alarm is normally part of this device, so that when problems arise the anaesthetic team are instantly aware (Milton 2009).

Rapid Perioperative Care, First Edition. Paul Wicker and Sara Dalby.

Capnograph: Monitoring of carbon dioxide using capnography is essential to monitor the patient's breathing. During ventilation, it is possible for the reservoir bag to leak, disconnect, receive high pressure or have other problems. The capnograph will be able to detect any changes in ventilation or breathing, especially when CO_2 levels increase rapidly (Reich 2011).

Vapour analyser: Vapour analysers are used especially when volatile anaesthetic agents are used, and also during the use of oxygen and carbon dioxide. The most common form of oxygen analysers are called paramagnetic oxygen analysers. Oxygen and nitric oxide are strong paramagnetic gases and are attracted into a magnetic field within the vapour analyser. Other types of vapour analysers are also used, including the mercury vapour analyser which is able to analyse the presence of toxic gases and also vapour detection (Langton & Hutton 2009).

Infusion devices: Infusion devices are checked before anaesthesia to ensure the alarm settings and infusion limits are working and set to appropriate levels. This is especially important when anaesthetic drugs such as analgesics and muscle relaxants are infused. The infusion site should be easily visible for the anaesthetic team and secure to prevent it being disconnected.

Alarms: Anaesthetists and anaesthetic practitioners normally set alarms on monitors at suitable upper or lower levels, which can then inform the anaesthetic team of errors or problems for the patient. It is important the alarms are loud enough to be heard by the anaesthetic team when anaesthesia commences. An example of a monitor with an alarm is the airway pressure monitor, which is used during intermittent positive pressure ventilation while the patient is anaesthetised (Reich 2011). When the alarm sounds, it can indicate high pressure in the airway, disconnection of the airway tubes or leaks in the tubing (Reich 2011). There are normally hospital rules and regulations which indicate the maintenance and setting up of the alarms during anaesthesia.

Monitors during and after anaesthesia

Monitoring devices as well as clinical observation ensure the patient has continuous assessment of their physiological health and the depth of anaesthesia. Examples of clinical observations of the patient during anaesthesia include signs of hypoxia, responses to surgical stimuli and unusual movements of the chest wall (AAGBI 2007). The anaesthetist or practitioner may also check the blood pressure, pulse rate and rhythm, level of breathing, urine output and any blood loss due to surgery.

There are many monitoring devices available during the stages of anaesthesia, and these can include induction and maintenance, recovery and additional monitoring depending on the surgery and the health of the patient. If a monitor is unavailable, the anaesthetist is required to record this information in the patient's notes, as there is a lack of monitors and there may be problems resulting from the induction of anaesthesia.

There are several monitors used during induction of the patient and also following the maintenance of anaesthesia during the surgical procedure. The most important monitors include (AAGBI 2007, Milton 2009, O'Neill 2010):

1. *Pulse oximeter*: This is attached to a finger, toe or earlobe and measures the oxygen levels in the bloodstream.
2. *Non-invasive blood pressure monitor*: Normally attached to the arm, this measures the patient's blood pressure and also identifies any issues related to hypotension or hypertension.
3. *Electrocardiograph*: This involves attaching two ECG electrodes to the upper part of the chest and the third electrode to the lower part of the left-hand side of the chest. The ECG monitors the patient's pulse and rhythm. The ECG monitor may also be connected to the airway gases (oxygen, carbon dioxide and anaesthetic gases) and may record the airway pressure via the oxygen analyser.

4. *Nerve stimulator*: This device is used to assess neuromuscular transmission when neuromuscular blocking agents block musculoskeletal activity. The nerve stimulator assesses the depth of the neuromuscular blockade, which ensures suitable levels of medication to decrease the incidence of side effects.
5. *Temperature monitor*: Temperature is usually monitored every 30 min throughout surgery to ensure the patient's temperature is held within normal limits, especially during long procedures and when warming devices are being used. Heat production in the body is often reduced during anaesthesia because anaesthetic drugs tend to reduce metabolic rate, relax muscles and increase heat loss from the body.

During recovery from anaesthesia, it is essential that monitoring of the patient is carried out regularly and consistently, until the patient is fully awake. The monitors used in recovery are very similar to those used in the operating theatre, including the pulse oximeter, blood pressure monitor, electrocardiograph, nerve stimulator, temperature probes and capnograph (ANZCA 2013). Other devices may also be used depending on the state of the patient and the surgery undertaken.

Normally the recovery area is immediately adjacent to the operating theatre, and so monitors will be removed in the operating room and reattached in the recovery room. However, if the patient is not well or has issues regarding pulse, blood pressure, temperature and so on, then monitoring of the patient will be needed during transfer. Examples of appropriate monitoring include oxygen saturation, arterial pressure and pulse and heart rhythm. Sometimes following surgery, intravascular or intracranial pressure monitoring may also be needed. Oxygen supply, expiration of CO_2, airway pressure, tidal volume and respiratory rate will also be monitored during transfer and in the recovery room, when the patient is on a ventilator (AAGBI 2007).

Elderly patients are also much more likely to need different monitors because of their age and their low physiological status. For example, elderly patients are likely to suffer from acute falls, dementia and cardiac conditions. It is therefore likely that in the future, even more monitors are likely to be used as the population ages (Kang *et al.* 2010).

The anaesthetist and anaesthetic assistant normally transfer the patient to the recovery room in order for close monitoring to continue in the recovery stage of the patient's perioperative care, so that monitoring is continued and the postoperative care of the patient is discussed with the recovery staff.

References and Further Reading

14. Preoperative Evaluation of the Anaesthetic Patient

References

Goodman T, Spry C (2014) *Perioperative Nursing*. Burlington MA, Jones and Bartlett Learning.
Mitchell M (2013) Anaesthesia type, gender and anxiety. *Journal of Perioperative Practice* **23** (3): 41–46.
Wicker P (2010) Preoperative Preparation of Perioperative Patients. In Wicker P, O'Neill J (eds) *Caring for the Perioperative Patient*. Chichester, Wiley-Blackwell.
Woodhead K, Fudge L (2012) *Manual of Perioperative Care: An Essential Guide*. Chichester, Wiley-Blackwell.

Further Reading

Green D, Ervine M, White S (2003) *Fundamentals of Perioperative Management*. London, Greenwich Medical Media.
Pudner R (2005) *Nursing the Surgical Patient*. Edinburgh, Elsevier Ltd.

Websites

Pre-operative Assessment and Patient Preparation: http://www.aagbi.org/sites/default/files/preop2010.pdf (accessed 27 December 2014)
Preoperative Evaluation and Preparation for Anaesthesia and Surgery: http://www.ncbi.nlm.nih.gov/pmc/articles/PMC2464262/ (accessed 27 December 2014)

Videos

Anaesthetic Pre-assessment of ASA 1: https://www.youtube.com/watch?v=VoLAiJeQmng (accessed 27 December 2014)
Anaesthetic Preoperative Assessment and the Preoperative Visit: https://www.youtube.com/watch?v=LzOFBh-tzXg (accessed 28 December 2014)
ODP Anaesthetic Machine Check: https://www.youtube.com/watch?v=bu5nXPe6w_U (accessed 28 December 2014)

15. Preparing Anaesthetic Equipment

References

Association of Anaesthetists of Great Britain and Northern Ireland (2012) *Checking Anaesthetic Equipment*. London, AAGBI.
Green D, Ervine M, White S (2003) *Fundamentals of Perioperative Management*. London, Greenwich Medical Media.
Higginson R, Parry A (2015) Laryngoscopes in Anaesthetic Practice: What's Available to ODPs? *Journal of Operating Department Practitioners* **3** (2): 72–76.
Hughes SJ, Mardell A (2012) *Oxford Handbook of Perioperative Practice*. Oxford, Oxford University Press.
Shaikh BA, Stacey S (2013) *Essentials of Anaesthetic Equipment*, 4th ed. London, Elsevier.

Further Reading

Cassidy CJ, Smith A, Arnot-Smith J. (2011) Critical Incident Reports Concerning Anaesthetic Equipment: Analysis of the UK National Reporting and Learning System (NRLS) Data from 2006–2008. *Anaesthesia* **66**: 879–888.

Rapid Perioperative Care, First Edition. Paul Wicker and Sara Dalby.

Magee P (2012) Checking Anaesthetic Equipment: AAGBI 2012 Guidelines. *Journal of the Association of Anaesthetists of Great Britain and Northern Ireland* **67** (6): 571–574.
Wicker P, Smith B (2006) Checking the Anaesthetic Machine. *Journal of Perioperative Practice* **16** (12): 585–590.

Websites

Core Competencies for Anaesthetic Assistants: http://www.nes.scot.nhs.uk/media/4239/anaesthetic_core_competencies_2011.pdf (accessed 24 December 2014)
The Royal College of Anaesthetists: http://www.rcoa.ac.uk/ (accessed 24 December 2014)

Videos

Anaesthetic Machine Check Part 1 – UK 2012: https://www.youtube.com/watch?v=07xAC81ACqk (accessed 24 December 2014)
Anaesthetic Machine Check Part 2 – UK 2012: https://www.youtube.com/watch?v=qAid8c6-KNc (accessed 24 December 2014)
Anaesthesia Equipment and Products: https://www.youtube.com/watch?v=55sYMLx6n1M (accessed 24 December 2014)
Anaesthetic Equipment: https://www.youtube.com/watch?v=9TBHy_dyCFI&list=PL095EE9A0A00D487A (accessed 24 December 2014)

16. Checking the Anaesthetic Machine

References

Al-Shaikh B, Stacey S (2002) *Essentials of Anaesthetic Equipment*, 2nd ed. London, Churchill Livingstone.
Association of Anaesthetists of Great Britain and Northern Ireland (2012) *Checklist for Anaesthetic Equipment*. Available at http://www.aagbi.org/sites/default/files/checklist_for_anaesthetic_equipment_2012.pdf (accessed 16 February 2015)
Cheng CJC, Bailey AR (2002) Flow Reversal through the Anaesthetic Machine Back Bar: An Unusual Assembly Fault. *Anaesthesia* **57** (1): 82–101.
Chilton R, Thompson R (2012) Anaesthetic Care. In Woodhead K, Fudge L (eds) *Manual of Perioperative Care: An Essential Guide*. Chichester, John Wiley & Sons.
Hughes SJ, Mardell A (2012) *Oxford Handbook of Perioperative Practice.* Oxford, Oxford University Press.
Kumar B (1998) *Working in the Operating Department.* New York, Churchill Livingstone.
Wicker P, Smith B (2008) Checking the Anaesthetic Machine. *Journal of Perioperative Practice* **18** (8): 354–359.

Further Reading

Gurudatt CL (2013) The Basic Anaesthetic Machine. *Indian Journal of Anaesthesia* **57** (5): 438–445.
Hartle A, Anderson E, Bythell V, Gemmell L, Jones H, McIvor D, *et al.* (AAGBI) (2012) Checking Anaesthetic Equipment 2012: Association of Anaesthetists of Great Britain and Ireland. *Journal of Anaesthesia* **67** (6): 660–668.
Umesh G, Manjunath P (2013) Anaesthesia Machine: Checklist, Hazards, Scavenging. *Indian Journal of Anaesthesia* **57** (5): 533–540.

Websites

Anaesthetic Machine: http://en.wikipedia.org/wiki/Anaesthetic_machine (accessed 17 February 2015)
The Anaesthetic Machine: http://info.mhra.gov.uk/learning/AnaestheticMachines/player.html (accessed 17 February 2015)
Guide for Novice Trainees: http://www.e-lfh.org.uk/e-learning-sessions/rcoa-novice/content/started/theatre.html (accessed 17 February 2015)

Videos

Anaesthetic Machine Check Part 1 – UK 2012: https://www.youtube.com/watch?v=07xAC81ACqk (accessed 17 February 2015)
Anaesthetic Machine Check Part 2 – UK 2012: https://www.youtube.com/watch?v=qAid8c6-KNc (accessed 17 February 2015)

The Anaesthetic Machine Check: https://www.youtube.com/watch?v=DojLuUsoEBg (accessed 17 February 2015)
Anaesthesia Operating Room Setup: https://www.youtube.com/watch?v=oXn0wqGB6So (accessed 17 February 2015)

17. Anatomy and Physiology: The Cardiovascular System

References

Clancy J, McVicar A (2009) *Physiology and Anatomy*, 3rd ed. London, Hodder Arnold
Marieb EN (2006) *Essentials of Human Anatomy and Physiology*, 8th ed. San Francisco, Pearson Education.
Tortorra GJ, Derrickson B (2011) *Principles of Anatomy & Physiology*, 13th ed. Hoboken, John Wiley & Sons.
Wicker P (2010) *Perioperative Homeostasis*. In Wicker P, O'Neill J (eds) *Caring for the Perioperative Patient*. Chichester, Wiley-Blackwell.

Further Reading

Aresti NA, Malik AA, Ihsan KM, Aftab SME, Khan WS (2014) Perioperative Management of Cardiac Disease. *Journal of Perioperative Practice* **24** (1–2): 9–14.
Parry A (2011) Management and Treatment of Local Anaesthetic Toxicity. *Journal of Perioperative Practice* **21** (12): 404–409.

Websites

Cardiovascular System: http://www.innerbody.com/anatomy/cardiovascular/upper-torso (accessed 23 January 2015)
Inner Body – Cardiovascular System: http://www.innerbody.com/image/cardov.html (accessed 23 January 2015)
Live Science – Circulatory System: http://www.livescience.com/22486-circulatory-system.html (accessed 23 January 2015)

Videos

Cardiovascular System Anatomy: https://www.youtube.com/watch?v=Sc3IN99sRrI (accessed 23 January 2015)
Cardiovascular System – Heart Fundamentals:
https://www.youtube.com/watch?v=Y335KJ-EuDw (accessed 23 January 2015)
The Circulatory System: https://www.youtube.com/watch?v=NJzJKvkWWDc (accessed 23 January 2015)
Introduction to the Cardiovascular System: https://www.youtube.com/watch?v=DAXa4eR1s0M (accessed 23 January 2015)

18. Anatomy and Physiology: The Lungs

References

Clancy J, McVicar A (2009) *Physiology and Anatomy*, 3rd ed. London, Hodder Arnold.
Marieb EN (2006) *Essentials of Human Anatomy and Physiology*, 8th ed. San Francisco, Pearson Education.
Pudner R (2010) *Nursing the Surgical Patient*, 3rd ed. Edinburgh, Elsevier Ltd.
Wicker P (2010) Perioperative Homeostasis. In Wicker P, O'Neill J (eds) *Caring for the Perioperative Patient*. Chichester, Wiley-Blackwell.

Further Reading

Francis C (2009) *Respiratory Care*. Oxford, Blackwell.
Kendrick AH, Newall C. (2011). Anatomy and Physiology of the Respiratory System. Available at http://www.artp.org.uk/download.cfm/docid/89E2B9CB-A73A-4072-81B92B2CC9217EBE (accessed 14 January 2015)
Tortora GJ (2008) *Principles of Anatomy and Physiology*, 12th ed. Chichester, John Wiley & Sons.

Websites

Anatomy and Function of the Normal Lung: http://www.thoracic.org/clinical/copd-guidelines/for-patients/anatomy-and-function-of-the-normal-lung.php (accessed 14 January 2015)

Lung Anatomy: http://www.innerbody.com/anatomy/respiratory/lungs (accessed 14 January 2015)

Lung Cancer: http://www.cancer.ca/en/cancer-information/cancer-type/lung/anatomy-and-physiology/?region=on (accessed 14 January 2015)

Videos

Anatomy and Physiology of the Lungs: https://www.youtube.com/watch?v=mMQsZimjayI (accessed 14 January 2015)

Lung Anatomy: https://www.youtube.com/watch?v=Aw9OJLTlClQ (accessed 14 January 2015)

The Lungs and Pulmonary System: https://www.youtube.com/watch?v=SPGRkexl_cs&list=PLZ_Kc5EesQi05Oi7PoSF9qgZgD3ETwWPX (accessed 14 January 2015)

Meet the Lungs: https://www.youtube.com/watch?v=qGiPZf7njqY (accessed 14 January 2015)

Respiratory System: https://www.youtube.com/watch?v=B1w3s9m3hlg (accessed 14 January 2015)

19. General Anaesthesia

References

Association of Anaesthetists of Great Britain and Ireland (AAGBI) (2007) Recommendations for Standards of Monitoring during Anaesthesia and Recovery: Guideline, 4th ed. London: AAGBI.

Conway N, Ong P, Bowers M, Grimmett N (2014) *Operating Department Practice*, 2nd ed. Oxford, Innovation House.

Gan TJ (2006) Risk Factors for Postoperative Nausea and Vomiting. *Anesthesia and Analgesia Journal* **102** (6): 1884–1898.

Mitchell M (2013) Anaesthesia Type, Gender and Anxiety. *Journal of Perioperative Practice* **23** (3): 41–46.

O'Neill J (2010) Patient Care during Anaesthesia. In Wicker P, O'Neill J (eds) *Caring for the Perioperative Patient*. Chichester, Wiley-Blackwell

Young D, Griffiths J (2006) Clinical Trials of Monitoring in Anaesthesia, Critical Care and Acute Ward Care: A Review. *British Journal of Anaesthesia* **97**(1): 39–45.

Further Reading

O'Donnell (2012) *Anaesthesia: A Very Short Introduction*. Oxford, Oxford University Press.

Smith T, Pinnock C, Lin T (2009) *Fundamentals of Anaesthesia*, 3rd ed. Cambridge, Cambridge University Press.

Stone J, Fawcett W (2014) *Anaesthesia at a Glance*. Chichester, Wiley-Blackwell.

Websites

Awareness during General Anaesthesia: http://www.rcoa.ac.uk/document-store/awareness-during-general-anaesthesia (accessed 18 January 2015)

General Anaesthesia: http://en.wikipedia.org/wiki/General_anaesthesia (accessed 18 January 2015)

General Anaesthesia: http://emedicine.medscape.com/article/1271543-overview (accessed 18 January 2015)

Largest Ever Study of Awareness during General Anaesthesia: http://www.aagbi.org/news/largest-ever-study-awareness-during-general-anaesthesia-identifies-risk-factors-and-consequence (accessed 18 January 2015)

Videos

General Anaesthetic: https://www.youtube.com/watch?v=_hof4z9MYTI (accessed 18 January 2015)

Putting a Patient into Sleep: General Anaesthesia: https://www.youtube.com/watch?v=kGRCjhtuWSE (accessed 18 January 2015)

Learn to Intubate during General Anaesthesia: https://www.youtube.com/watch?v=CrLJwwSnUws (accessed 18 January 2015)

General Anaesthesia Induction Routine: https://www.youtube.com/watch?v=HHoBLuvu3Mo (accessed 18 January 2015)

General Anaesthesia Procedure Video: https://www.youtube.com/watch?v=PWR1vTovcPU (accessed 18 January 2015)

20. Local Anaesthesia

References

Becker DE, Reed KL (2006) Essentials of Local Anesthetic Pharmacology. *Anesthesia Progress Journal* **53** (3): 98–109. Available at http://www.ncbi.nlm.nih.gov/pmc/articles/PMC1693664/ (accessed 21 January 2015)

Reis A (2009) Sigmund Freud (1856–1939) and Karl Köller (1857–1944) and the Discovery of Local Anesthesia. Available at http://www.scielo.br/scielo.php?pid=s0034-70942009000200013&script=sci_arttext&tlng=en (accessed 20 January 2015)

Torpy JM, Lynm C (2011) Local Anesthesia. *Journal of the American Medical Association* **306** (12): 1395.

Wicker P, Bocos A (2010) Perioperative Pharmacology. In Wicker P, O'Neill J (eds) *Caring for the Perioperative Patient*. Chichester, Wiley-Blackwell.

Further Reading

Clancy J, McVicar A (2009) *Physiology and Anatomy*, 3rd ed. London, Hodder Arnold.

Manley K, Bellamn L (2000) *Surgical Nursing: Advancing Practice*. Edinburgh, Churchill Livingstone.

Ueno T, Tsuchiya H, Mizogami M, Takakura K (2008) Local Anesthetic Failure Associated with Inflammation: Verification of the Acidosis Mechanism and the Hypothetic Participation of Inflammatory Peroxynitrite. *Journal of Inflammation Research* **2008** (1): 41–48.

Websites

Local Anaesthetics: http://www.frca.co.uk/SectionContents.aspx?sectionid=235 (accessed 21 January 2015)

Local and Regional Anaesthesia: http://emedicine.medscape.com/article/1831870-overview (accessed 21 January 2015)

Practical Local Anaesthesia: http://www.patient.co.uk/doctor/Practical-Local-Anaesthesia.htm (accessed 21 January 2015)

Videos

Injection of Local Anaesthetic: https://www.youtube.com/watch?v=Uxav0kAWU14 (accessed 21 January 2015)

Local Anaesthesia Pharmacology: https://www.youtube.com/watch?v=kM4hTdSvTEo (accessed 21 January 2015)

Local Anaesthetics – Esters and Amides: https://www.youtube.com/watch?v=celQcBocaWY (accessed 21 January 2015)

Local Anaesthetics – Pharmacology and Toxicity: https://www.youtube.com/watch?v=BrlWUPG0fnc (accessed 21 January 2015)

Pharmacology – Local Anaesthetic: https://www.youtube.com/watch?v=K_qjguv2Wtg (accessed 21 January 2015)

21. Regional Anaesthesia

References

Burkard J, Lee Olson R, Vacchiano CA (2005) Regional Anesthesia. In Nagelhout JJ, Zaglaniczny KL (eds) *Nurse Anesthesia*, 3rd ed. Philadelphia, Saunders, pp. 977–1030.

Hadzic A (2007) *Textbook of Regional Anaesthesia and Acute Pain Management*. New York, McGraw Hill.

McConachie I (2014) *Anesthesia and Perioperative Care of the High Risk Patient*. Cambridge, Cambridge University Press.

Wedel DJ, Horlocker TT (2005) Nerve Blocks. In Miller RD (ed) *Miller's Anesthesia*, 6th ed. Philadelphia, Elsevier, pp. 1685–1715.

Further Reading

Euliano TY, Gravenstein JS (2004) *Essential Anaesthesia: From Science to Practice*. Cambridge, Cambridge University Press.

Hadzic A (2006) *Regional Anaesthesia and Acute Pain Management*. Maidenhead, McGraw-Hill Education.

Scott NB, Kehlet H (1988) Regional Anaesthesia and Surgical Morbidity. *British Journal of Surgery* **75** (4): 299–304. Available at http://europepmc.org/abstract/MED/3282596 (accessed 25 January 2015)

Websites

Bier Block: http://www.ifna-int.org/ifna/e107_files/downloads/lectures/H16BierBlock.pdf (accessed 25 January 2015)

Epidural Techniques:
http://www.ifna-int.org/ifna/e107_files/downloads/lectures/H12Epidural.pdf (accessed 25 January 2015)

Regional Anaesthesia and Patients with Abnormalities of Coagulation: http://www.aagbi.org/sites/default/files/rapac_2013_web.pdf (accessed 25 January 2015)

Videos

Caudal Anaesthesia: http://www.youtube.com/watch?v=I0hwZGcmuic (accessed 25 January 2015)

Epidural Anaesthesia: http://www.youtube.com/watch?v=rM1aQC-HAX0 (accessed 25 January 2015)

Spinal Anaesthesia Technique before Surgery: http://www.youtube.com/watch?v=LpLIK2XmbVc (accessed 25 January 2015)

What Is an Epidural? http://www.youtube.com/watch?v=uNDcf3Vw1vo (accessed 25 January 2015)

22. Rapid Sequence Induction

References

McConachie I (2014) *Anesthesia and Perioperative Care of the High Risk Patient*, 3rd ed. Cambridge, Cambridge University Press.

Nolan J, Soar J (2012) *Anaesthesia for Emergency Care*. Oxford, Oxford University Press.

Simpson W (2013) *Primary FRCA: OSCEs in Anaesthesia*. Cambridge, Cambridge University Press.

Yentis S, Hirsch N, Smith G (2009) *Anaesthesia and Intensive Care A–Z*, 4th ed. Edinburgh, Elsevier Ltd.

Further Reading

Aitkenhead AR, Moppett IK, Thompson JP (2013) *Textbook of Anaesthesia*. New York, Churchill Livingstone/Elsevier.

Braude D (2009) *Rapid Sequence Intubation and Rapid Sequence Airway: An Airway 911 Guide*. Albuquerque, New Mexico Health Sciences Center.

El-Orbany M, Connolly LA (2010) Rapid Sequence Induction and Intubation: Current Controversy. *Journal of Anesthesia and Analgesia* **110** (5): 1318–1325.

Stewart JC, Bhananker S, Ramaiah R (2014) Rapid-Sequence Intubation and Cricoid Pressure. *International Journal of Critical Illness and Injury Science* **4**: 42–49. Available at http://www.ijciis.org/text.asp?2014/4/1/42/128012 (accessed 5 June 2016)

Websites

Rapid Sequence Intubation: http://lifeinthefastlane.com/ccc/rapid-sequence-intubation/ (accessed 28 January 2015)

Rapid Sequence Intubation in Adults:
http://www.uptodate.com/contents/rapid-sequence-intubation-in-adults (accessed 28 January 2015)

Rapid Sequence Induction: Its Place in Modern Anaesthesia: http://ceaccp.oxfordjournals.org/content/early/2013/09/18/bjaceaccp.mkt047.full (accessed 28 January 2015)

Videos

Endotracheal Intubation: RSI with Rocuronium/Ketamine: https://www.youtube.com/watch?v=kTd7km_jnKw (accessed 28 January 2015)

Rapid Sequence Induction: https://www.youtube.com/watch?v=DvFFL2Jctu4 (accessed 28 January 2015)

Rapid Sequence Induction with Cricoid Pressure and without Ventilation: https://www.youtube.com/watch?v=NAQ42rVybpI (accessed 28 January 2015)
Rapid Sequence Intubation – Part 1 (up to Part 7): https://www.youtube.com/watch?v=5c8S2VaG4ZA (accessed 28 January 2015)

23. Total Intravenous Anaesthesia

References

Aitkenhead AR, Moppett IK, Thompson JP (2014) *Smith & Aitkenhead's Textbook of Anaesthesia*, 6th ed. Edinburgh, Elsevier Ltd.
Nimmo AF, Cook T (2014) *Total Intravenous Anaesthesia: Report and Findings of the 5th National Audit Project*. London, National Association of Academic Anaesthesia. Available at http://nap5.org.uk/download.php/?fn=NAP5%20Chapter%2018.pdf&mime=application/pdf&pureFn=NAP5%20Chapter%2018.pdf (accessed 1 February 2015)
Reves JG, Glass PSA, Lubarsky DA, MvEvoy MD, Martinez-Ruiz R (2007) Intravenous Anesthetics. In Miller RD (ed) *Miller's Anesthesia*. Philadelphia, Churchill Livingston, pp. 719–768.
Smith B, Rawling P, Wicker P, Jones C (2007) *Core Topics in Operating Department Practice: Anaesthesia and Critical Care*. Cambridge, Cambridge University Press.
Wicker P, O'Neill J (2010) *Caring for the Perioperative Patient*. Chichester, Wiley-Blackwell.
Yentis S, Hirsch N, Smith G (2009) *Anaesthesia and Intensive Care A–Z*, 4th ed. Edinburgh, Elsevier Ltd.

Further Reading

Hornuss C, Praun S, Villinger J, Dornauer A, Moehnle P, Dolch M, *et al.* (2007) Real-Time Monitoring of Propofol in Expired Air in Humans Undergoing Total Intravenous Anesthesia. *Journal of Anesthesiology* **106** (4): 665–674.
Sukhminder JSB, Sukhwinder KB, Jasbir K (2010) Comparison of Two Drug Combinations in Total Intravenous Anesthesia: Propofol–Ketamine and Propofol–Fentanyl. *Saudi Journal of Anaesthesia* **4** (2): 72–79.
Yuill G, Simpson M (2002) An Introduction to Total Intravenous Anaesthesia. *British Journal of Anaesthesia* **2** (1): 24–26.

Websites

A Comparison of Total Intravenous Anaesthesia (TIVA) to Conventional General Anaesthesia for Day Care Surgery: https://ispub.com/IJA/22/1/6033 (accessed 30 January 2015)
Guaranteeing Drug Delivery in Total Intravenous Anaesthesia: http://www.aagbi.org/sites/default/files/tiva_info.pdf (accessed 30 January 2015)
Total Intravenous Anaesthesia (TIVA): http://www.ebme.co.uk/articles/clinical-engineering/95-total-intravenous-anaesthesia-tiva (accessed 30 January 2015)

Videos

Dr. Rutledge Talks about Total Intravenous Anaesthesia: https://www.youtube.com/watch?v=ryPRQqtAflU (accessed 30 January 2015)
Tivatek TIVA Anaesthesia Benefits: https://www.youtube.com/watch?v=BqgDqeDKJbc (accessed 30 January 2015)
TIVA Total Intravenous Anesthesia Mini-Gastric Bypass: https://www.youtube.com/watch?v=eNgRrrkdMbs (accessed 30 January 2015)
Total Intravenous Anaesthesia Made Even Safer: https://www.youtube.com/watch?v=2leAS5lCSYw (accessed 30 January 2015)

24. Airway Management

References

Cook TM, MacDougall-Davis SR (2012) Complications and Failure of Airway Management. *British Journal of Anaesthesia* **109** (S1): i68–i85.
Nolan JP, Kelly FE (2011) Airway Challenges in Critical Care. *British Journal of Anaesthesia* **66**: 81–92.

Quasim I (2010) Advanced Airway Management. In Smith FG, Yeung J (eds) *Core Topics in Critical Care Medicine*. Cambridge, Cambridge University Press.
Smith B, Rawling P, Wicker P, Jones C (2007) *Core Topics in Operating Department Practice: Anaesthesia and Critical Care*. Cambridge, Cambridge University Press.
Yentis SM, Hirsch NP, Smith GB (2013) *Anaesthesia and Intensive Care A to Z: An Encyclopaedia of Principles and Practice*, 5th ed. Edinburgh, Elsevier Ltd.

Further Reading

Cook T, Woodall N, Frerk C (2011) Major Complication of Airway Management in the United Kingdom. *The Royal College of Anaesthetists and the Difficult Airway Society*. Available at http://www.rcoa.ac.uk/system/files/CSQ-NAP4-Full.pdf (accessed 4 February 2015)
Horton CL, Brown CA, Raja AS (2014) Trauma Airway Management. *The Journal of Emergency Medicine* **46** (6): 814–820.
Ross AK, Ball DR (2009) Equipment for Airway Management. *Journal of Anaesthesia and Intensive Care Medicine* **10** (10): 471–475.

Websites

Airway Management: https://ambulance.qld.gov.au/docs/02_cpp_airway.pdf (accessed 4 February 2015)
The Laryngeal Mask: http://www.frca.co.uk/article.aspx?articleid=238 (accessed 4 February 2015)
Sedation Airway Management: http://www.sgna.org/issues/sedationfactsorg/patientcare_safety/airwaymanagement.aspx (accessed 4 February 2015)

Videos

Advanced Airway Management Techniques: https://www.youtube.com/watch?v=eOfeLj8_43A (accessed 4 February 2015)
Airway Management – i-gel Training: https://www.youtube.com/watch?v=ao-Sb_OuIE8 (accessed 4 February 2015)
Airway Management with Simple Adjuncts – Respiratory Medicine: https://www.youtube.com/watch?v=U4FrtssdyEQ (accessed 4 February 2015)
Basic Airway Management: https://www.youtube.com/watch?v=etPa9oxVWyU (accessed 4 February 2015)
Preoperative Airway Management Training: https://www.youtube.com/watch?v=HJddgaDaFNk (accessed 4 February 2015)

25. General Anaesthetic Pharmacology

References

Bergendahl H, Lönnqvist PA, Eksborg S (2006) Clonidine in Paediatric Anaesthesia: Review of the Literature and Comparison with Benzodiazepines for Anesthetic Premedication. *Acta Anaesthesiologica Scandinavica* **50** (2): 135–143.
Bozkurt P (2007) Premedication of the Pediatric Patient – Anesthesia for the Uncooperative Child. *Current Opinion in Anaesthesiology Journal* **20** (3): 211–215.
Cox RG, Nemish U, Ewen A, Crowe MJ (2006) Evidence-Based Clinical Update: Does Premedication with Oral Midazolam Lead to Improved Behavioural Outcomes in Children? *Canadian Journal of Anaesthesia* **53** (12): 1213–1219.
English W (2002). Post-Operative Shivering, Causes, Prevention and Treatment (Letter). *Update in Anaesthesia*. Available at http://web.squ.edu.om/med-lib/med_cd/e_cds/health%20development/html/clients/WAWFSA/html/acrobat/Update15.pdf (accessed 7 February 2015)
Naguib M, Gottumukkala V, Goldstein PA (2007) Melatonin and Anesthesia: A Clinical Perspective. *Journal of Pineal Research* **42** (1): 12–21.

Further Reading

Dewachter P, Mouton-Faivre C, Emala CW (2009) Anaphylaxis and Anesthesia: Controversies and New Insights. *Journal of Anesthesiology* **111** (5): 1141–1150.
Nair PN, White E (2014) Care of the Eye during Anaesthesia and Intensive Care. *Journal of Anaesthesia and Intensive Care Medicine* **15** (1): 40–43.

Websites

Induction Agents:

http://www.frca.co.uk/Documents/107%20-%20IV%20induction%20agents.pdf (accessed 5 June 2016)

Inhalational Anaesthetic Drugs: http://www.frca.co.uk/documents/pharminhal.pdf (accessed 5 June 2016)

IV Induction Agents: http://www.anesthesiologynews.com/download/Induction_ANSE10_WM.pdf (accessed 5 June 2016)

Videos

General Anaesthesia – Fundamentals and Pharmacology: https://www.youtube.com/watch?v=JHp_4uRyvi8 (accessed 7 February 2015)

General Anaesthetics: https://www.youtube.com/watch?v=UR5YvTZopMA (accessed 7 February 2015)

Popular Anaesthetic and Pharmacology Videos: https://www.youtube.com/watch?v=K_qjguv2Wtg&list=PLAAzPx97Xpa1tuMkqlkCB7R80rAFNgiJ7 (accessed 7 February 2015)

26. Intraoperative Fluid Management

References

Ait-Oufella H, Maury E, Lehoux S, Guidet B, Offenstadt G (2010) The Endothelium: Physiological Functions and Role in Microcirculatory Failure during Severe Sepsis. *Intensive Care Medicine* **36**: 1286.

Bamboat ZM, Bordeianou L (2009) Perioperative Fluid Management. *Journal of Clinics in Colon and Rectal Surgery* **22** (1): 28–33.

Bundgaard-Nielsen M, Secher NH, Kehlet H (2009) Liberal' vs. 'Restrictive' Perioperative Fluid Therapy – a Critical Assessment of the Evidence. *Acta Anaesthesiologica Scandinavica* **53**: 843–851.

Chappell D, Dörfler N, Jacob M, Rehm M, Welsch U, Conzen P (2010). Glycocalyx Protection Reduces Leukocyte Adhesion after Ischemia/Reperfusion. *Shock* **34**: 133–139.

Chappell D, Heindl B, Jacob M, *et al.* (2011) Sevoflurane Reduces Leukocyte and Platelet Adhesion after Ischemia Reperfusion by Protecting the Endothelial Glycocalyx. *Anesthesiology* **115**: 483–491.

Contant CM, Hop WC, van't Sant HP, Oostvogel HJ, Smeets HJ, Stassen LP, *et al.* (2007) Mechanical Bowel Preparation for Elective Colorectal Surgery: A Multicentre Randomised Trial. *Lancet* **370**: 2112–2117.

Kuper M, Gold SJ, Callow C, Quraishi T, King S, Mulreany A, *et al.* (2011) Intraoperative Fluid Management Guided by Oesophageal Doppler Monitoring. *British Medical Journal* **11** (342): d3016.

Lamke LO, Nilsson GE, Reithner HL (1977) Water Loss by Evaporation from the Abdominal Cavity during Surgery. *Acta Chirurgica Scandinavica* **143**: 279–284.

Lobo DN, MacAfee DA, Allison SP (2006) How Perioperative Fluid Balance Influences Postoperative Outcomes. *Best Practice and Research Clinical Anaesthesiology Journal* **20**: 439–455.

Further Reading

Wicker P, O'Neill J (2010) *Caring for the Perioperative Patient*. Chichester, Wiley-Blackwell.

Yentis S, Hirsch N, Smith G (2009) *Anaesthesia and Intensive Care A–Z*. Edinburgh, Elsevier Ltd.

Websites

Intraoperative Fluids: http://bja.oxfordjournals.org/content/early/2012/05/31/bja.aes171.full (accessed 5 June 2016)

Perioperative Fluid Management: http://www.ncbi.nlm.nih.gov/pmc/articles/PMC2780230/ (accessed 5 June 2016)

Videos

Fluids and Electrolytes Part 1: https://www.youtube.com/watch?v=vvGyHBWcQQU (accessed 12 February 2015)

Fluids and Electrolytes Part 2: https://www.youtube.com/watch?v=G7lDP6ygGBE (accessed 12 February 2015)

Perioperative Fluid Management: https://www.youtube.com/watch?v=eyL2l1TCDjo (accessed 12 February 2015)

Perioperative Fluid Therapy: https://www.youtube.com/watch?v=LFz43_fKkIM (accessed 12 February 2015)

27. Monitoring Perioperative Patients

References

Association of Anaesthetists of Great Britain and Ireland (AAGBI) (2007) *Recommendations for Standards of Monitoring during Anaesthesia and Recovery*, 4th ed. London, AAGBI.

Australian and New Zealand College of Anaesthetists (2013) Recommendations on Monitoring during Anaesthesia. Available at http://www.anzca.edu.au/resources/professional-documents/pdfs/ps18-2013-recommendations-on-monitoring-during-anaesthesia.pdf (accessed 14 February 2015)

Kang HG, Mahoney DF, Hoenig H, Hirth VA, Bonato P, Hajjar I, *et al.* (2010) In situ monitoring of health in older adults: technologies and issues. *Journal of the American Geriatric Society* **58** (8): 1579–1586.

Langton JA, Hutton A (2009) Respiratory Gas Analysis. *Continuing Education in Anaesthesia, Critical Care and Pain Journal* **9** (1): 19–23. Available at http://ceaccp.oxfordjournals.org/content/9/1/19.short (accessed 16 February 2015)

Milton S (2009) Circulation and Invasive Monitoring. *Journal of Perioperative Practice* **19** (7): 213–220.

O'Neill (2010) Patient Care during Anaesthesia. In Wicker P, O'Neill J (eds) *Caring for the Perioperative Patient*. Chichester, Wiley-Blackwell.

Reich DL (2011) The History of Anesthesia and Perioperative Monitoring. In *Monitoring in Anesthesia and Perioperative Care*. Cambridge, Cambridge University Press.

Further Reading

Deschamps A, Denault A (2008) Analysis of Heart Rate Variability: A Useful Tool to Evaluate Autonomic Tone in the Anesthetized Patient? *Canadian Journal of Anaesthesiology* **55** (4): 208–213.

Reich DL (2011) *Monitoring in Anesthesia and Perioperative Care*. Cambridge, Cambridge University Press. Available at http://ebooks.cambridge.org/ebook.jsf?bid=CBO9780511974083 (accessed 14 February 2015)

Thompson JP, Mahajan RP (2006) Monitoring the Monitors – beyond Risk Management. *British Journal of Anaesthesia* **97**: 1–3.

Websites

Critical Care and Perioperative Monitoring: http://www.hindawi.com/journals/tswj/2014/737628/ (accessed 14 February 2015)

Patient Monitoring Devices: http://www.smiths-medical.com/products/patient-monitoring/ (accessed 14 February 2015)

Perioperative Management of the Geriatric Patient: http://emedicine.medscape.com/article/285433-overview (accessed 14 February 2015)

Recommendations for Standards of Monitoring during Anaesthesia and Recovery: http://www.aagbi.org/sites/default/files/standardsofmonitoring07.pdf (accessed 14 February 2015)

Videos

Anaesthesia Monitoring:
https://www.youtube.com/playlist?list=PLEH-ayhgmxpoDH7zSgEmlQ47pveXEUKlz (accessed 14 February 2015)

Monitoring General Anaesthesia: https://www.youtube.com/watch?v=YBbI3oYa3sU (accessed 14 February 2015)

Monitor General Anaesthesia: https://www.youtube.com/watch?v=_hpTN5c5MAA (accessed 14 February 2015)

Reading Anaesthesia Machine Monitor: https://www.youtube.com/watch?v=-O5Uo2S8P18 (accessed 14 February 2015)

SECTION 3

Surgical Specialities

Sara Dalby

28 Laparoscopic Surgery

Since the early 1990s, there have been significant developments in the techniques for reducing the level of surgical intervention. Laparoscopic surgery is considered the most significant advancement in surgery over the last decade. Laparoscopic surgery has proved beneficial with regards to decreased length of hospital stay, less pain, lower infection rates, faster return to daily activities and improved cosmetic result (Ulmer 2010). Due to these benefits, both patients and surgeons continue to opt for laparoscopic surgery. It has now become common practice in a number of specialities, including colorectal, upper gastrointestinal (GI), urology, endocrine, gynaecology and hepatobiliary. The introduction of the principles of enhanced recovery support the use of laparoscopic techniques due to reduced recovery times.

Basic principles of laparoscopic surgery

Laparoscopic surgery enables surgeons to carry out surgery without the need to make large incisions for exposure. In order to have space to operate, it is necessary to inflate the area; depending on the area and technique, a Veress needle or port will be placed and gas introduced. Additional ports can then be placed safely under direct vision. The camera holder should ensure the tips of instruments are within sight of the operating surgeon at all times to minimise the risk of injury. Specialised laparoscopic instruments are then utilised to carry out the operative procedure.

Equipment

In this economic climate, the cost of healthcare has become a hot topic. Laparoscopic surgery is expensive: costs include stack systems, instruments (disposable vs. reusable), staple guns, haemostats, harmonic and ligature. To validate these, there needs to be savings elsewhere such as early discharge, reduced analgesia requirement and earlier return to daily activities.

An awareness of how the equipment functions and how to problem solve is important to optimise the procedure. The theatre practitioners should have a working knowledge of the stack system, attachments and normal settings.

In addition to the stack system, the scrub practitioner will need specific laparoscopic equipment such as ports. Ports provide an entry into the cavity to insufflate and introduce instruments. They come in a variety of sizes and may be bladed or unbladed. The selection depends on a number of factors; for example, for a laparoscopic cholecystectomy, the method used to create a pneumoperitoneum and the size of the scope or instruments influence the size of the port (Whalan 2008).

It is important for the scrub nurse to check the integrity of the insulation surrounding the laparoscopic instruments to reduce the incidence of insulation failure which could occur when using electrosurgery, potentially causing damage to adjacent tissue and structures off-screen (Goodman and Spry 2014).

Rapid Perioperative Care, First Edition. Paul Wicker and Sara Dalby.

Difficulties for surgeons

There are a number of technical difficulties encountered by operating surgeons:

- Three-dimensional operating transposed as two-dimensional images, hindering depth perception
- Limited vision
- Reliance on the assistant to provide vision
- Reduced tactile sensation (although this develops over time)
- Nonstandard methods of haemostasis
- Handling of laparoscopic instruments differs from open surgery (Hamlin *et al.* 2010).

Conversion to open

As laparoscopic surgery is becoming more common practice, training and education for all members of the multidisciplinary team are important. The laparoscopic practitioner will need education but will also be expected to provide training to others in new equipment and techniques.

The two major categories of patient injuries during laparoscopic surgery are mechanical injury and thermal injuries. Complications include bleeding, perforation, lacerations, infections, dehiscences and occlusions; equipment failure may be attributed to some of these complications (Clarke 2009). With the expansion of laparoscopic surgery, practitioners need to learn new technology and instrumentation, as well as any techniques and potential challenges associated with the new technology to ensure patient safety.

The theatre teams should ensure that all the additional instruments and equipment are readily available should it be necessary to convert to open and that practitioners are up to date with the equivalent open cases. Haemorrhage is a common cause of conversion.

Further developments and innovations

Advancements in laparoscopic surgery are often dictated by the limitations of technical instrumentation. There is always new and developing technology which can affect laparoscopic surgery and the laparoscopic practitioner's role in the future. The question to ask about any new technology is whether clinicians are adhering to important clinical principles; with any new technique, the complication rate is expected to be higher for surgeons early in their learning curve.

Further innovations include:

- *Ports*: As people are striving for increasingly less invasive surgery techniques which use only one small incision linked with the development of suitable products, single-port laparoscopic cholecystectomies have been devised – laparoscopic surgery through a 2–3 cm periumbilical incision. The potential benefits are less pain, faster recovery and improved cosmetic result. Such developments may also result in changes in instruments. Surgeons may select a flexible port to counteract some of the known frustrations of single-port surgery: conflicting instruments, limited manoeuvrability and air leakage (Romanelli *et al.* 2009, Saber *et al.* 2010).
- *Instruments*: With the continued expansion of laparoscopic surgery, the instrumentation needed to carry out the increasingly intricate procedure has become more specialised; the goal of increased specialisation of instruments is to reduce risk and increase patient safety. An understanding of the uses, maintenance and decontamination of these instruments is an important part of a theatre practitioner's role. Due to single-incision procedures, bendable articulating instruments are required due to the space reduction and limited range of motion. As well as developments for instruments, there have been developments made to laparoscopes; they can be rigid or flexible, may have no operating channels or may have connectors for suction, instruments and irrigation. For laparoscopic practitioners,

an understanding of the laparoscope and an ability to adapt are essential when camera holding to ensure the surgical team have an appropriate operative view (Moran *et al.* 2010, Ulmer 2010).

- *Haemostasis*: In an effort to improve methods of haemostasis laparoscopically, several companies have developed novel energy sources that coagulate, ligate and frequently transect vessels and tissue bundles. Laparoscopic liver resections are becoming more popular; however, the laparoscopic approach is reserved for small segment resections due to a fear of significant blood loss. The expansion of laparoscopic liver resections depends on surgical ability and technological advances to address bleeding and haemostasis with any new approach (Mohammed *et al.* 2010).
- *NOTES (Natural Orifice Transluminal Endoscopic Surgery)*: The rationale for gaining access to the abdominal cavity through natural openings will further reduce pain and wound and pulmonary complications, and improve cosmesis, early ambulation and discharge. Transgastric, transvaginal, transvesical and transcolic methods can be used for NOTES. There are difficulties to this method, such as access, closure, infection, suturing technology, orientation, physiology and training. The instruments needed for surgeons to carry out NOTES need more developing, and clinicians need advanced training.
- *Robotic surgical techniques*: These techniques are revolutionising the way surgery is performed in an effort to improve patient outcomes. Advances in computer capabilities make it possible for surgeons to carry out surgery without even touching patients. It is ideal for more complex procedures as da Vinci robots increase dexterity and precision by eliminating surgeon's tremor and allowing a three-dimensional vision of the operative environment (Jayaraman *et al.* 2010). The dexterity of the Endowrist design allows precise control of technically challenging tasks such as fine suturing. An evaluation of the quality of the anastomosis, learning curves and impact of experience on performance should be assessed. Benefits for the patient are smaller incisions, better cosmesis, reduced blood loss, reduced tissue loss and faster return to work, *but* current literature is limited (Mabrouk *et al.* 2009). When robotics are used within the theatre department, it would be the laparoscopic practitioner's role to ensure equipment availability and care, assist intraoperatively with the robotic procedures, provide patient and staff education and assist with research (Ulmer, 2010). Issues with emergencies include indirect patient contact and when robotic instruments need to be removed.

The developments are continuing, and patient outcomes will influence future laparoscopic practices; this will result from audit and research to establish new practices and findings. Audits of patient outcomes may establish any trends to support practices. Assess that quality is above the essential standards and that patients receive services which meet standards of safety and quality (CQC 2010). Any new technology or surgical techniques will require auditing to assess patient outcomes and assess the complication rate.

It is imperative from a patient safety perspective that changes are implemented appropriately and introduced to the perioperative department in a correct manner, training is provided, support is given and competencies are completed and kept up to date.

As well as advancements in surgical techniques, there may be advancements in other areas such as endoscopy or diagnostics, which means that other nonsurgical treatments may be more pertinent. Science and technology are advancing at a rapid rate, in some cases reducing the need for surgery due to advancements in radiology and endoscopy as well as biotechnology and gene therapy; but innovations are in various stages of development, so therefore patients will still need surgical interventions.

29 Vascular Surgery

Atherosclerosis is a disease that affects arteries, causing fatty plaques to form in the arterial wall, which can narrow the vessel lumen. Atherosclerosis can cause coronary artery disease, cerebrovascular disease and peripheral vascular disease. The symptoms of atherosclerosis are secondary to limitation of flow (narrowing), thrombosis and embolism (Bradbury and Cleveland 2012).

Vascular risk factors

- Non-modifiable risk factors:
  - Age
  - Family history (age of parent with heart attack or stroke)
  - Nationality (increased risk in African Caribbean population)
- Major modifiable risk factors:
  - Hypertension
  - Smoking
  - Cholesterol
  - Exercise
  - Alcohol
  - Diabetes
  - Homocysteine.

Aneurysms

An aneurysm is an abnormal dilatation of a blood vessel more than 1.5 times the normal diameter. They are most common in arteries. Aneurysms may rupture (resulting in bleeding), or thrombose or give off distal emboli which will both cause distal ischaemia. Aneurysms are classified by their site, aetiology and morphology and whether are true or false (pseudoaneurysm) (Wieczorek 2011).

Different sites in which aneurysms occur are:

- *Abdominal aortic aneurysms (AAAs)*: Five percent of men over 70 years have AAAs. Patients who are asymptomatic should be considered for repair with an aneurysm of 5.5 cm, and if the procedure is deemed to have a less than 5% mortality. These may also extend into the chest as thoraco-AAAs and more commonly are infrarenal aneurysms.
  - *Symptomatic AAAs*: Patients in pain should be considered for elective repair as pain is an indication of a potential future rupture. They can be repaired through an open approach with a prosthetic graft or an endovascular aneurysm repair (EVAR). This procedure involves placing a graft inside an aneurysm via a femoral arteriotomy or percutaneously under radiological guidance.

Rapid Perioperative Care, First Edition. Paul Wicker and Sara Dalby.

  - *Ruptured AAA*: This is a life-threatening emergency. The choice of method of repair depends on patient- and aneurysm-specific factors that in turn depend on the size and site of rupture. Swift diagnosis and surgical intervention are essential.
- *Peripheral aneurysms*: Any peripheral artery can be affected by an aneurysm; the site of disease affects the aetiology, clinical features and subsequent treatment.
- Popliteal aneurysms
- Iliac aneurysms
- Femoral aneurysms. (Lin *et al.* 2010, Wieczorek 2011, Sayers 2013)

Lower limb ischaemia

Lower limb ischaemia can be classified as asymptomatic, intermittent claudication, rest pain and ulceration gangrene (Bradbury and Cleveland 2012). The main cause is atherosclerosis; however, in younger patients, other potential causes for lower limb ischaemia include:

- Aortic dissection
- Aneurysms
- Accelerated atherosclerosis caused by hyperhomocysteinaemia, hyperlipidaemia and AIDS
- Buerger's disease
- Popliteal entrapment
- Fibromuscular dysplasia
- Persistent sciatic artery
- Cystic adventitial disease.

Investigations may include:

- Ankle-brachial pressure index (ABPI)
- Duplex ultrasound
- Angiography (this can be both diagnostic and therapeutic)
- Computed tomography (CT) angiography
- Magnetic resonance (MR) angiography
- Intravascular ultrasound (Lin *et al.* 2010, Bradbury and Cleveland 2012).

Chronic lower limb arterial disease presents as either intermittent claudication or critical limb ischaemia (Bradbury and Cleveland 2012).

Patients with chronic limb ischaemia present with some of the following symptoms:

- Cool extremities
- Pallor, especially on elevation
- Thin and dry skin
- Brittle and crumbly nails
- Muscle wasting
- Pulses are weak or absent.

Intermittent claudication causes tight cramp-like pain on exertion in the calf muscle due to the reduced blood supply; it is uncomfortable, but it is a relatively benign condition. Its management is risk factor modification, statin and antiplatelet therapy and exercise (known as *best medical therapy*); following this, patients may require angioplasty, stenting or bypass surgery. Critical lower limb ischaemia threatens part or all of the limb; it causes constant recurring rest pain for two weeks or ulceration or gangrene of the foot. Initial treatment is endovascular to perform an angioplasty, with surgical intervention if this fails (Lin *et al.* 2010, Bradbury and Cleveland 2012, Sayers 2013).

Acute limb ischaemia is an emergency; if untreated, the limb becomes unsalvageable, and it is necessary to carry out an amputation to save the patient's life. Time is key in this instance, and interventions include urgent surgery such as embolectomy or bypass, amputation, endovascular therapy such as suction thrombectomy, and angioplasty with or without stenting. Diabetics are prone to ulceration and infection due to vascular disease and neuropathy, and this progression of tissue necrosis may require surgical intervention in the form of amputation (Lin *et al.* 2010).

Amputations

Amputation is one of the oldest operations and is a life-saving procedure in severe trauma, vascular disease and tumours. It is the last resort in management of non-salvageable critical limb ischaemia or extensive necrosis or gangrene which without amputation would lead to death. The aim is to preserve as much limb as possible while choosing a level with viable tissue and the best chance of successful healing. The level of amputation depends on:

- The status of joints
- Local blood supply
- Patient's age
- Patient's general health.

An important part of postoperative management is to encourage wound healing and early rehabilitation. A good amputation stump allows successful use of a prosthesis and better quality of life (Wieczorek 2011, Bradbury and Cleveland 2012, Sayers 2013).

Arterial disease of the upper limb

Occlusive arterial disease is significantly lower in the upper limb; however, when affected, the arm can be difficult to treat. The common site of disease is the left subclavian artery, which may cause:

- Arm claudication
- Subclavian steal syndrome
- Athero-embolism to the hand.

Management is normally balloon angioplasty and stenting, as surgical access can be difficult.

Carotid embolisation

Plaques form within the arteries; part of the surface breaks off and embolises to the brain. Embolism from diseased carotid arteries results in:

- Amaurosis fugax or permanent monocular blindness if it enters the ophthalmic artery
- Hemiparesis and hemisensory loss on the opposite side if it enters the middle cerebral artery; if the dominant hemisphere is affected, the patient may also suffer from dysphasia.

The goal of surgical intervention is to prevent strokes. Carotid artery embolisms may be asymptomatic or cause amaurosis fugax, a transient ischaemic attack or strokes. A carotid endartectomy is performed to remove the atheromatous plaque, leaving the inside of the artery smooth. A patch is often used to prevent narrowing of the lumen. This operation can be done under local or general anaesthetic (Lin *et al.* 2010, Wieczorek 2011).

Venous disease

Varicose veins are dilated superficial veins in the lower limb which cause discomfort to the individual, particularly when standing for extended periods of time, with pain alleviated once the leg is raised. Treatment can be conservative with compression stockings, regular exercise, weight reduction, avoidance of constricting clothing and, if possible, reduction of standing time. Surgical options include stripping the long saphenous vein and avulsions of multiple varicosities, laser removal or sclerotherapy. These are usually day case procedures. Varicose veins can recur, and the cosmetic outcome may be poor (Liem and Moneta 2010, Wieczorek 2011, McCollum and Chetter 2013).

30 Cardiothoracic Surgery

Cardiac surgery

Common investigations for cardiac disease

The investigations which may be required for diagnosis include:

- Blood tests: Hb, C-reactive protein, blood cultures and erythrocyte sedimentation rate
- Specialist blood tests (i.e. cardiac enzymes)
- Chest x-ray
- Electrocardiogram
- Stress test and myocardial perfusion imaging
- Echocardiography
- Cardiac catheterisation
- Cardiac isotope scanning
- Coronary angiography
- Evaluation of aortic and cardiac disease by magnetic resonance (MR) and computed tomography (CT) (Schwartz *et al.* 2010, Bojar 2011, Seifert 2011).

Acquired heart disease

Coronary heart disease, also known as ischaemic heart disease, is a term used for all conditions which involve the blockage or narrowing of coronary arteries by atherosclerosis (Bojar 2011).

The clinical manifestations of coronary artery disease include:

- Angina
- Acute coronary syndrome
- Myocardial infarction
- Mitral valve incompetence
- Arrhythmias due to ischaemia, such as atrial fibrillation or heart block
- Ventricular aneurysm
- Heart failure (Schwartz *et al.* 2010).

First-line treatment is to encourage patients to modify risk factors, such as smoking cessation, strict diabetic control and losing weight if obese. This has the benefit of potentially slowing disease progression so there is no requirement for intervention, and it reduces the risk of re-occlusion following surgery. The next step is medical therapy to reduce myocardial oxygen demand.

For more severe cases, the patient may need coronary artery interventions such as:

- Percutaneous transluminal coronary angioplasty (PTCA) and stenting; this expands stenosed or recanalises occluded coronary arteries.
- Coronary artery bypass grafting (CABG), in which the occluded arteries are bypassed to provide a new source of blood flow (Schwartz *et al.* 2010, Anderson and Zakkar 2013).

Rapid Perioperative Care, First Edition. Paul Wicker and Sara Dalby.

The decision to carry out a CABG should be based on patient benefit versus risk. Indications for CABG include:

- Failure of medical therapy with chronic stable angina
- Left main stem disease
- Post-infarct angina
- Unstable angina
- Symptomatic three-vessel disease
- Failed PTCA
- Acute myocardial infarction with cardiogenic disease
- Kawasaki disease
- Congenital abnormalities
- Coronary disease affiliated with other cardiac procedures
- Reoperation for recurrent symptoms. (Seifert 2011)

Postoperative complications of a CABG include bleeding, neurological dysfunction, wound infection, arrhythmias, poor cardiac output state and mortality (Anderson and Zakkar 2013).

Congenital cardiac disease

Congenital heart disease involves abnormalities which can be categorised as repairable or palliative. It is classified depending on specific presentation, physiology, anatomy, outcome, type of correction and technical aspects. Causes are multifactorial and may include rubella, maternal diabetes mellitis, maternal alcohol abuse, maternal drug and radiation treatment and genetic and chromosomal abnormalities (Anderson and Zakkar 2013).

Congenital heart disorders include:

- Types where repair is the option:
  - Atrial septal defect
  - Aortic stenosis
  - Truncus arteriosus
  - Total anomalous pulmonary venous connection
  - Patent ductus arteriosus
  - Aortic coarctation
  - Cor triatriatum
  - Aortic pulmonary window
- Defects requiring palliation:
  - Tricuspid atresia
  - Left heart hypoplasia
- Defects which may be repaired or palliated:
  - Ebstein's anomaly
  - Transposition of the great arteries
  - Double-outlet right ventricle
  - Taussig–Bing syndrome
  - Tetralogy of Fallot
  - Ventricular septal defect
  - Interrupted aortic arch
  - Atrioventricular canal defects (Karamlou *et al.* 2010).

Surgical management aims to palliate the adverse effects, correct the defects mechanically or do both in sequence.

When palliating congenital heart disorders, if the pulmonary blood flow is reduced, the aim is to increase pulmonary flow by creating a shunt between the arterial circulation and the pulmonary artery. If the pulmonary blood flow is too great, the aim is to reduce the flow by using an external band to artificially narrow the main pulmonary artery (Karamlou *et al.* 2010).

Surgical correcting of congenital cardiac disorders depends on identifying the lesion or lesions, then carrying out corrective surgery to restore normal function and flow to the heart. It may be categorised as mechanically straightforward or complex.

Valvular heart disease

Valvular disease can cause valvular stenosis, valvular regurgiutation or both. The clinical signs and symptoms of valvular heart disease during a clinical examination will reveal stenosis which is restricted blood flow across the valve, or regurgiutation when the valve allows backflow (Schwartz *et al.* 2010).

- *Infective or subacute infective endocarditis*: This affects mainly aortic and mitral valves and tricuspids in intravenous drug users; there is often an underlying abnormality of the valve.
- *Rheumatoid heart disease*: Progressive valve damage may be as a consequence of rheumatoid fever in childhood.
- *Degenerative*: The most common is stenosis of the aortic valve in older patients. An ineffective aortic valve is associated with Marfan's syndrome and ankylosing spondylitis.

Valve replacement can involve either mechanical valves (which are durable but patients require permanent anticoagulation) or tissue valves (which do not generally require anticoagulation therapy but are more prone to structural failure). Valve repair is becoming increasingly used, especially for patients with mitral or tricuspid valve insufficiency (Schwartz *et al.* 2010).

Selection of a procedure (repair or replace) depends on a number of factors:

- Stage of disease
- Mitral valve anatomy
- Patient's ability to tolerate anticoagulation therapy
- If there is calcification disease
- History of thromboembolism and dysrhythmia (Seifert 2011).

Indications for valve surgery are when the risks of surgery are the least but the potential benefits are optimum:

- For aortic or mitral stenosis, surgical intervention is required when patients become symptomatic.
- For aortic or mitral valve regurgitation, surgical intervention should occur when there is left ventricular dilatation in patients whom are asymptomatic (Price and El Khoury 2014).

Valve-related risks and complications:

- Prosthetic failure
- Anticoagulation-related haemorrhage
- Prosthetic valve endocarditis
- Paravalvular leak
- Thromboembolism (Seifert 2011, Anderson and Zakkar 2013).

Thoracic surgery

Neoplastic (Cancerous) lung tumours

Lung cancer is one of the most prevalent cancers in the United Kingdom. The risk factors for lung cancer include smoking, second-hand smoke exposure and industrial compound exposure such as asbestos (Nason *et al.* 2010).

PRESENTING SYMPTOMS General cancer symptoms:

- Fatigue
- Anaemia
- Weight loss.

The local symptoms of a lung cancer include:

- Haemoptysis
- Chest pain
- Cough
- Shortness of breath
- Dysphagia
- Arm symptoms from brachial plexis invasion
- Hoarse voice
- Wheezing
- Superior vena cava obstruction (Nason *et al.* 2010, Hunt and Tan 2013).

Metastatic symptoms may include:

- Pathological fractures
- Bone pain
- Cerebral metastases.

DIAGNOSTIC INVESTIGATIONS FOR LUNG TUMOURS

- Bloods, for example urea–electrolytes and calcium for SIADH (syndrome of inappropriate antidiuretic hormone secretion) and hypercalcaemia
- Chest x-ray
- CT or MR imaging of the thorax
- Bronchoscopy
- Mediastinoscopy
- Positron emission tomography (PET) scan
- Liver ultrasound
- Bone scan
- Brain CT or MR imaging if there is a suspicion of metastases (Nason *et al.* 2010, Hunt and Tan 2013).

Types of pathology include:

- Squamous cell carcinoma
- Small cell carcinoma
- Adenocarcinoma
- Bronchoalveolar carcinoma
- Large cell carcinoma (Nason *et al.* 2010, Hunt and Tan 2013).

The treatment is for the resection of operable tumours; for more advanced tumours, chemotherapy or radiotherapy may be appropriate. Laparoscopic thoracic surgery can be used as a diagnostic tool for pleural disease or treatment of conditions such as cysts or effusions, biopsies or resections. Thoracotomy is performed to enable operating on the patient's lungs for both benign and malignant conditions. A pneumonectomy is the complete removal of the lung, usually due to malignancy (Blanchard 2011, Hunt and Tan 2013). Complications of lung resections include respiratory infection, bleeding, bronchopleural fistula and persistent air leak.

Benign lung tumours

The most common benign tumours are hamartomas and carcinoid. On chest x-ray, they are well defined; however, they may be difficult to define, and therefore biopsy is needed to confirm diagnosis. If obtaining a biopsy is difficult, the lesion may be resected, particularly when there is a suspicion it may be cancerous. However, clinical signs such as calcification, a well-defined edge and slow growth are typical of benign tumours (Hunt and Tan 2013).

31 Orthopaedics and Trauma

Orthopaedic specialities cover all joints and bones within the body and are divided into upper limb, lower limb and spinal. Patients can present either with wear-and-tear conditions (e.g. osteoarthritis in an elective setting) or with fractures following a trauma. Treatment may be categorised as conservative or operative; patient factors including comorbidities and lifestyle are important to consider before determining the appropriate management.

Investigations

Pain is usually the main symptom for patients seeking an orthopaedic examination. Following history taking and clinical examination, the patient may require further investigations to confirm or rule out the differential diagnosis. These include:

- Imaging such as x-rays, arthrography, tomography, computed tomography (CT), magnetic resonance imaging (MRI), ultrasound and isotope scanning
- Nerve conduction tests and electromyography (EMG) to evaluate nerves
- Blood tests, including markers of inflammation and disease specific such as rheumatoid factor
- Aspiration of synovial fluid looking for white blood cells and inflamed or infected joints or cultures to identify organisms
- Arthroscopy may be performed on a joint to directly carry out a diagnostic examination. During an arthroscopy, interventions such as a meniscectomy (to manage a meniscus tear during a knee arthroscopy) may be carried out to address the patient's pain (McRae 2008, McKinley and Ahmed 2012).

Orthopaedic specialities

Orthopaedic specialities can be divided into upper limb, lower limb and spinal. The upper limb speciality can be divided into shoulder, elbow and the hands:

- Shoulder, common problems of
  - Rotator cuff tears
  - Anterior dislocation
  - Impingement syndrome
  - Acromioclavicular osteoarthritis and rheumatoid arthritis
  - Adhesive capsulitis (frozen shoulder)
  - Calcific tendinitis
- Elbow, disorders of
  - Arthritis of the elbow
  - Olecranon bursitis
  - Tennis and golfer's elbow

Rapid Perioperative Care, First Edition. Paul Wicker and Sara Dalby.

- The hands, disorders of
  - Carpel tunnel syndrome
  - Trigger finger
  - Ganglion
  - Rheumatoid arthritis or osteoarthritis
  - Dupuytrens contracture
  - Ulnar nerve entrapment.

Spinal is normally presented as lower back pain; there are a number of causes for this presentation:

- Mechanical causes
  - Spondylosis
  - Spondylolisthesis
  - Lumbar disc prolapse
  - Spinal canal stenosis
  - Ligament injuries
- Infection
  - Bacterial discitis
  - Tuberculosis of the spine
- Metabolic bone disease
  - Paget's disease
  - Osteoporosis
- Inflammatory disorders
  - Ankylosing spondylitis
  - Arthritis
- Tumours of the bone
  - Myeloma
  - Metastases
- Referred pain
  - Pancreatitis
  - Ruptured aortic aneurysm
  - Pyelonephritis
  - Peptic ulceration.

The lower limb speciality can be divided into hip, knee and ankle and foot:

- Hip
  - Osteoarthritis (may present as referred pain in the groin, thigh or knee)
- Knee
  - Osteoarthritis
  - Haemarthrosis
  - Meniscal tears
  - Recurrent dislocated patella
  - Anterior cruciate ligament injuries
  - Posterior cruciate ligament injuries
- Ankle and foot
  - Hallux varus
  - Lesser toe deformities
  - Arthritic disease
  - Tendon disorders

  - Heel pain
  - Hyperkeratotic pathologies (Heggeness *et al.* 2010, Brunton and Chhabra 2012, Kadakia and Irwin 2012, Lauerman and Baumbusch 2012, McKinley and Ahmed 2012, McPherson 2012).

Conservative management

- Physical therapy
  - Physiotherapy
  - Occupational therapy
  - Chiropractors and osteopaths
  - Hydrotherapy
- Aids and appliances
  - Walking aids
  - Appliances
- Medications
  - Nonsteroidal anti-inflammatory drugs (NSAIDs)
  - Steroids
  - Antibiotics
  - Anticoagulants (McKinley and Ahmed 2012; McPherson 2012).

Operative management

Most elective orthopaedic procedures are carried out on patients who are otherwise healthy but for whom a full health assessment is still necessary. If the patient is found to have a chest infection or hypertension, elective surgery should be postponed. For trauma patients, this may not be the case; however, they need to be optimised in the timeframe available, in particular regarding blood loss and dehydration.

- Operations on tendons
  - Tenotomy
  - Tendon lengthening
  - Tendon transposition
  - Tendon release
  - Tenodesis
  - Tendon repair
- Operations on bones
  - Osteotomy
  - Osteosynthesis
  - Bone grafting
  - Lengthening bones
  - Exostectomy
  - Draining infection
- Operations on joints
  - Arthrodesis
  - Arthrotomy
  - Arthroplasty
  - Synovectomy
  - Arthrolysis
  - Arthroscopy
  - Aspiration

  - Manipulation under anaesthetic
  - Repair
  - Replacement or reconstruction
  - Plication and capsulorrhaphy
- Operations on nerves
  - Decompression
  - Repair
  - Neurolysis
  - Grafting
- Operations on skin
  - Repair
  - Graft
  - Plastic operations (Dandy and Edwards 2009, Springfield 2009, Heggeness *et al.*, 2010).

Fractures

For fractures, the priorities are to realign the bone without deformity and restore function for the patient to continue with their daily lives.

As closed reduction and fixation of a fracture may be indicated, the displaced fracture is manipulated into the correct position. Caution needs to be exercised to ensure there is no damage to vessels or nerves. Once the fracture has been reduced to ensure it does not become displaced, the patient may require a plaster cast or external fixation.

For open fractures, there is an increased risk of infection, all foreign bodies need to be removed including any nonviable tissue and the wound must be washed thoroughly. Antibiotics are commenced to try to reduce the incidence of infection. The wound needs to be assessed to ensure there is no major arterial injury or any neurological injuries. Fixation of the fracture depends on the site, chance of infection and quality of fixation needed. When there is a high risk of infection, an external fixator may be chosen (Springfield 2009).

Trauma presentations may include periprosthetic fractures; the patient presents with a fracture and has a primary or revision prosthesis on the same extremity. Depending on the extent of the fracture and position, either the treatment can be plating and cabling once the fracture is reduced, leaving the implants from arthroplasty in situ, or, if complex, there may be a need to carry out an endoprosthesis in which a measured resection of the femur is taken and rebuilt with segmental constructs.

A number of factors affect the healing of a fracture:

- Patient's age
- Mobility at the fracture site
- Type of bone
- Infection
- Separation at the bone ends
- Disturbance of blood supply
- Joint involvement
- Properties of the bone involved
- Bone pathology.

Most fractures occur from trauma; however, pathological fractures occur in abnormal or diseased bone, where minimal stress can result in a fracture. The following are conditions responsible for pathological fractures:

- Osteoporosis
- Osteomalacia
- Paget's disease

- Osteitis
- Osteogenesis imperfecta
- Simple bone tumours and cysts
- Primary malignant bone tumours
- Secondary malignant bone tumours (McRae 2008).

Joint replacements

Joints are predisposed to wear and tear, and osteoporosis presents as painful stiff joints. Nonsurgical management is an option, including analgesics, physiotherapy and weight loss. However, it may be deemed necessary to list the patient for elective surgery on their joints, such as a total hip replacement. Prostheses have been improved and developed to be functional for 15–20 years. The main reasons for failure of a joint replacement are infection and loosening of the prosthesis (Miles and Skinner 2010). Joint replacements can be cemented or cementless; cemented ones are used in older adult patients (Springfield 2009). In patients with severe knee deformities having joint replacements, custom-designed cutting-blocks arthroplasty is utilised; using CT scans, blocks can be custom designed for femoral and tibial resection to ensure that the implants fit the anatomy and that the mechanics of the knee are accurate.

Specialist equipment

For surgical interventions, a number of implants are utilised, including plates, screws, guide wires and prostheses. It is essential that the practitioners have a knowledge of the potential implants required and that they are checked prior to the patient being anaesthetised.

There are a number of factors to consider when utilising implants. Due to bone being more flexible than metal plates, it can predispose the bone to fracturing at the end of the plate, termed a *stress riser*. Also, when drilling holes into the bone, there is a weakening effect; this is overcome to some extent with the introduction of a screw. The introduction of 'foreign material' in the form of a prosthesis or metal may leave the patient more susceptible to infection, so patients are usually given prophylactic antibiotics in an attempt to reduce the risk (Dandy and Edwards 2009).

The 'ideal' material for a prosthesis is insoluble, nontoxic and strong, with the main materials being metal, plastic or ceramic depending on the patient. Once utilised, the implant may require fixation by cement, screws, bone ingrowth or being a 'snug fit'. The National Joint Registry (NJR 2016) collects information on joint replacement surgery which is used to monitor implant performance.

Orthopaedics is a varied speciality, and the management of the complaint varies depending on the presentation (elective or traumatic), patient factors and conservative or surgical management.

32 Gynaecology Surgery

Gynaecology presenting symptoms

A full history should be carried out when a patient presents with gynaecological symptoms. The history should focus on:

- Menstrual cycle (last menstrual period (LMP), lengths of menses and cycle, menorrhagia, dysmenorrhoea and intermenstrual bleeding)
- Post-coital bleeding, deep or superficial dyspareunia (if sexually active)
- Age at menarche and menopause (if applicable)
- Obstetric history
- Any previous gynaecological surgery
- Cervical screening history (results and timing)
- Previous pelvic infections or sexually transmitted infections (STIs) (Oats and Abraham 2010).

Examination and diagnostic tests

There are a variety of examinations and tests which can be utilised to help diagnose the presenting symptoms:

- Abdominal examination
- Pelvic examination (speculum, swabs, smear and bimanual exam)
- Pelvic ultrasound (transabdominal or transvaginal)
- Colposcopy
- Computed tomography (CT)
- Magnetic resonance imaging (MRI)
- Laparoscopy
- Hysterosalpingography
- Hysteroscopy
- Endometrial biopsy (pipette or curettage) (Cain *et al.* 2010, Oats and Abraham 2010).

Gynaecological infections

A number of potential infections may lead to gynaecological problems. These include:

Lower Genital Tract Infections

- Vaginitis
  - Bacterial vaginosis
  - Vulvovaginal candidiasis
  - Trichomonas vaginalis

Rapid Perioperative Care, First Edition. Paul Wicker and Sara Dalby.

- Genital ulcer syndromes
  - Genital herpes
  - Syphilis
  - Chancroid
  - Lymphogranuloma venereum
  - Granuloma inguinale
- Molluscum contagiosum
- Vulvar condylomas
- Bartholin's cysts and abscesses

Upper Genital Tract Infections

- STI-related pelvic inflammatory disease (PID)
  - Chlamydial infection
  - Gonococcal genital infection
  - Subacute salpingitis
  - Chronic genital infection (chronic PID)
    - Pyosalpinx
    - Hydrosalpinx
    - Chronic pelvic cellulitis
- Tuberculous infection of the genital tract (Cain *et al.* 2010, Oats and Abraham 2010, Monga and Dobbs 2011, Kennedy and McVeigh 2013).

Pelvic floor dysfunction

Pelvic floor disorders can be divided into three categories:

1. Female urinary incontinence and voiding dysfunction
2. Pelvic organ prolapse
3. Disorders of defecation (Cain *et al.* 2010).

Factors affecting pelvic floor problems:

- Congenital factors
  - Determine fascial strength, elasticity and resistance to trauma. Weak endopelvic fascia can predispose a woman to increased risk of stress incontinence and prolapse.
  - Rare in African Caribbean population.
- Acquired factors
  - *Childbirth*: vaginal delivery; forceps or vacuum delivery in particular increases the incidence of stress incontinence and prolapse.
  - *Lifestyle*: obesity, constipation, chronic cough, heavy lifting, increased age and previous pelvic surgery are all factors which increase the risk.

In addition to the normal gynaecological tests, additional specialised investigations may be required:

- For urinary incontinence or voiding problems
  - Cystoscopy, multichanneled urodynamics and/or fluoroscopic evaluation of the urinary tract
- For defecatory dysfunction
  - Defecography, anal manometry and endorectal ultrasound (Cain *et al.* 2010).

Management of pelvic organ prolapse

There are a number of nonsurgical and surgical procedures to manage pelvic organ prolapse:

- Physiotherapist-led pelvic-floor muscle exercises
- Pessaries (ring, shelf and Gellhorn)
- Vaginal surgery
    - Colporrhaphy (anterior and posterior vaginal wall repair)
    - Sacrospinous fixation
    - Uterosacral ligament suspension
    - Colpocleisis
- Abdominal surgery
    - Sacrocolpopexy (Monga and Dobbs 2011, Kennedy and McVeigh 2013).

Management of stress urinary incontinence

The nonsurgical and surgical techniques which can be used to manage a patient with stress urinary incontinence are:

- Lifestyle intervention
- Medication review and adjustment, if applicable
- Pelvic-floor muscle training
- Devices (i.e. to support the bladder neck)
- Bladder retraining
- Anticholinergics
- Vaginal oestrogens
- Surgery
    - Retropubic colposuspension
        - Burch procedure
        - Marshall–Marchetti–Krantz procedure
    - Tape procedures
        - TransObturator tape (TOT or TVT-O)
        - Tension-free transvaginal tape (TVT)
    - Collagen (Cain *et al.* 2010).

Pelvic neoplasms

There are a number of gynaecological sites which can be affected by neoplasms:

- Cervix
    - Benign cervical lesions
        - Cervical polyps
        - Nabothian cysts
        - Posttrauma malformation of the cervix (i.e. delivery-related cervical tear, or secondary to previous surgery)
        - Cervical condylomata
        - Cervical ectropion
    - Cervical cancer

      Patients may present with abnormal vaginal bleeding (particularly post-coital) or vaginal discharge. A biopsy of the tumour and further imaging are utilised to aid in diagnosis. Factors which increase risk are early age of first intercourse and multiple sexual partners due to increased risk of human papilloma virus.
        - Squamous lesions of the cervix
        - Glandular lesions of the cervix

- Sarcoma
- Melanoma
- Lymphoma
- Metastatic

Treatment for cervical cancer may be chemoradiation or surgery.

Surgical management offers variable procedures depending on the extent of the cancer and if there is an interest in preserving fertility:

- Radical hysterectomy
- Radical trachelectomy with intact uterus
- Radical trachelectomy after prior supracervical hysterectomy (Cain *et al.* 2010, McEwen 2011, Monga and Dobbs 2011).
- Uterine corpus
  - Benign uterine diseases, some of which can be managed conservatively in the first instance; however, some may need localised or complete resection:
    - Dysfunctional uterine bleeding
    - Endometrial polyps
    - Adenomyosis
    - Endometriosis: uterine leiomyomas (fibroids) (Oats and Abraham 2010, Kennedy and McVeigh 2013)
- Endometrial cancer
  - Patients may be asymptomatic or present with abnormal vaginal bleeding. To aid with diagnosis, a biopsy is taken. If it is unsuccessful or shows hyperplasia, or if an ultrasound of the endometrium shows increased endometrial thickness in postmenopausal women, a hysteroscopy and curettage may be carried out.
  - Factors which put a patient at increased risk of type 1 endometrial cancer: obesity, diabetes, oestrogen-producing tumour, anovulatory cycles, polycystic ovarian syndrome, hypertension and unopposed oestrogen used in hormone replacement therapy.
  - Type 2 endometrial cancer is not oestrogen driven. Women with a family history of hereditary non-polyposis colonic cancer are at increased risk of endometrial cancer.
  - Treatment is surgical. The aim is to removal all disease and may involve: total abdominal hysterectomy, bilateral salpingo-oophorectomy, omentectomy, peritoneal cytology, pelvic and para-aortic lymph node sampling and resection of any gross disease. The patient may also have postoperative adjuvant radiotherapy or chemotherapy depending on the histology and stage of disease (Cain *et al.* 2010, McEwen 2011, Kennedy and McVeigh 2013).
- Ovarian cancer
  - *Epithelial ovarian cancer*: It tends to have a late presentation and be asymptomatic. Common symptoms include abdominal bloating and changes in bowel function. For advanced cases, the symptoms include: weight loss, anorexia, nausea, vomiting, abdominal distension from ascites and possibly bowel obstruction. Diagnosis requires tissue samples from a laparotomy. They are usually serous, endometrial or mucinous.

    Treatment for early-stage cancer may include: total abdominal hysterectomy, bilateral salpingo-oophorectomy, collection of peritoneal washings and lymph node biopsies, and omentectomy. For patients wanting fertility, a unilateral salpingo-oophorectomy may be carried out, but they require careful follow-up. For advanced stages, 'debulking' surgery is carried out with the aim to remove all primary and metastatic disease. Depending on the stage and extent of disease, patients will also require chemotherapy and/or radiotherapy.
  - *Non-epithelial ovarian cancers*: In contrast to epithelial tumours, which are relatively slow growing, these tumours grow rapidly, and patients present with acute pelvic pain, menstrual irregularities and bladder and bowel pressure symptoms. Surgical

  intervention to remove the tumour is the optimal treatment; patients may also require chemotherapy and potentially radiotherapy.
  - *Germ cell tumours*: One-third of these are malignant.
  - *Sex cord stromal tumours*: Mostly benign, except granulosa cell tumours and Sertoli–Leydig cell tumours (Oats and Abraham 2010, McEwen 2011, Monga and Dobbs 2011, Kennedy and McVeigh 2013).
- Vulvovaginal lesions
  - *Benign vulvar lesions*: Patients often present with itching and pain.
    - Atrophic vulvovaginitis
    - Vulvar contact dermatitis
    - Lichen sclerosis, lichen planus and lichen simplex
    - Paget's disease of the vulva
  - *Vulvar intra-epithelial neoplasia (premalignant)*: Can be treated surgically, with laser ablation or medical treatment (imiquimod), with close surveillance.
  - *Vulvar cancer*: Patients present with irritation, pruritus and a lump, ulceration or skin change on the vulva. Less commonly, they have bleeding, pain, discharge or dysuria. Treatment for a small primary lesion is excision if it is small enough to be completely removed with a good margin. If the margins are unsatisfactory, then local radiation is required. For larger primary lesions, preoperative radiation with chemotherapy is followed by wide excision of the tumour bed. The groin nodes are also surgically excised (Cain *et al.* 2010, McEwen 2011).
- *Vaginal cancer*: Patients present with painless vaginal bleeding or discharge, with some patients having no symptoms but being detected by cervical screening. Treatment differs depending on stage and location but can include laser ablation and brachytherapy, surgical excision, radiotherapy, chemotherapy and pelvic exenteration (Oats and Abraham 2010).

33 Plastic Surgery

An adaptable surgical speciality, plastic surgery covers the entire body. It uses diverse and specific techniques depending on the patient presentation to manage the best clinical outcome. The focus of plastic surgery is to restore both function and form for patients following trauma, surgery or congenital abnormalities by using a variety of reconstructive techniques. Among the techniques utilised to achieve reconstruction are skin grafting, muscle flaps, bone grafting, tissue expansion, replantation and free tissue transfer with microsurgery.

Scope of plastic surgery

Reconstructive plastic surgeons treat a number of conditions:

- Trauma
  - Soft-tissue loss (skin, tendons, nerves and muscle)
  - Hand and lower limb injury
  - Burns
- Cancer
  - Skin
  - Head and neck
  - Breast
  - Soft-tissue sarcoma
- Congenital
  - Clefts and craniofacial malformations
  - Skin, giant nevi and vascular malformations
  - Urogenital
  - Hand and limb malformations
- Miscellaneous
  - Bell's (facial) palsy
  - Pressure sores or complex wound closure
  - Aesthetic surgery
  - Chest wall reconstruction (Goodacre 2013: 403).

Wounds

Skin acts as a barrier and plays an important role in homeostasis. Disruption due to trauma may be due to a penetrating or non-penetrating force. To properly treat the wound, it should be assessed and classified to determine the most appropriate management. Wound healing needs to be optimised with a multifactorial approach to produce the best outcome, including ensuring a good blood supply to the affected area (Watson 2012).

Rapid Perioperative Care, First Edition. Paul Wicker and Sara Dalby.

Grafts

Grafts of any type involve transfer of tissues from a donor site without their blood supply; therefore, the tissues need to re-vascularise once placed on the new site. Tendons, nerves, skin, bone and fat can all be utilised as grafts.

Modern skin graft techniques can be divided into:

- *Split-thickness skin grafts* are of varying thickness and are the simplest method of superficial reconstruction. They have poor durability and tend to contract over time, but they have a high reliability of graft take.
- *Full-thickness skin grafts* have the least amount of contraction when healing, best cosmetic appearance and highest durability. However, the wound bed on which the graft will be placed needs to be well vascularised and without any damage such as radiation or bacterial colonisation. These grafts tend to be used for smaller areas of skin where elasticity is important, such as the hands and face.
- *Composite skin grafts* use skin and underlying tissue such as cartilage to repair a deep defect. This technique is used with nasal reconstruction to repair a deep defect with donor tissue taken from the ear margin. (Losee *et al.* 2010, Dreger 2011, Watson 2012, Goodacre 2013).

Other grafts

- Nerve grafts are commonly taken from the sural nerve and can be used when there is a traumatic deficit or in cases of re-animation.
- Tendon grafts are utilised in cases of injury or reconstructionm and the palmaris longus or plantaris tendons can be used (Goodacre 2013).

Flaps

Flaps are tissues transferred with a blood supply that is mobilised from its current site to the donor site. It has the benefit of bringing its own vascular supply and can consist of any tissue. There are different types which are categorised depending on their blood supply, their size and how they are manipulated to cover the transfer site:

- Random flaps
- Axial flaps
- Pedicled flaps
- Free flaps
- Composite flaps
- Perforator flaps (Losee *et al.* 2010, Dreger 2011, Watson 2012, Goodacre 2013)

Tissue expansion

Tissue expansion is used when extra skin is required to close a large area. This is often done in cases of large lesion excisions. A tissue expander is an empty balloon connected to a tube that is implanted subcutaneously adjacent to the defect. Over time, the balloon is inflated with saline, which distends the skin, providing extra tissue that can later be used for closure of the tissue deficit. Surgery is scheduled when there is enough surplus skin to reconstruct the defect. Tissue expansion is beneficial because the expanded skin has similar qualities to the area being excised. Known complications include infection and erosion of the skin, and the complication rate is 30–40% (Losee *et al.* 2010, Goodacre 2013, Kamolz and Spendel 2013).

Burns

Burn injuries can fluctuate from trivial to severe and life-threatening. They can be caused by a number of factors, including flames, hot fluids or steam, electricity, chemicals or irradiation. Burns cause tissue destruction, increase the metabolic rate and increase capillary permeability. The effects of the burn depend on its size, with larger burns having a more significant effect. The classification of burns is by depth and is determined by reviewing the appearance, mechanisms and sensation. Prognosis depends on age and general health; the extent, site and depth of the burn; and if there is an associated respiratory injury. It is important to cleanse and debride the burn and minimise the risk of infection. It may be possible to restore the skin within three months; however, this is not definitive treatment (Kamolz 2013, Shahrokhi 2013, Tyler and Ghosh 2013).

After surgery, physiotherapy is necessary to mobilise joints, the donor sites need aftercare, splints may be used to prevent contractures, pressure garments may be utilised to prevent hypertrophic scars and further reconstructive surgery may be necessary (Gauglitz 2013, Tyler and Ghosh 2013).

Reconstructive surgery

Reconstructive surgery can be categorised into procedures that treat tissue loss, deformity and loss of function, which may be due to a number of reasons. In composite loss following the resection of a deep tumour, plastic surgeons may be involved in the reconstruction post excision. For patients who have suffered a trauma, the plastic surgeon may be required to assess tissues which are viable and the deficits to establish how and when the affected area can be reconstructed after removing the devitalised tissue and any potential debris to optimise the site. Reconstructive surgery incorporates a number of specialities and procedures such as:

- Facial reconstruction after fracture
  - Mandible fractures
  - Orbital fractures
  - Zygoma and zygomaticomaxillary complex fractures
  - Naso-orbital-ethmoid fractures
  - Frontal sinus fractures
  - Nasal fractures
  - Panfacial fractures
- Ear reconstruction
- Nasal reconstruction
- Lip reconstruction
- Eyelid reconstruction
  - Upper eyelid
  - Lower eyelid
  - Ptosis
- Skull and scalp reconstruction
  - Scalp reconstruction
  - Calvarial reconstruction
- Head and neck reconstruction
  - Tumour-ablative surgery
  - Mandible and midface
  - Oesophagus and hypopharynx
  - Recipient vessels in the head and neck for free flaps

- Facial reanimation
  - Neural techniques
  - Muscle transposition techniques
  - Innervated free tissue transfer
  - Ancillary procedures
- Breast reconstruction
  - Partial breast reconstruction
  - Implant-based reconstruction
  - Total autologous tissue reconstruction
  - Implant and autologous tissue reconstruction
  - Accessory procedures
  - Radiation-related considerations
- Trunk and abdominal reconstruction
  - Thoracic wall
  - Abdominal wall
  - Partial defects of the abdominal wall
- Extremity reconstruction
  - Posttraumatic reconstruction
  - Reconstruction after oncologic resection
  - Diabetic ulceration
  - Lymphedema
- Pressure sore treatment
- Reconstructive transplant surgery (Losee *et al.* 2010, Dreger 2011).

Congenital abnormalities

Congenital abnormalities are defects present at birth which result in a failure of development of an area of the body; they require intervention from a plastic surgeon to reconstruct the body to as near to normal appearance and function as possible. The following conditions are addressed with reconstructive techniques:

- Paediatric plastic surgery
  - Cleft lip and palate
    - Unilateral cleft lip
    - Bilateral cleft lip
    - Cleft palate
  - Craniofacial anomalies
    - Craniofacial clefts
    - Craniosynostosis
    - Atrophy and hypoplasia
    - Hyperplasia, hypertrophy and neoplasia
  - Vascular anomalies
    - Hemangiomas
    - Vascular malformations
  - Congenital melanocytic nevi (Losee *et al.* 2010).

34 Urology

Urology is a surgical speciality which includes the male and female urinary tract (kidney, ureter, bladder and urethra) and the male reproductive organs (scrotum, prostate and penis).

Common urological symptoms

A number of symptoms are common to a urological presentation:

- *Dysuria*: Pain when passing urine
- *Pain*: The location of this depends on the organ involved:
  - *Kidney*: Usually a dull ache in the flank
  - *Bladder*: Suprapubic
  - *Ureter*: Loin to groin, usually severe colicky pain
- *Haematuria*: Can be visible or non-visible (microscopic); both are a potential sign of malignancy – needs investigation in accordance with national guidelines.
- Lower urinary tract symptoms
  - Storage symptoms
    - Urgency
    - Frequency
  - Voiding symptoms
    - Hesitancy
    - Straining
    - Weak stream
    - Intermittency (stops and starts)
    - Nocturia
    - Terminal dribbling
  - Post-micturition symptoms
    - Sensation of incomplete voiding
    - Post-micturition dribbling
- Erectile dysfunction
- Urinary incontinence
  - Urge incontinence
  - Stress urinary incontinence
  - Overflow incontinence
  - Mixed incontinence (combination of above) (Stewart and Finney 2012, Fowler 2013b).

Investigations

To aid in the diagnostics, the following investigations can be used:

- *Blood tests*: Urea, creatinine, calcium, electrolytes, alkaline phosphatase (ALP) and prostate-specific antigen (PSA)

Rapid Perioperative Care, First Edition. Paul Wicker and Sara Dalby.

- *Urine sample*: For a ward test of urine (urinalysis), and to be analysed for microscopy, culture and sensitivities. Use cytology if underlying urothelial malignancy is suspected.
- *X-ray*: To look for abnormal calcification in the urinary tract.
- *Ultrasound*: Used to identify dilatation of the urinary tract (hydronephrosis and hydroureter), renal masses and calculi. However, ultrasound cannot visualise the mid-third of the ureter, so a normal scan does not exclude stones with 100% certainty. Commonly used to investigate scrotal pathology.
- *Computed tomography (CT)*: Non-contrast CT is the gold standard for diagnosing renal tract calculi. CT-IVU (intravenous urogram) is used to investigate haematuria, and a pre- and post-contrast CT is used to differentiate benign and malignant renal masses.
- *Contrast studies*: Retrograde and anterograde uretero-pyelography.
- Urodynamic studies
- Angiography
- Magnetic resonance imaging (MRI)
- Isotope studies (Marley 2011, Stewart and Finney 2012, Fowler 2013b).

Common diagnoses

- Urinary tract infections
    - Pyelonephritis
    - Acute cystitis
    - Prostatitis
    - Epididymo-orchitis
    - Tuberculosis of the bladder
    - Schistosomiasis
- Upper urinary tract: kidneys and ureters
    - Malignancy
        - *Renal cell carcinoma (RCC), also known as renal cell adenocarcinoma*: Clear cell, papillary, chromophobe, collecting duct and medullary subtypes
        - Transitional cell carcinoma (TCC)
        - *Nephroblastoma (Wilms tumour)*: Childhood urological malignancy
    - Stone disease
    - Retroperitoneal fibrosis
    - Congenital abnormalities
        - Cysts
        - Horseshoe and pelvic kidney
        - Ureteric duplication
        - Congenital pelviureteric junction obstruction
        - Megaureter
        - Vesicoureteric reflux
- Lower urinary tract
    - Urinary retention
    - Bladder cancer: TCC, squamous cell carcinoma and adenocarcinoma
    - Interstitial cystitis
- Prostate gland
    - Prostatitis
    - Benign prostatic hyperplasia (BPH)
    - Prostate cancer
- Penis and male urethra
    - Phimosis
    - Paraphimosis

  - Urethral stricture
  - Peyronie's disease
  - Priapism
- Testes and scrotum
  - Testicular torsion
  - Undescended testes
  - Testicular cancer
  - Scrotal swellings (La Rochelle *et al.* 2010, Stewart and Finney 2012, Eardley 2013a,b, Fowler 2013a, Hamdy 2013, Neal and Shaw 2013).

Urological surgery

Urology surgery can be divided into endoscopic procedures, robotic and laparoscopic procedures and open procedures.

Endoscopic procedures

- *Cystoscopy*: Visualisation of the urethra, and prostate in men; positioning of the ureteric orifices bilaterally; and normality of the bladder mucosa. Can be performed with a rigid or flexible scope. Used to diagnose urethral stricture, bladder stones and carcinoma of the urethra and bladder. It can help assess prostatic size, especially if there is a prominent middle lobe, and gauge whether the lateral lobes are occlusive or not. During a cystoscopy, the surgeon can perform multiple procedures:
  - Biopsy suspicious lesions
  - Diathermy bleeding points or small bladder tumours
  - Bladder washout
  - Catheterise the ureter, for x-ray studies or to insert an indwelling ureteric stent to bypass an obstruction from a stone or tumour.
- *Ureteroscopy*: Semi-rigid ureteroscopy is used to visualise the inside of the ureter to the renal pelvis. Flexible ureteroscopy is used to visualise the renal pelvis and calyces. Suspicious ureteric lesions can be biopsied, and holmium laser can be used to fragment small stones and extract them with a basket by passing the instruments through the working channel of the scope.
- Transurethral resections are performed with a resectoscope. An electric current passes through a loop at the end of the scope, and this cuts and removes tissue, cauterising the tissue to limit bleeding. The loop is then switched to a roller ball, and a lower electric current is passed through this to coagulate the area and achieve haemostasis.
  - *Transurethral resection of prostate*: Performed on patients with acute and chronic retention as a result of prostatic hypertrophy.
  - *Transurethral resection of bladder tumour*: Used to completely resect bladder tumours.

Robotic and laparoscopic procedures

The da Vinci robot is used a lot in urological surgery. It allow better visualisation, better dexterity because the instruments can move in all directions and improved precision compared with laparoscopic surgery.

- *Radical prostatectomy*: This is complete removal of the prostate for localised adenocarcinoma. An extended lymph node dissection may also be undertaken at the time of surgery if the patient is deemed to be at high risk of lymph node metastasis.
- *Partial nephrectomy*: Nephron-sparing surgery; this is used to remove malignant renal tumours (RCCs) 4 cm or smaller. It is occasionally used for larger tumours if the patient has impaired renal function normally or bilateral tumours.

- *Nephrectomy*: Complete removal of the kidney for malignancy or because it is a non-functioning kidney due to congenital abnormality or secondary to chronic obstruction. Indications for removal include persisting pain or recurrent infections.
- *Nephro-ureterectomy*: This is the removal of the kidney and ureter all the way down to the vesicouretric junction due to TCC of the renal pelvis or ureter.
- *Pyeloplasty*: Surgical reconstruction of the renal pelvis. Commonly performed due to pelviureteric junction obstruction. The abnormal pelviureteric junction is removed, and the renal pelvis is anastomosed to the proximal ureter. The procedure improves the drainage of urine and reduces the pelvic dead space.

Open procedures

- *Circumcision*: Performed for religious reasons, phimosis, recurrent balanitis and cancer of the penis
- *Hydrocelectomy*: Performed for patients with symptomatic hydroceles
- *Orchidopexy*: Indicated for a patient with an undescended or ectopic testicle or to resolve testicular torsion
- *Urethroplasty*: Repair of an abnormal urethra (e.g. due to a stricture or fistula)
- *Urinary diversions*: If the bladder needs to be removed, there needs to be an alternative pathway created for urination. A conduit may be created by detaching the ureters from the bladder and connecting this to a detached bowel segment, brought out as a stoma (urostomy).
- *Cystoplasty*: This is bladder augmentation commonly performed in patients who have poor bladder compliance (non-stretchy) or a small bladder capacity to allow continence and prevent renal failure from resulting hydronephrosis. A section of bowel is anastomosed into the bladder to increase its volume and reduce pressure. *Neuropathic indications*: Spina bifida, spinal cord injury and tethered spinal cord. *Non-neuropathic indications*: Detrusor over-activity, radiation cystitis, chronic cystitis and genitourinary tuberculosis.
- *Cystectomy*: Removal of the bladder (and prostate in men), obturator, external and internal iliac lymph nodes and potentially the urethra. Usually performed for malignancy invading the bladder muscle. Women will have a simultaneous hysterectomy (La Rochelle *et al.* 2010, Marley 2011, Stewart and Finney 2012, Eardley 2013a,b, Fowler 2013a, Hamdy 2013, Neal and Shaw 2013).

All of the robotic and laparoscopic procedures can also be performed open but rarely are in current practice.

35 Breast Surgery

Not all patients presenting with breast disease will require surgical intervention. However, for patients with breast cancer, surgery is required to remove the tumour.

Breast clinic

Patients presenting with breast symptoms are normally referred to a specialised breast clinic, where a triple assessment is made for a quick diagnosis using:

- History taking and clinical examination
- Imaging (mammogram +/– ultrasound)
- Fine-needle aspiration (Pearsall 2011, Sainsbury 2013).

Specific evaluation of breast patients

A number of specific items can be highlighted during the history which are important in distinguishing between benign and malignant diseases:

- Patient's age
- Age at onset of menstruation
- Age of menopause
- History of menstrual irregularities
- Age at first pregnancy
- Number of pregnancies
- History of breastfeeding
- Duration and use of oral contraceptives or hormone replacement medications
- Past history of breast complaints and interventions
- Previous history of radiation exposure
- Family history of breast, ovarian and prostate cancer (Dixon 2012, Sainsbury 2013).

When evaluating patients who present with a breast lump, the practitioner needs to assess the patient to establish:

- When and how it was found
- If it has changed
- If it is painful
- Timing in relation to menstrual cycle
- Nipple discharge
- Nipple or skin retraction
- Other associated skin changes
- Fatigue
- Weight loss
- Bone pain
- Breathlessness (Dixon 2012, Sainsbury 2013).

Rapid Perioperative Care, First Edition. Paul Wicker and Sara Dalby.

Factors which increase the risk of breast cancer

A number of factors increase an individual's chances of breast cancer:

- Age
- Dietary fat
- Alcohol consumption
- Reproductive or hormone history
- Personal or family history of breast cancer
- History of radiation exposure
- History of benign breast disease (Pearsall 2011).

Management of high-risk patients

If a patient is determined as being high risk, they can be incorporated into a surveillance programme. Clinical examinations, mammograms and sometimes magnetic resonance imaging (MRI) scans are performed for patients with a family history and a personal history of breast cancer, and they are carried out at defined intervals (Sainsbury 2013).

Chemotherapy and radiotherapy are used in some cases with surgery in women who have high-risk tumours or involved lymph nodes, resulting in prolonged survival.

Surgery for women with breast cancer can be breast conserving, which involves a wide local excision of the tumour and a cuff of healthy tissue, or a mastectomy. At the same time, most women with breast tumours will undergo a procedure on the axilla to help stage their disease. This is called a *sentinel node biopsy* and involves giving a radioactive dye to the breast. The dye will drain to the first lymph node that the cancer would spread to, and this can be identified and removed. If this node contains evidence of cancer, the patient will need a further procedure to remove all lymph nodes in that axilla – an axillary clearance (Sainsbury 2013).

In rare cases where women carry a gene that predisposes them to breast cancer (BRCA), a prophylactic mastectomy may be offered. Even following surgery, there may be some breast tissue in situ; therefore, all risk cannot be removed.

Breast disease

Benign breast disease

Mastalgia (breast pain): Usually occurs at the beginning of the menstrual cycle, with the pain escalating until just before menstruation.

Breast lumpiness and lumps: It is sometimes difficult to determine between the general lumpiness of breast tissue and an isolated lump. The age of the patient and whether the lump is painful can influence the clinician's diagnosis.

- *Lumpiness*: This is commonly part of normal breast tissues as they develop and differs on an individual basis. It may be localised which makes it difficult to determine if a lump is present.
- *Discrete single lump*: The benign causes are trauma, breast cysts, fibroadenoma and localised fibroadenosis. (Sainsbury 2013)

Nipple discharge: Pathologic discharge is unilateral from one duct which may be clear, brownish or bloody. Normally, green or milky discharge is harmless. However, management depends on if there is a lump, there is a bloody discharge or it is from a single duct. Cytology may reveal malignancy, but a negative result does not necessarily exclude carcinoma (Sainsbury 2013).

Breast abscess: Breastfeeding women get cracks in the nipple through which bacteria access the breast tissue, causing cellulitis and a build-up of pus (Dixon 2012).

Breast cancer

Breast cancers are usually associated with fibrous tissue proliferation, causing the surrounding tissues to contract and resulting in dimpling and nipple inversion. Breast cancer can be classified as either invasive cancer or carcinoma in situ. These can also be classified regarding whether they involve the ducts or lobes of the breast. The most common is ductal carcinoma in situ (DCIS) or ductal adenocarcinoma.

For most of the 20th century, patients who presented with breast cancer had a radical mastectomy, which is extremely invasive surgery removing the breast, chest muscle and lymph nodes. Since the 1980s, less radical surgeries have been developed with the aim of preserving breast tissue.

The aim of surgery is local control and breast tissue conservation, which encompasses complete removal of the tumour and local radiotherapy with or without chemotherapy. The factors which determine the specific surgical intervention include cell characteristics, stage and patient choice. For the removal of the lump in the early stages, breast-conserving surgery in the form of a wide local excision is performed with better cosmesis. However, depending on the size of the lesion, location of lesion and size of the breast, a mastectomy may be more appropriate for local control. It is important to perform assessment of the axillary nodes; therefore, an axillary node clearance or node sampling is necessary to plan postoperative management and prognosis (Hindle *et al.* 2011, Pearsall 2011, Sainsbury 2013).

As with other surgical specialities, there has been a move to incorporate minimally invasive surgery; this has been possible due to developments in diagnosing the disease in the early stages. Minimally invasive techniques for the axilla have also been developed. The sentinel lymph node is the first lymphatic node that the primary breast tumour drains to. Therefore, sentinel lymph node biopsy was established; it has increased in frequency, and rates of complications such as lymphoedema, limited arm movements and haematoma of primary surgery patients have been reduced (Bafford *et al.* 2010, Sainsbury 2013).

Surgery and radiotherapy manage the breast cancer locally, with chemotherapy given if lymph nodes have evidence of cancer. Some patients may present with metastatic disease. Common sites of metastatic deposits include the bones which cause bone pain or pathological fractures. Pleural and lung metastases may cause symptomatic pleural effusions which can be aspirated (Dixon 2012).

Reconstruction surgery can be performed to help provide a positive body image for the patient. Reconstruction can be performed during the same operation as the mastectomy, or it can be delayed. Options for reconstruction include a latissimus dorsi flap, a TRAM (transverse rectus abdominus muscle) flap or reconstruction with expanders and prosthesis to produce symmetry for the patient (Sainsbury 2013).

Unusual presentations of breast cancers:

- Paget's disease
- Occult breast cancer presenting as axillary metastases
- Breast cancer during pregnancy
- Non-epithelial tumours
- Male breast cancer (Dixon 2012, Sainsbury 2013).

Surgical procedures

- Fine-needle aspiration
- Trucut biopsy of breast
- Incision and drainage of breast abscess
- Mastectomy
- Latissimus dorsi reconstruction
- Sentinel lymph node biopsy
- Lumpectomy and wide local excision

- Breast augmentation
- Breast reduction (Pearsall 2011, Adam and Wilkinson 2014, De Andrade and Dirkensen 2014, Scott-Conner 2014)

Imaging

- Mammography
- Ultrasound
- MRI (Dixon 2012, Sainsbury 2013)

Tissue diagnosis

- Fine-needle aspiration with cytology
- Wide-bore core biopsy
- Surgical biopsy (Dixon 2012, Sainsbury 2013)

Complications of mastectomy

- Flap necrosis
- Haematoma
- Wound infection
- Seroma
- Arm and shoulder stiffness
- Nerve paresis
- Swollen arm

Risk factors for tumour recurrence

Patients are followed up post surgery, with the following being risk factors of recurrence:

- Younger age
- Positive surgical margin
- Clinical tumour size
- Omission of radiotherapy
- Lymphovascular invasion (Anderson *et al.* 2009).

36 Endocrine Surgery

Most surgical endocrine disorders are genetic, neoplastic or autoimmune. Endocrine surgery involves the thyroid, parathyroid and adrenals. This chapter also includes a brief overview of gastrointestinal disorders.

Thyroid

Tests for thyroid function:

- Serum thyroid hormones
- Thyroid autoantibodies
- Thyroid imaging: chest and thoracic x-rays, ultrasound, computed tomography (CT), magnetic resonance imaging (MRI), positron emission tomography (PET) and isotope scanning
- Fine-needle aspiration cytology (Lal and Clark 2010, Krukowski 2013).

Common thyroid disorders are:

- *Hyperthyroidism (overproduction of T3 and T4, causing thyrotoxicosis)*: The three main causes of thyrotoxicosis are:

  Diffuse toxic goitre – Graves' disease: This is caused by an autoimmune process resulting in abnormal autoantibodies which attack thyroid-stimulating hormone (TSH) receptors. It is more prevalent in females and occurs between 20 and 40 years of age. The thyroid is enlarged but not nodular.

  Multinodular toxic goitre – Plummer's syndrome: This is a nodular goitre which has been present for several years and may become overactive; cardiac arrhythmias and heart failure are common associated factors. The goitre may cause tracheal compression.

  Toxic solitary nodule or adenoma: A single nodule becomes overactive (Lal and Clark 2010, Al-Shoumer and Gharib 2013, Krukowski 2013, Lee *et al.* 2014).

- If a patient presents with thyrotoxicosis, it is necessary to ascertain the cause. Initial treatment for all causes is controlled with medication, followed by definitive treatment of radioactive iodine or surgery for either a solitary toxic node to remove the lobe or total thyroidectomy for Graves' disease and toxic goitre. Following total thyroidectomy, thyroxine replacement therapy will be required; and, for subtotal thyroidectomy, thyroid function tests will need to be monitored for hypothyroidism or recurrence of hyperthyroidism (McHenry and Lo 2013).
- *Hypothyroidism (underproduction of T3 and T4 which can cause myxoedema)*: This requires medical hormone replacement (Krukowski 2013).
- *Enlarged thyroid (goitre)*: This presents as a neck swelling, and it may be smooth or nodular. Large goitres cause discomfort, stridor and dysphagia (due to tracheal and oesophageal compression). It can be caused by pregnancy, iodine deficiency, genetic abnormalities, Graves' disease and Plummer's syndrome.

  It is necessary to determine thyroid function by performing thyroid function tests and to exclude malignancy by ultrasound and fine-needle biopsy (of prominent nodules). Chest x-ray or CT thorax may be used to assess for retrosternal extension of the thyroid.

Rapid Perioperative Care, First Edition. Paul Wicker and Sara Dalby.

The indications for a thyroidectomy include: changes in cosmetic appearance leading to suspected or confirmed malignancy on biopsy; pressure symptoms, such as discomfort, dysphagia and stridor; or, more rarely, for the control of hyperthyroidism following failed medical management (Krukowski 2013, Lee *et al.* 2014).

- *Thyroid nodules*: These solitary thyroid nodules have a number of causes: cyst, primary malignant tumour, metastatic deposit, functioning adenoma, non-functioning adenoma, dominant nodule of a multinodular goitre and localised Hashimoto's disease. One in 10 solitary thyroid nodules are malignant, with risk factors including radiation exposure, iodine deficiency and family history of thyroid carcinoma. If the diagnosis is unconfirmed and there is a concern of malignancy, the affected lobe is removed, an intraoperative frozen section can be undertaken and, if malignant, a total thyroidectomy is performed (Lal and Clark 2010).
- *Thyroid cancer*: The patient will present with a painless lump in the neck which is revealed on examination as a solitary thyroid nodule. Local invasion of nerves may cause stridor, hoarse voice and fixity of the lump. The first sign of disease may be enlarged cervical lymph nodes. Spread can be to lung, bone or brain. There are a number of different malignancies:

  Papillary: These account for over two-thirds of thyroid malignancies, and they are diagnosed with ultrasound and fine-needle aspiration cytology. Treatment is surgical removal with either total thyroid lobectomy or total thyroidectomy; cervical lymph nodes may be resected. Distal metastases may be treated with radioactive iodine.

  Follicular: These account for 20% of thyroid malignancies; diagnosis depends on the presence or absence of extracapsular or venous invasion. Treatment is the same as with papillary tumours.

  Medullary: These are derived from C cells which produce calcitonin that is detected in the bloodstream. Some cases are inherited. It may be associated with other endocrine disorders. Treatment is total thyroidectomy and thyroid replacement treatment.

  Anaplastic: Clinical features of anaplastic malignancies include a goitre, which may have been present for some time but has recently enlarged. Presents as hard woody mass with fixation and is diagnosed with a biopsy. It requires surgical removal and adjuvant radiotherapy.

  Lymphoma: This is rare, with long-standing Hashimoto's thyroiditis as the only known risk factor. Diagnosed with histology (Lal and Clark 2010, Krukowski 2013, Lee *et al.* 2014).

- *Thyroiditis*

  Hashimoto's thyroiditis: This is an autoimmune disease which is thought to occur due to a number of mechanisms where follicular destruction and cellular infiltration of the thyroid may be seen. On examination, patients usually have a firm and irregular goitre. Patients may have raised levels of autoantibodies. Management is with hormone replacement therapy to reduce TSH levels.

  De Quervain's thyroiditis: This is caused by a viral infection which causes inflammation. Patients report acute pain in the neck, a temperature and tender goitre. It is normally self-limiting with full recovery; less than 1% may remain hypothyroid.

  Riedel's thyroiditis: This is a rare condition which causes fibrosis to the surrounding soft tissues in the neck. The patient has a fast increasing goitre which causes oesophageal and trachea compression. Again, it is normally self-limiting, but it may require steroids or surgery (Lal and Clark 2010, Farwell and Braverman 2013, Lee *et al.* 2014).

Parathyroid

Hyperparathyroidism is a common cause of hypercalcaemia. There are three subtypes:

1. Primary hyperparathyroidism
2. Secondary hyperparathyroidism
3. Tertiary hyperparathyroidism.

Primary hyperparathyroidism is the commonest presentation for surgical intervention. By removing the overactive parathyroid gland, the patient will be cured. There are four parathyroids, paired on either side of the thyroid. Either a focused parathyroidectomy may be performed when one parathyroid has been shown on imaging to be enlarged, or a bilateral neck exploration may be undertaken. Intraoperative parathyroid hormone (PTH) monitoring and frozen section are used to help determine if the correct parathyroid has been removed (Lal and Clark 2010, Silverberg and Bilezikian 2013, Ibanet *et al.* 2014).

Adrenal disorders

- *Primary hyperaldosteronism*: This manifests in two types: idiopathic hyperaldosteronism and Conn's syndrome. Conn's syndrome is more common and is a benign aldosterone-secreting tumour which requires surgery.
- *Virilising tumours*: These cause overproduction of sex steroid hormones. Half of these are aggressive adrenocortical cancer and require urgent surgical excision.
- *Cushing's syndrome*: This has a number of causes; patients present with trunk and face obesity, excessive facial hair, muscle weakness, hypertension and osteoporosis. If due to an adrenal adenoma, the treatment is adrenalectomy.
- *Phaeochromocytoma*: This is a tumour in the adrenal medulla or the paraganglionic tissues next to the sympathetic chain. Treatment requires the stabilisation of hypertension prior to surgery, following which excision of the tumour is required. (Lal and Clark 2010, Lennard 2013, Aspinall *et al.* 2014).

Gastrointestinal endocrine tumours

- *Insulinoma*: These make up 70% of all pancreatic endocrine tumours. They secrete insulin and as a consequence cause hypoglycaemia which causes hypoglycaemic attacks, the main reason for diagnosis. Surgical removal is curative.
- *Gastrinoma*: This is the second commonest tumour, and it causes excess secretion of gastric acid leading to severe peptic ulceration (Zollinger–Ellison syndrome). A well-localised tumour can be surgically removed.
- *Carcinoid tumours*: These tumours are often submucosal, and they are found in some resected appendixes as an incidental finding which may lead to a right hemicolectomy.
- *VIPoma*: These tumours secrete vasoactive intestinal peptide, resulting in Verner–Morrison syndrome. This is managed with surgery if there is no proven metastatic spread, in which case the management is chemotherapy (Lennard 2013, Cisco and Norton 2014).

37 Colorectal Surgery

Colorectal surgical procedures vary from large bowel resections to hemorrhoidectomies. The procedures are carried out for a variety of reasons but predominantly inflammatory bowel disease or cancer.

The colon can be divided into four parts: right colon (caecum, ascending colon), transverse, left colon (descending, sigmoid) and rectum. The major functions of the colon are absorption, storage, propulsion and digestion (Dunlop 2012b, Carlson and Epstein 2013).

Investigations

There are a number of potential investigations which may be pertinent to help with the patient diagnosis following history taking and examination, including:

- Bloods, including full blood count (FBC), liver function test (LFT) and urea–electrolytes (UE)
- Diagnostic endoscopic procedures such as sigmoidoscopy or colonoscopy depending on indication
- Abdominal x-ray
- Computed tomography (CT) (chest, abdomen and pelvis) (Dunn and Rothenberger 2010, Dunlop 2012b, Carlson and Epstein 2013).

Colorectal disorders

A number of inflammatory bowel conditions may require surgical interventions:

- *Ulcerative colitis (UC)*: Chronic inflammatory disease which involves the whole or part of the colon. The inflammation is confined to the mucosa. In the majority of instances, it affects the rectum but is not proximal to the ileocaecal valve.

  The common presenting features include:
  - Bloody diarrhoea, causing anaemia, electrolyte disturbances and hypoproteinaemia
  - Rectal bleeding
  - Abdominal pain
  - Fever
  - Weight loss.
- Patients who have UC are at an increased risk of colorectal cancer and require surveillance with regular colonoscopy.

  UC is treated medically in the majority of patients. In patients who fail to respond to medical therapy or have a malignant change, surgical treatment may be required. An elective proctocoloectomy, which is the removal of the entire colon and rectum, results in a permanent end ileostomy. For younger patients, a proctocolectomy with a formation of an ileo-anal pouch is an alternative to a permanent stoma (Carlson and Epstein 2013; Dunlop 2012b; Dunn and Rothenberger 2010).

Rapid Perioperative Care, First Edition. Paul Wicker and Sara Dalby.

- *Crohn's disease*: Another chronic inflammatory bowel disease which can affect anywhere in the gastrointestinal (GI) tract from mouth to anus. It commonly affects the small bowel, especially the terminal ileum and the colon. After repeated attacks on the same area, fibrosis will occur in the inflamed area, resulting in narrowing and causing signs of obstruction. Progressive disease may result in adhesions, intraabdominal abscesses and formation of fistulas.

  Symptoms include:
  - A history of months of mild diarrhea
  - Intermittent fevers
  - Abdominal pain, particularly right iliac fossa
  - Weight loss
  - Perianal problems (perianal abscess, fissure or fistula)
- The patient may be offered medical treatment similar to that of patients with ulcerative colitis, but surgery such as a small bowel resection may be required (Carlson and Epstein 2013, Dunn and Rothenberger 2010, Tavakkolizadeh *et al.* 2010, Dunlop 2012b).
- Diverticular disease results in pouching of the mucosa outwards through the bowel wall, most commonly in the sigmoid colon. Risk factors include chronic constipation, slow transit and lack of fibre.

  Faeces and undigested food stuff get stuck within the neck of the diverticulum, leading to inflammation which can cause diarrhoea and bleeding; and in extreme cases inflammation may result in perforation, a subsequent diverticular abscess or peritonitis. There may also be fistulation through to adjacent organs.

  Diverticular disease can be asymptomatic.

  Acute diverticulitis typical presentation:
  - Gradual onset of left lower quadrant pain
  - Loose motions, bleeding PR
  - Low-grade fever
  - If inflammatory process has spread to adjacent organs, other symptoms include constipation, diarrhoea, anorexia, nausea, vomiting and dysuria.
- Treatment for uncomplicated diverticular disease includes avoiding constipation, so increasing fluid intake, increasing dietary fibre and the use of laxatives are beneficial. Mild cases of acute diverticulitis can be managed with antibiotics and clear fluids. Perforated disease associated with peritonitis requires a laparotomy. An anastomosis is best avoided in the presence of inflammation, so a Hartmann's procedure with the formation of an end colostomy is common. Rectal bleeding due to diverticular haemorrhage can be life-threatening and needs transfusion, identification of the source and therapeutic intervention (Dunn and Rothenberger 2010, Tavakkolizadeh *et al.* 2010, Dunlop 2012b, Carlson and Epstein 2013).
- Volvulus occurs when a loop of bowel twists or rotates around its mesentery which causes luminal obstruction and vascular occlusion. The twist impairs blood supply and so can result in gangrene and perforation, leading to high mortality and morbidity; therefore, early diagnosis is important.

  Intestinal volvulus is associated with specific conditions:
  - Previous abdominal surgery
  - Chronic constipation
  - Parkinson's disease
  - Neurological disorders
  - Diabetes
  - Infectious and ischaemic colitis
- Patient presentation:
  - Abdominal pain
  - Distension
  - Severe or absolute constipation

- Volvulus of the sigmoid colon may be managed non-surgically by introducing a flatus tube for decompression; however, recurrence is common, so a resection may be required. A volvulus involving small bowel or the caecum requires a laparotomy. (Dunn and Rothenberger 2010, Hill 2013).

Colorectal cancer

Colorectal polyps

These include adenomas which can be pre-malignant, malignant polyps which are early cancers, and non-adenoma pus polyps which have no malignant potential.

Most polyps are asymptomatic, but they can present with rectal bleeding or mucus discharge or are found as part of bowel screening or investigations for other symptoms. The histology is important as adenomas may develop into a carcinoma. If a polyp is found, the patient requires a full colonoscopy and any additional polyps must be removed.

Familial adenomatous polyposis is an autosomal dominant condition in which multiple polyps develop, with a progression to cancer. These patients may undergo an elective colectomy to reduce their risk (Dunn and Rothenberger 2010, Dunlop 2012b, Carlson and Epstein 2013).

Cancer

Colorectal cancer affects people mostly in the Western world. A number of factors increase the incidence of colorectal cancer:

- Increased age
- Family history
- Diets high in fat and low in fibre
- Inflammatory bowel disease.

Cancer screening and surveillance have been integrated into patient care, with screening used to identify patients who have asymptomatic colon cancer and surveillance used to monitor identified high-risk patients.

Common presentation:

- Bleeding
- Change of bowel habit
- Unplanned weight loss
- Abdominal pain
- Acute onset of intestinal obstruction
- Perforation.

The majority of patients with colorectal cancer will have a resection to remove the tumour which is potentially curative (Hewitt Richards *et al.* 2010). Curative surgery requires removal of the primary tumour with negative margins and complete oncologic lymphadenectomy. The histology of the specimen, in particular the lymph nodes, will determine the patient's future management (Mourneau *et al.* 2013).

Traditionally, resections were carried out with open procedures; however, there has been a shift to perform laparoscopic resections due to short-term benefits, including faster recovery, shorter length of stay and reduced postoperative pain. The surgical procedure and approach will be determined by the localisation and tumour stage (Berardi *et al.* 2009).

Colonic cancer, especially of the rectum or left colon, can present as large bowel obstruction. It is usually due to a large tumour and has a poor prognosis. The surgical intervention depends on the location of the obstruction.

Perforation of colon cancer has a poor prognosis and high recurrence rate. If feasible, the perforated section should be resected, but in the instance of peritonitis an anastomosis should not be formed (Dunlop 2012b).

Anal, perianal and rectal disorders

Anal disorder presentation:

- Rectal bleeding
- Itching
- Pain on defecation
- Perianal swelling or discharge
- Tenesmus
- Prolapse
- Discharge
- Loss of weight
- Altered bowel habit (Clark 2013).

Patients who present with anal or perianal symptoms require a thorough history and clinical examination, including a per rectal examination. Specialist tests that are needed may include: endo-anal ultrasound, contrast enema, defecography, endoscopy or an examination under anaesthesia.

Benign Diseases

- Anorectal abscess and fistula
- Haemorrhoids
- Pilonidal disease
- Pelvic floor dysfunction
- Benign tumours

Anal Neoplasms

- Squamous cell carcinoma
- Basal cell carcinoma
- Bowen's disease
- Epidermoid carcinoma (Dunn and Rothenberger 2010, Dunlop 2012a, Clark 2013, Lunniss and Nugent 2013)

Procedures

- Minor
    - Haemorrhoidectomy
    - Treatment of perianal fistulas
    - Treatment of anal fissures
    - Perianal abscess – incision and drainage
    - Removal of anal skin tags
- Intermediate
    - Formation of a stoma
    - Reversal of a loop stoma
    - Trans-anal endoscopic microsurgery (TEMS)
    - Rectal prolapse surgery

- Major
  - Right hemicolectomy
  - Left hemicolectomy
  - Anterior resection
  - Abdominoperineal resection
  - Sigmoid colectomy
  - Hartmann's procedure
  - Reversal of Hartmann's procedure (Dunn and Rothenberger 2010, Tavakkolizadeh *et al.* 2010, Dunlop 2012a, Carlson and Epstein 2013, Clark 2013, Lunniss and Nugent 2013)

Colon tests and investigations

- Faecal occult blood testing
- Flexible sigmoidoscopy
- Colonoscopy
- Barium enema
- Computed tomography (CT) colonography
- CT abdomen (Dunn and Rothenberger 2010, Carlson and Epstein 2013)

Indications for resections

- Failure to respond to conservative or medical treatment in any condition
- Diverticula causing perforation, obstruction or bleeding
- Infective conditions causing bleeding or perforation
- Inflammatory conditions
- Neoplastic conditions
- Trauma
- Vascular complications (Carlson and Epstein 2013)

Factors to consider with anastamosis

- Appropriate bowel prep if required
- Antibiotic prophylaxis
- Early pedicle ligation to identify resection line
- Good blood supply (most important)
- Minimal disparity of bowel lumen
- Anastomosis should not be under tension.
- Avoid anastomosis if:
  - Perforation
  - Inflammation
  - Ischaemia
  - Obstruction
  - Sepsis. (Dunn and Rothenberger 2010)

Complications of colonic resection

- Haemorrhage
- Anastomotic leak
- Local and systematic sepsis
- Increased frequency or urgency of bowel movements

- Hernias
- Damage to sexual function
- Ureteric damage
- Pneumonia
- Deep vein thrombosis and pulmonary embolism
- Myocardial infarction (Korner *et al.* 2009)

38 Upper Gastrointestinal Surgery

Oesophagus

Symptoms

Patients with oesophageal problems commonly present with a number of symptoms:

- Dysphagia
- Odynophagia
- Weight loss
- Pain in back or epigastrium
- Reflux symptoms
- Cough (Alderson 2013).

INVESTIGATIONS FOR OESOPHAGEAL CLINICAL SYMPTOMS There are a number of potential investigations depending on the clinical presentation of the patient. In almost all cases, if pathology in the oesophagus is suspected, direct visualisation is indicated.

- Oesophago-gastro-duodenoscopy (OGD) and biopsies
- Water-soluble or barium swallow
- Manometry and pH studies
- Blood tests, full blood count, urea and electrolytes, liver function tests and clotting studies
- Chest x-ray
- Computed tomography (CT) chest and abdomen
- Endoluminal ultrasound
- Bronchoscopy
- PET scan (Hardwick 2012, Couper 2014).

Dysphagia

The main clinical presentation of a patient who has a problem with their oesophagus is dysphagia. If it is progressive, this may be a sign that it is a malignant growth or stricture, whereas non-progressive suggests a functional disorder.

Dysphagia of the oesophagus can be categorised as being caused:

- In the lumen
  - Foreign body
- In the wall
  - Carcinoma
  - Achalasia
  - Scleroderma
  - Stricture (inflammatory)
  - Plummer–Vinson

Rapid Perioperative Care, First Edition. Paul Wicker and Sara Dalby.

  - Post radiotherapy
  - Atresia (congenital)
- Outside of the lumen
  - Mediastinal lymphadenopathy
  - Bronchial carcinoma.

Some neurological conditions may also cause dysphagia, such as bulbar palsy and myasthenia gravis (Jobe *et al.* 2010).

Oesophageal perforation

Two common causes include iatrogenic causes following therapeutic dilatation and Boerhaave's syndrome. Boerhaave's syndrome is oesophageal perforation due to vomiting against a closed glottis. Overwhelming mediastinal sepsis quickly ensues, and an emergency thoracotomy is often indicated. Less common causes include foreign bodies and ingestion of corrosive liquid (Shenfine and Griffin 2014).

Signs of oesophageal perforation include pain, sepsis, pneumothorax, air within the mediastinum and surgical emphysema.

Corrosive oesophagitis

This can occur from the ingestion of corrosive substances. Oesophageal strictures may form. Oesophageal dilatation is often required, and in extreme cases surgery is indicated (Shenfine and Griffin 2014).

Gastro-oesophageal reflux (GORD)

An incompetent physiological gastro-oesophageal sphincter can give rise to the reflux of gastric acid up the oesophagus. Causes include anything that can physically disrupt the sphincter such as hiatus hernia, obesity and pregnancy. Drugs can also lead to a relaxation of the sphincter; causes include smoking, caffeine and alcohol.

Chronic reflux can cause Barrett's oesophagus which may lead to stricture or malignancy, subsequently requiring surgical intervention. Drugs to reduce the acid production in the stomach such as proton pump inhibitors (PPIs) can significantly reduce the symptoms of GORD and may obviate the need for surgery (Findlay and Maynard 2014).

Hiatus hernia

These can be categorised into two types: sliding in which reflux is common and rolling in which reflux does not occur. Strangulation of the hernia is more likely to occur with the rolling type. Surgical intervention can be taken in the form of Nissens fundoplication, which is taken if conservative measures fail and the reflux is substantial (Findlay and Maynard 2014).

Oesophageal tumours

Can be categorised into benign; benign oesophageal tumours account for 2%, are often asymptomatic and are removed by local excision. Malignant tumours are more common.

- Benign
  - Leiomyoma
  - Polyp
  - Haemangioma
  - Granular cell tumour

- Malignant
  - Squamous cell carcinoma
  - Adenocarcinoma
  - Primary melanoma
  - Small cell carcinoma

The only potential cure for a malignant oesophageal cancer is surgical resection, in the form of an oesophagectomy. If surgery is not feasible, radiotherapy +/– chemotherapy may be used, but results are variable. Oesophageal stenting may be another possible course of action (Jobe *et al.* 2010).

Peptic ulceration

Peptic ulcers can occur in the stomach, the duodenum, and to a lesser extent the oesophagus. Causes include the use of NSAIDs, smoking and alcohol and *Helicobacter pylori* infection. Symptoms often include epigastric pain. Patients are managed with conservative treatment initially to reduce acid production with medication such as proton pump inhibitors, and they are advised to address risk factors. The mainstay of investigation is direct visualisation with OGD. Surgical intervention is now very rare but includes vagotomy and even partial gastrectomy (Primrose and Underwood 2013).

Gastric neoplasia

Benign gastric neoplasms may originate from epithelial or mesenchymal tissue.

- Adenomatous polyps
- *Gastrointestinal stromal tumours (GISTs)*: Small and asymptomatic, these can be left alone; however, larger ones need to be under surveillance or possibly resected.

Gastric carcinomas are divided into four main types:

- Adenocarcinoma, which makes up approximately 90%
- Lymphoma
- Carcinoid
- Gastrointestinal stromal tumours (Hardwick 2014).

Common presenting features are:

- Weight loss
- Pain
- Nausea and vomiting
- Abdominal discomfort
- Dysphagia
- Upper gastrointestinal (GI) bleeding.

An early diagnosis is imperative for a cure, with the only curative treatment being surgical resection with neoadjuvant chemotherapy (Primrose and Underwood 2013).

Miscellaneous disorders of the stomach

Other disorders of the stomach which may require surgical intervention include:

- Menetrier's disease
- Gastritis
- Dieulafoy's lesion
- Bezoars. (Hardwick 2012)

Miscellaneous disorders of the duodenum

Additional duodenal disorders which may need surgical intervention include:

- Duodenal obstruction
- Duodenal diverticula
- Duodenal trauma
- Surgery for obesity (Hardwick 2012).

Acute upper GI bleeding

This is a life-threatening emergency; the commonest presentations are hematemesis and melena. A substantial amount of bleeding may result in the patient with the following symptoms:

- Fainting
- Pallor
- Sweating
- Tachycardia
- Hypotension
- Tachypnoea.

The most frequent causes are:

- Peptic ulceration
- Oesophageal varices
- Gastroduodenal erosions (unlikely to cause significant bleeding)
- Malignancy.

Management of a patient presenting with GI bleeding and shock needs to be simultaneous with treatment incorporating prompt resuscitation and investigation to diagnose the source of bleeding. The initial intervention may be endoscopic to inject adrenaline into an ulcer, to clip a bleeding artery, for diathermy bleeding or for banding of varicies. Failing endoscopic intervention, surgical intervention in the form of laparotomy with direct control of bleeding may be required (Wayman 2014).

39 Hepato-Pancreato-Biliary Surgery

Hepato-pancreato-biliary surgery involves the treatment of surgical conditions in the liver, pancreas and biliary system.

Liver disease

Liver disease is a common presentation, and it manifests in a number of clinical features, such as jaundice in biliary obstruction. However, patients with liver disease can present with jaundice without biliary obstruction, and with portal hypertension, low serum albumin and clotting disorders in patients with chronic hepatic failure.

- A patient with chronic biliary obstruction has jaundice with usually (but not always) abnormal liver function tests (LFTs). These can be categorised as surgical (i.e. dilated) ducts or medical (i.e. undilated) ducts usually due to medication.
- The most common cause of portal hypertension is cirrhosis due to alcohol disease. Surgical intervention may be needed if there is a variceal haemorrhage which cannot be stopped endoscopically.
- Chronic hepatic failure usually occurs in patients with a degree of liver failure, normally due to liver cirrhosis as a consequence of liver disease. A surgeon may be asked to assist with the management of a patient with ascites (Geller *et al.* 2010, Koti *et al.* 2013).

Liver tumours

Benign tumours: These are rare and can be categorised as solid or cystic lesions.

- Liver cysts
- Liver cell adenoma
- Focal nodular hyperplasia
- Hepatic adenomas

They may require surgical intervention for prevention of haemorrhage, for relief of symptoms or to exclude malignancy if there is a risk of malignancy or any diagnostic uncertainty.

Malignant tumours: Due to improved screening, there has been an increase in the number of resectable primary and secondary liver tumours. The resectability depends upon functional ability and anatomical position.

- Hepatocellular carcinoma
- Cholangiocarcinoma
- Liver metastases: commonest areas are primary colon, breast, lung, pancreas and stomach (Geller *et al.* 2010, Garden 2012, Koti *et al.* 2013).

Rapid Perioperative Care, First Edition. Paul Wicker and Sara Dalby.

Liver cysts

Liver cysts can be divided into:

- Simple lesion
- Hydatid cyst
- Neoplastic cysts
- They tend to non-symptomatic, usually being diagnosed incidentally. Simple cysts which are not causing the patients any problems are usually left and monitored. Symptomatic cysts should be treated by external drainage, cyst deroofing or cyst removal–liver resection (Geller *et al.* 2010).

Liver infections

Classified as bacterial, fungal or parasitic, the main categories are:

- Viral hepatitis
- Ascending cholangitis
- Pyogenic liver abscess
- Amoebic liver abscess
- Hydatid disease (Geller *et al.* 2010, Garden 2012, Koti *et al.* 2013).

Liver trauma

Liver injuries are graded I–VI, ranging from small haematomas to complete hepatic avulsion. If the patient is haemodynamically stable, then a non-operative management course is preferred. However, it may be necessary for surgical intervention in patients with blunt liver trauma in order to control major haemorrhage. In this instance, packing of the liver with swabs may control bleeding; in severe cases, a liver resection may be required (Koti *et al.* 2013).

Biliary tract

Patients presenting to surgical units with conditions affecting the biliary tract are very common. Most patients present with benign conditions related to the presence of gallstones. Rarely, patients present with malignant conditions manifesting in the biliary tract.

Gallstones are caused by excess cholesterol in bile, bile stasis or increased bilirubin.

Complications of Gallstones

- Gallbladder
  - *Biliary colic*: A spasmodic pain in the right upper quadrant caused by contraction of the gallbladder or common bile duct (CBD) as it tries to expel a stone. Treatment of this condition in the acute setting is primarily symptomatic. The definitive surgical treatment for recurrent biliary colic is a cholecytectomy (removal of the gallbladder).
- *Acute cholecystitis*: An infection of the gallbladder characterised by constant right upper quadrant pain and fever. In the acute setting, treatment is with antibiotics, analgesia and fluids. Traditionally, patients were brought back to have their gallbladder removed electively once the infection had settled. However, the latest guidance advises cholecystectomy within 72 h of onset of symptoms.
- Common bile duct
  - *Biliary colic*: See above.
  - *Obstructive jaundice*: If a stone within the CBD becomes stuck, it will prevent the drainage of bile, making the patient become jaundiced. Patient presenting with an

obstructing CBD stone will require endoscopic retrograde cholangiography (ERCP) to identify the point of obstruction and remove the stone.
  - *Cholangitis*: Occasionally, an obstructing stone within the CBD can cause a serious infection of the biliary tract called cholangitis. This condition is characterised by right upper quadrant pain, fever and jaundice (Charcot's triad). Management is with IV antibiotics, fluids and analgesia. Patient will also require an emergency inpatient ERCP to relieve the blockage and will ultimately require a cholecystectomy to prevent future attacks.
  - *Pancreatitis*: Just before the CBD enters the duodenum, it joins with the pancreatic duct. An obstruction at this junction can cause an inflammatory reaction in the pancreas known as pancreatitis (see the "Pancreatic Disease" section).
- Small intestine
  - *Gallstone ileus*: A rare compilation of gallstones where a stone passes out of the CBD into the duodenum and gets stuck within the small bowel (most commonly at the ileocaecal valve), causing small bowel obstruction. Should this occur, patients may require a laparotomy to remove the stone and relieve the obstruction (Oddsdottir *et al.* 2010, Garden 2012, Conlon 2013).

Biliary strictures

A number of conditions can be associated with benign biliary strictures; the most common causes are inflammation or due to an injury to the bile duct. Causes include:

- Traumatic
- Congenital
- Bile duct injuries
- Radiotherapy
- Post-inflammatory
- Primary sclerosing cholangitis
- Sphincter of Oddi stenosis (Oddsdottir *et al.* 2010, Conlon 2013).

Gallbladder tumours

Cancers of the gallbladder or bile duct are uncommon malignancies. Treatment in stage I and II is removal. In patients with stage III, the spread may be into the right lobe of the liver; this may need to be removed as well as the gallbladder.

- Benign tumours
- Gallbladder cancer (Oddsdottir *et al.* 2010, Conlon 2013)

Biliary tract cancers

Cancers of the gallbladder or bile ducts (cholangiocarinoma) are uncommon malignancies. Signs and symptoms include abnormal LFTs, abdominal pain, painless jaundice and weight loss.

Complete surgical resection is the only curative intervention. Unfortunately, cancers of the biliary tract are often asymptomatic until an advanced stage of disease, and fewer than 33% are operable at the point of diagnosis. In patients with unresectable tumours, chemotherapy and radiotherapy may help slow the progression of disease (Oddsdottir *et al.* 2010, Garden 2012, Conlon 2013).

Pancreatic disease

Pancreatitis is inflammation of the pancreas, and it can be acute or chronic.

Acute pancreatitis

Gallstones and alcohol excess account for up to 80% of cases of acute pancreatitis. Other common causes include medications (particularly steroids), trauma, metabolic disorders, infection, and genetic and autoimmune conditions.

Patients with acute pancreatitis typically present with severe epigastric pain radiating through to the back associated with a raised serum amylase. A computed tomography (CT) scan may be necessary to confirm the diagnosis or assess its severity. Multiple different scoring systems exist to classify the severity of acute pancreatitis, but most cases can be broadly divided into mild or severe (Fisher *et al.* 2010, McKay and Carter 2012).

Mild acute pancreatitis: The majority of attacks are mild and are characterised by minimal organ disruption and an uneventful recovery. No surgical intervention is required, and treatment is primarily supportive.

Severe pancreatitis: This is associated with significant pancreatic necrosis and a systemic inflammatory response. Patients can become critically ill and develop multi-organ failure. Treatment is again primarily supportive, although surgery may be required in the presence of significant pancreatic or peripancreatic necrosis or collections, especially if these become infected. Open surgical debridement has largely been replaced by minimally invasive techniques such as transgastric endoscopy necrosectomy and minimally invasive retroperitoneal necrosectomy (Bhattacharya 2013).

Chronic pancreatitis

Following repeated or severe attacks of acute pancreatitis, patients may develop chronic pancreatitis. The most common cause is alcohol abuse. Chronic pancreatitis is characterised by a chronic persistent pain with intermittent acute inflammatory exasperations (acute-on-chronic pancreatitis). The subclinical morphological derangement and fibrotic changes caused by chronic inflammation can lead to exocrine and endocrine failure of the gland and predispose patients to developing pancreatic cancer (Fisher *et al.* 2010, Bhattacharya 2013).

Indications for surgical intervention include intractable pain, complications to adjacent organs (i.e. distal CBD stenosis) or if pancreatic cancer is suspected. Surgical treatment aims to provide pain relief, treat complications and preserve exocrine and endocrine pancreatic function. The three surgical options are a Whipple's pancreatoduodenectomy, pylorus-preserving pancreatoduodenectomy and duodenum-preserving pancreatic head resection (Beger's procedure) (McKay and Carter 2012).

Pancreatic carcinoma

- *Pancreatic ductal adenocarcinoma*: This is the most common type of pancreatic cancer, accounting for 85% of cases. It is difficult to treat, surgical intervention is high risk and the survival rate is low predominantly due to late diagnosis. Risk factors for pancreatic cancer include family history, smoking, poor diet, diabetes, genetics and chronic pancreatitis. Presenting features include anorexia, weight loss, malaise, epigastric discomfort, pain and jaundice. Complete surgical resection represents the only possible cure. Unfortunately, pancreatic cancer is often asymptomatic until an advanced stage. As a result, many patients present with inoperable disease due to the presence of distant metastases or early encasement of the superior mesenteric vessels.

For those able to undergo surgery, the operation chosen depends upon the location of the tumour. For tumours in the head, neck or body of the pancreas, the most common operation is a *pylorus-preserving* or *non-pylorus-preserving* (Whipple's) *pancreatoduodenectomy*. This operation removes en bloc the distal portion of the stomach, duodenum, gallbladder, CBD and head of pancreas. For cancers in the tail of the pancreas, a left/distal pancreatectomy may be performed (Fisher *et al.* 2010, McKay and Carter 2012).

- *Cystic tumours of the pancreas*: These are a rare group of tumours which arise from the pancreatic duct tissue. They are predominantly incurable, but sometimes operable; they are important as a differential diagnosis for pancreatic cysts. Presenting symptoms are mild pain in the upper abdomen, weight loss, palpable mass and nausea and vomiting. Surgical treatment is a laparotomy and excision.
- *Neuroendocrine tumour*: These are uncommon, generally slow-growing tumours. Surgical resection is the only prospective cure.
- *Periampullary tumour*: This tumour originates near the ampulla of Vater. The tumour cells can arise from the pancreas, distal bile duct or duodenum. Surgery treatment is either a pylorus-preserving or Whipple's pancreatoduodenectomy (Bhattacharya 2013).

References and Further Reading

28. Laparoscopic Surgery

References

Care Quality Commission (CQC) (2010) *Position Statement and Action Plan for Safe and Effective Care 2010–2015*. London, CQC.

Clarke JR (2009) Designing Safety into the Minimally Invasive Surgical Revolution: A Commentary Based on the Jaques Perissat Lecture of the International Congress of the European Association for Endoscopic Surgery. *Surgical Endoscopy* **23** (1): 216–220.

Goodman T and Spry C (2014) *Essentials of Perioperative Nursing*, 5th ed. Burlington MA, Jones and Bartlett Learning.

Hamlin L, Richardson-Trench M and Davies M (2010) *Perioperative Nursing: An Introductory Text*. Sydney, Elsevier Australia.

Jayaraman S, Quan D, Al-Ghamdi I, El-Deen F and Schlachta CM (2010) Does Robotic Assistance Improve Efficiency in Performing Complex Minimally Invasive Surgical Procedures? *Surgical Endoscopy* **24**: 584–588.

Mabrouk M, Frumovitz M, Greer M, Sharma S, Schmeler KM, Soliman PT and Ramirez PT (2009) Trends in Laparoscopic and Robotic Surgery among Gynecologic Oncologists: A Survey Update. *Gynaecological Oncology* **112** (3): 501–505.

Mohammad AH, Underwood T, Taylor MG, Hamdan K, Elberm H and Pearce NW (2010) Bleeding and Haemostasis in Laparoscopic Liver Surgery. *Surgical Endoscopy* **24**: 572–577.

Moran EA, Bingener J and Gostout CJ (2010) Functional and Comparative Evaluation of Flexible Monopolar Endoscopic Scissors. *Surgical Endoscopy* **24**: 1769–1773.

Romanelli JR, Roshek TB, Lynn DC and Earle DB (2009) Single-Port Laparoscopic Cholecystectomy: Initial Experience. *Surgical Endoscopy* **24**: 1374–1379.

Saber AA, El-Ghazaly TH, Lain A and Dewoolkar AV (2010) Single-Incision Laparoscopic Placement of an Adjustable Gastric Band versus Conventional multiport Laparoscopic Gastric Banding: A Comparative Study. *The American Surgeon* **76** (12): 1328–1332.

Ulmer BC (2010) Best Practices for Minimally Invasive Procedures. *AORN Journal* **91** (5): 558–575.

Walters L and Eley S (2011) Robotic-Assisted Surgery and the Need for Standardized Pathways and Clinical Guidelines. *AORN Journal* **93**: (4) 455–463.

Whalan C (2008) Laparoscopic Surgery. In Whalan C (ed) *Assisting at Surgical Operations: A Practical Guide*. Cambridge, Cambridge University Press, pp. 103–117.

Further Reading

Hunter JG and Jobe BA (2010) Minimally Invasive Surgery, Robotics, and Natural Orifice Transluminal Endoscopic Surgery. In Brunicardia FC, Andersen DK, Billiar TR, Dunn DL, Hunter JG, Matthews JB and Pollock RE (eds) *Schwartz's Principles of Surgery*, 9th ed. New York, McGraw-Hill, pp. 359–378.

Websites

Association of Laparoscopic Surgeons of Great Britain and Ireland: www.alsgbi.org

British Hernia Society: www.britishherniasociety.org

European Association for Endoscopic Surgery and other interventional techniques: http://www.eaes-eur.org/home.aspx

29. Vascular Surgery

References

Bradbury AW and Cleveland TJ (2012) Vascular and Endovascular Surgery. In Garden OJ, Bradbury AW, Forsythe JLR and Parks RW (eds) *Principles and Practice of Surgery*, 6th ed. London, Elsevier, pp. 345–378.

Liem TK and Moneta GL (2010) Venous and Lymphatic Disease. In Brunicardia FC, Andersen DK, Billiar TR, Dunn DL, Hunter JG, Matthews JB and Pollock RE (eds) *Schwartz's Principles of Surgery*, 9th ed. New York, McGraw-Hill, pp. 777–802.

Lin PH, Kougias P, Bechara C, Cagiannos C, Huynh TT and Chen CJ (2010) Arterial Disease. In Brunicardia FC, Andersen DK, Billiar TR, Dunn DL, Hunter JG, Matthews JB and Pollock RE (eds) *Schwartz's Principles of Surgery*, 9th ed. New York, McGraw-Hill, pp. 701–776.

McCollum P and Chetter I (2013) Venous Disorders. In Williams NS, Bulstrode CJK and O'Connell PR (eds) *Bailey & Love's Short Practice of Surgery*, 26th ed. Kent, CRC Press, pp. 901–922.

Sayers R (2013) Arterial Disorders. In Williams NS, Bulstrode CJK and O'Connell PR (eds) *Bailey & Love's Short Practice of Surgery*, 26th ed. Kent, CRC Press, pp. 877–900.

Wieczorek P (2011) Vascular Surgery. In Rothrock JC (ed) *Alexander's Care of the Patient in Surgery*, 14th ed. St. Louis, Elsevier Mosby, pp. 969–1001.

Further Reading

Beard JD, Gaines PA and Loftus I (2014) *Vascular and Endovascular Surgery: A Companion to Specialist Surgical Practice*, 5th ed. Oxford, Saunders Elsevier.

Scott-Conner CEH (2014) *Scott-Conner & Dawson Essential Operative Techniques and Anatomy*, 4th ed. Philadelphia, Lippincott Williams & Wilkins.

Websites

European Society for Vascular Surgery: www.esvs.org
Vascular Society: www.vascularsociety.org.uk

30. Cardiothoracic Surgery

References

Anderson JR and Zakkar M (2013) Cardiac Surgery. In Williams NS, Bulstrode CJK and O'Connell PR (eds) *Bailey & Love's Short Practice of Surgery*, 26th ed. Kent, CRC Press, pp. 823–849.

Blanchard B (2011) Thoracic Surgery. In Rothrock JC (ed) *Alexander's Care of the Patient in Surgery*, 14th ed. St. Louis, Elsevier Mosby, pp. 936–968.

Bojar RM (2011) *Manual of Perioperative Care in Adult Cardiac Surgery*, 5th ed. Oxford, Wiley-Blackwell.

Hunt I and Tan C (2013) The Thorax. In Williams NS, Bulstrode CJK and O'Connell PR (eds) *Bailey & Love's Short Practice of Surgery*, 26th ed. Kent, CRC Press, pp. 850–876.

Karamlou TB, Welke KF and Ungerleider RM (2010) Congenital Heart Disease. In Brunicardia FC, Andersen DK, Billiar TR, Dunn DL, Hunter JG, Matthews JB and Pollock RE (eds) *Schwartz's Principles of Surgery*, 9th ed. New York, McGraw-Hill, pp. 591–626.

Nason KS, Maddaus MA and Luketich JD (2010) Chest Wall, Lung, Mediastinum and Pleura. In Brunicardia FC, Andersen DK, Billiar TR, Dunn DL, Hunter JG, Matthews JB and Pollock RE (eds) *Schwartz's Principles of Surgery*, 9th ed. New York, McGraw-Hill, pp. 513–590.

Price J and El Khoury G (2014) Aortic Valve Repair. In Moorjani N, Ohri SK and Wechsler AS (eds) *Cardiac Surgery: Recent Advances and Techniques*. Boca Raton, CRC Press.

Schwartz CF, Crooke GA, Grossi EA and Galloway AC (2010) Acquired Heart Disease. In Brunicardia FC, Andersen DK, Billiar TR, Dunn DL, Hunter JG, Matthews JB and Pollock RE (eds) *Schwartz's Principles of Surgery*, 9th ed. New York, McGraw-Hill, pp. 627–664.

Seifert PC (2011) Cardiac Surgery. In Rothrock JC (ed) *Alexander's Care of the Patient in Surgery*, 14th ed. St. Louis, Elsevier Mosby, pp. 1002–1084.

Further Reading

Chikwe J, Cooke DT and Weiss A (2013) *Cardiothoracic Surgery*, 2nd ed. Oxford, Oxford University Press.

Jeffery RR (2012) Cardiothoracic Surgery. In Garden OJ, Bradbury AW, Forsythe JLR and Parks RW (eds) *Principles and Practice of Surgery*, 6th ed. London, Elsevier, pp. 379–398.
Moorjani N, Ohri SK and Wechsler AS (2014) *Cardiac Surgery: Recent Advances and Techniques*. Boca Raton, CRC Press.

Websites

European Association for Cardiothoracic Surgery: www.eacts.org
Society for Cardiothoracic Surgery in Great Britain and Ireland: http://www.scts.org/default.aspx

31. Orthopaedic and Trauma Surgery

References

Brunton LM and Chhabra AB (2012) Hand, Upper Extremity and Microvascular Surgery. In Miller MD, Thompson SR and Hart JA (eds) *Review of Orthopaedics*, 6th ed. Philadelphia, Elsevier Saunders, pp. 517–588.
Dandy DJ and Edwards DJ (2009) *Essential Orthopaedics and Trauma*, 5th ed. London, Churchill Livingstone Elsevier.
Heggeness MH, Gannon FH, Weinberg J, Ben-Galim P and Reitman CA (2010) Orthopaedic Surgery. In Brunicardia FC, Andersen DK, Billiar TR, Dunn DL, Hunter JG, Matthews JB and Pollock RE (eds) *Schwartz's Principles of Surgery*, 9th ed. New York, McGraw-Hill, pp. 1557–1608.
Kadakia AR and Irwin TA (2012) Disorders of the Foot and Ankle. In Miller MD, Thompson SR and Hart JA (eds) *Review of Orthopaedics*, 6th ed. Philadelphia, Elsevier Saunders, pp. 429–516.
Lauerman WC and Baumbusch CC (2012) Spine. In Miller MD, Thompson SR and Hart JA (eds) *Review of Orthopaedics*, 6th ed. Philadelphia, Elsevier Saunders, pp. 589–622.
McKinley JC and Ahmed I (2012) Orthopaedic Surgery. In Garden OJ, Bradbury AW, Forsythe JLR and Parks RW (eds) *Principles and Practice of Surgery*, 6th ed. London, Elsevier, pp. 476–490.
McPherson EJ (2012) Adult Reconstruction. In Miller MD, Thompson SR and Hart JA (eds) *Review of Orthopaedics*, 6th ed. Philadelphia, Elsevier Saunders, pp. 353–428.
McRae R (2008) *Pocketbook of Orthopaedics and Fractures*, 2nd ed. London: Churchill Livingstone Elsevier.
Miles J and Skinner J (2010) Surgery of the Hip. In Briggs T, Miles J and Aston W (eds) *Operative Orthopaedics: The Stanmore Guide*. London, Edward Arnold Ltd.
National Joint Registry (NJR) (2016) About the NJR. Available at http://www.njrcentre.org.uk/njrcentre/AbouttheNJR/tabid/73/Default.aspx (accessed 1 February 2016)
Springfield D (2009) Orthopaedics. In Brunicardia FC, Andersen DK, Billiar TR, Dunn DL, Hunter JG, Matthews JB and Pollock RE (eds) *Schwartz's Principles of Surgery*, 9th ed. New York, McGraw-Hill, pp. 1130–1168.

Further Reading

Bowen B (2011) Orthopaedic Surgery. In Rothrock JC (ed) *Alexander's Care of the Patient in Surgery*, 14th ed. St. Louis, Elsevier Mosby, pp. 719–817.
Briggs T, Miles J and Aston W (2010) *Operative Orthopaedics: The Stanmore Guide*. London, Edward Arnold Ltd.

Websites

Association of Trauma and Military Surgery: http://www.atms.org.uk/default.aspx
British Orthopaedic Association: www.boa.ac.uk
British Orthopaedic Foot and Ankle Society: www.bofas.org.uk

32. Gynaecological Surgery

References

Cain JM, ElMasri WM, Gregory T and Kohn EC (2010) Gynaecology. In Brunicardia FC, Andersen DK, Billiar TR, Dunn DL, Hunter JG, Matthews JB and Pollock RE (eds) *Schwartz's Principles of Surgery*, 9th ed. New York, McGraw-Hill, pp. 1475–1514.

Kennedy S and McVeigh E (2013) Gynaecology. In Williams NS, Bulstrode CJK and O'Connell PR (eds) *Bailey & Love's Short Practice of Surgery*, 26th ed. Kent, CRC Press, pp. 1392–1406.

McEwen DR (2011) Gynaecologic and Obstetric Surgery. In Rothrock JC (ed) *Alexander's Care of the Patient in Surgery*, 14th ed. St. Louis, Elsevier Mosby, pp. 419–477.

Monga A and Dobbs S (2011) *Gynaecology*, 19th ed. London, Hodder & Stoughton Ltd.

Oats J and Abraham S (2010) *Fundamentals of Obstetrics and Gynaecology*, 9th ed. London, Mosby Elsevier.

Further Reading

Impey L and Child T (2012) *Obstetrics and Gynaecology*, 4th ed. Chichester, Wiley-Blackwell.

Symonds IM and Arulkumaran S (2013) *Essential Obstetrics and Gynaecology*, 5th ed. Oxford, Churchill Livingstone.

Websites

British Society for Gynaecological Endoscopy: http://bsge.org.uk

Royal College of Obstetricians and Gynaecologists: www.rcog.org.uk

33. Plastic Surgery

References

Dreger V (2011) Plastic and Reconstructive Surgery. In Rothrock JC (ed) *Alexander's Care of the Patient in Surgery*, 14th ed. St. Louis, Elsevier Mosby, pp. 885–935.

Gauglitz GG (2013) Long-Term Pathophysiology and Consequences of a Burn Including Scarring, HTS, Keloids and Scar Treatment. In Jeschke MG, Kamolz L-P and Shahrokhi S (eds) *Burn Care and Treatment: A Practical Guide*. London, Springer, pp. 157–166.

Goodacre T (2013) Plastic and Reconstructive Surgery. In Williams NS, Bulstrode CJK and O'Connell PR (eds) *Bailey & Love's Short Practice of Surgery*, 26th ed. Kent, CRC Press, pp. 401–416.

Kamolz L-P (2013) Acute Burn Injury. In Jeschke MG, Kamolz L-P and Shahrokhi S (eds) *Burn Care and Treatment: A Practical Guide*. London, Springer, pp. 57–66.

Kamolz L-P and Spendel S (2013) Burn reconstruction techniques. In Jeschke MG, Kamolz L-P and Shahrokhi S (eds) *Burn Care and Treatment: A Practical Guide*. London, Springer, pp. 167–181.

Losee JE, Gimbel M, Rubin JP, Wallace CG and Wei F-C (2010) Plastic and Reconstructive Surgery. In Brunicardia FC, Andersen DK, Billiar TR, Dunn DL, Hunter JG, Matthews JB and Pollock RE (eds) *Schwartz's Principles of Surgery*, 9th ed. New York, McGraw-Hill, pp. 1647–1708.

Shahrokhi S (2013) Initial Assessment, Resuscitation, Wound Evaluation and Early Care. In Jeschke MG, Kamolz L-P and Shahrokhi S (eds) *Burn Care and Treatment: A Practical Guide*. London, Springer, pp. 1–12.

Tyler M and Ghosh S (2013) Burns. In Williams NS, Bulstrode CJK and O'Connell PR (eds) *Bailey & Love's Short Practice of Surgery*, 26th ed. Kent, CRC Press, pp. 385–400.

Watson JD (2012) Plastic and Reconstructive Surgery. In Garden OJ, Bradbury AW, Forsythe JLR and Parks RW (eds) *Principles and Practice of Surgery*, 6th ed. London, Elsevier, pp. 281–302.

Further Reading

Stone E (2008) *The Evidence for Plastic Surgery*. Shrewsbury, tfm Publishing Ltd.

Websites

British Association of Plastic Reconstructive and Aesthetic Surgeons: www.bapras.org.uk

The British Association of Aesthetic Plastic Surgeons: http://baaps.org.uk

34. Urology

References

Eardley I (2013a) Testis and Scrotum. In Williams NS, Bulstrode CJK and O'Connell PR (eds) *Bailey & Love's Short Practice of Surgery*, 26th ed. Kent, CRC Press, pp. 1377–1391.

Eardley I (2013b) Urethra and Penis. In Williams NS, Bulstrode CJK and O'Connell PR (eds) *Bailey & Love's Short Practice of Surgery*, 26th ed. Kent, CRC Press, pp. 1359–1376.
Fowler CG (2013a) The Kidneys and Ureters. In Williams NS, Bulstrode CJK and O'Connell PR (eds) *Bailey & Love's Short Practice of Surgery*, 26th ed. Kent, CRC Press, pp. 1282–1308.
Fowler CG (2013b) Urinary Symptoms and Investigations. In Williams NS, Bulstrode CJK and O'Connell PR (eds) *Bailey & Love's Short Practice of Surgery*, 26th ed. Kent, CRC Press, pp. 1271–1281.
Hamdy F (2013) The Urinary Bladder. In Williams NS, Bulstrode CJK and O'Connell PR (eds) *Bailey & Love's Short Practice of Surgery*, 26th ed. Kent, CRC Press, pp. 1309–1339.
La Rochelle J, Shuch B and Belldegrun A (2010) Urology. In Brunicardia FC, Andersen DK, Billiar TR, Dunn DL, Hunter JG, Matthews JB and Pollock RE (eds) *Schwartz's Principles of Surgery*, 9th ed. New York, McGraw-Hill, pp. 1459–1474.
Marley HK (2011) Genitourinary Surgery. In Rothrock JC (ed) *Alexander's Care of the Patient in Surgery*, 14th ed. St. Louis, Elsevier Mosby, pp. 478–565.
Neal DE and Shaw GL (2013) The Prostate and Seminal Vesicles. In Williams NS, Bulstrode CJK and O'Connell PR (eds) *Bailey & Love's Short Practice of Surgery*, 26th ed. Kent, CRC Press, pp. 1340–1358.
Stewart LH and Finney SM (2012) Urological Surgery. In Garden OJ, Bradbury AW, Forsythe JLR and Parks RW (eds) *Principles and Practice of Surgery*, 6th ed. London, Elsevier, pp. 399–423.

Further Reading

Keane TE and Graham SD (2016) *Glenn's Urologic Surgery*, 8th ed. London, Wolters Kluwer.
Scott-Conner CEH (2014) *Scott-Conner & Dawson Essential Operative Techniques and Anatomy*, 4th ed. Philadelphia, Lippincott Williams & Wilkins.
Smith JA, Howards SS and Preminger GM (2012) *Hinman's Atlas of Urologic Surgery*, 3rd ed. London, Elsevier Saunders.

Websites

American Urological Association: www.auanet.org
British Association of Urological Surgeons: www.baus.org.uk

35. Breast Surgery

References

Adam LA and Wilkinson N (2014) Axillary Node Dissection. In Scott-Conner CEH (ed) *Scott-Conner & Dawson Essential Operative Techniques and Anatomy*, 4th ed. Philadelphia, Lippincott Williams & Wilkins.
Anderson SJ, Wapnir I, Dignam JJ, Fisher B, Mamounas EP, Jeong J-H, *et al.* (2009) Prognosis after Ipsilateral Breast Tumour Recurrence and Locoregional Recurrences in Patients Treated by Breast Conserving Therapy in Five National Surgical Adjuvant Breast and Bowel Project Protocols of Node-Negative Breast Cancer. *Journal of Clinical Oncology* **27**: 2466–2473.
Bafford A, Gadd M, Gu X, Lipsitz S and Golshan M (2010) Diminishing Morbidity with the Increased Use of Sentinel Node Biopsy in Breast Carcinoma. *American Journal of Surgery* **200**: 374–377.
De Andrade JP and Dirksen JL (2014) Surgery for Subreolar Abcess: Duct Excision. In Scott-Conner CEH (ed) *Scott-Conner & Dawson Essential Operative Techniques and Anatomy*, 4th ed. Philadelphia, Lippincott Williams & Wilkins.
Dixon JM (2012) The Breast. In Garden OJ, Bradbury AW, Forsythe JLR and Parks RW (eds) *Principles and Practice of Surgery*, 6th ed. London, Elsevier, pp. 302–324.
Pearsall EB (2011) Breast Surgery. In Rothrock JC (ed) *Alexander's Care of the Patient in Surgery*, 14th ed. St. Louis, Elsevier Mosby, pp. 588–609.
Sainsbury R (2013) The Breast. In Williams NS, Bulstrode CJK and O'Connell PR (eds) *Bailey & Love's Short Practice of Surgery*, 26th ed. Kent, CRC Press, pp. 798–822.
Scott-Conner CEH (2014) *Scott-Conner & Dawson Essential Operative Techniques and Anatomy*, 4th ed. Philadelphia, Lippincott Williams & Wilkins.

Further Reading

Dixon JM (2014) *Breast Surgery: A Companion to Specialist Surgical Practice*, 5th ed. London, Saunders Elsevier.

Hunt KK, Newman LA, Copeland EM and Bland KI (2010) The Breast. In Brunicardia FC, Andersen DK, Billiar TR, Dunn DL, Hunter JG, Matthews JB and Pollock RE (eds) *Schwartz's Principles of Surgery*, 9th ed. New York, McGraw-Hill, pp. 423–474.

Websites

Association of Breast Surgery: www.associationofbreastsurgery.org.uk
Breast Cancer UK: www.breastcanceruk.org.uk

36. Endocrine Surgery

References

Aspinall S, Bliss RD and Lennard TWJ (2014) The Adrenal Glands. In Lennard TWJ (ed) *Endocrine Surgery*, 5th ed. London, Saunders Elsevier, pp. 70–97.

Al-Shoumer KAS and Gharib H (2013) Hyperthyroidism: Toxic Nodular Goiter and Graves' Disease. In Randolph GW (ed) *Surgery of the Thyroid and Parathyroid Glands*, 2nd ed. Philadelphia, Elsevier Saunders, pp. 52–59.

Cisco RM and Norton JA (2014) Endocrine Tumours of the Pancreas. In Lennard TWJ (ed) *Endocrine Surgery*, 5th ed. London, Saunders Elsevier, pp. 125–146.

Farwell AP and Braverman LE (2013) Thyroiditis. In Randolph GW (ed) *Surgery of the Thyroid and Parathyroid Glands*, 2nd ed. Philadelphia, Elsevier Saunders, pp. 41–51.

Inabnet WB, Lee JA and Palmer BJA (2014) Parathyroid Disease. In Lennard TWJ (ed) *Endocrine Surgery*, 5th ed. London, Saunders Elsevier, pp. 1–40.

Krukowski ZH (2013) The Thyroid and Parathyroid Glands. In Williams NS, Bulstrode CJK and O'Connell PR (eds) *Bailey & Love's Short Practice of Surgery*, 26th ed. Kent, CRC Press, pp. 741–777.

Lal G and Clark OH (2010) Thyroid, Parathyroid and Adrenal. In Brunicardia FC, Andersen DK, Billiar TR, Dunn DL, Hunter JG, Matthews JB and Pollock RE (eds) *Schwartz's Principles of Surgery*, 9th ed. New York, McGraw-Hill, pp. 1343–1408.

Lee JC, Gundara JS and Sidhu SB (2014) The Thyroid Gland. In Lennard TWJ (ed) *Endocrine Surgery*, 5th ed. London, Saunders Elsevier, pp. 41–69.

Lennard TWJ (2013) The Adrenal Glands and Other Abdominal Endocrine Disorders. In Williams NS, Bulstrode CJK and O'Connell PR (eds) *Bailey & Love's Short Practice of Surgery*, 26th ed. Kent, CRC Press, pp. 778–797.

McHenry CR and Lo C-Y (2013) The Surgical Management of Hyperthyroidism. In Randolph GW (ed) *Surgery of the Thyroid and Parathyroid Glands*, 2nd ed. Philadelphia, Elsevier Saunders, pp. 85–94.

Silverberg SJ and Bilezikian JP (2013) Primary Hyperparathyroidism: Pathophysiology, Surgical Indications and Preoperative workup. In Randolph GW (ed) *Surgery of the Thyroid and Parathyroid Glands*, 2nd ed. Philadelphia, Elsevier Saunders, pp. 531–538.

Further Reading

Lennard TWJ (2012) Endocrine surgery. In Garden OJ, Bradbury AW, Forsythe JLR and Parks RW (eds) *Principles and Practice of Surgery*, 6th ed. London, Elsevier, pp. 325–344.

Wentzell J (2011) Thyroid and Parathyroid Surgery. In Rothrock JC (ed) *Alexander's Care of the Patient in Surgery*, 14th ed. St. Louis, Elsevier Mosby, pp. 566–587.

Websites

The American Association of Endocrine Surgeons: www.endocrinesurgery.org
British Association of Endocrine and Thyroid Surgeons: www.baets.org.uk

37. Colorectal Surgery

References

Berardi R, Maccaroni E, Onofri A, Giampieri R, Bittoni A, Pistelli M, *et al.* (2009) Multidisciplinary Treatment of Locally Advanced Rectal Cancer: A Literature Review. Part 1. *Expert Opinion on Pharmacotherapy* **10**: 2245–2258.

Billard Dunn KM and Rothenberger DA (2010) Colon, Rectum and Anus. In Brunicardia FC, Andersen DK, Billiar TR, Dunn DL, Hunter JG, Matthews JB and Pollock RE (eds) *Schwartz's Principles of Surgery*, 9th ed. New York, McGraw-Hill, pp. 1013–1072.

Carlson G and Epstein J (2013) The Small and Large Intestines. In Williams NS, Bulstrode CJK and O'Connell PR (eds) *Bailey & Love's Short Practice of Surgery*, 26th ed. Kent, CRC Press, pp. 1143–1180.

Clark S (2013) The Rectum. In Williams NS, Bulstrode CJK and O'Connell PR (eds) *Bailey & Love's Short Practice of Surgery*, 26th ed. Kent, CRC Press, pp. 1215–1235.

Dunlop MG (2012a) The Anorectum. In Garden OJ, Bradbury AW, Forsythe JLR and Parks RW (eds) *Principles and Practice of Surgery*, 6th ed. London, Elsevier, pp. 263–280.

Dunlop MG (2012b) The small and large intestine. In Garden OJ, Bradbury AW, Forsythe JLR and Parks RW (eds) *Principles and Practice of Surgery*, 6th ed. London, Elsevier, pp. 233–262.

Hewitt Richards C, Leitch FE, Horgan PG and McMillan DC (2010) A Systematic Review of POSSUM and Its Related Models as Predictors of Post-operative Mortality and Morbidity in Patients Undergoing Surgery for Colorectal Surgery. *Journal of Gastrointestinal Surgery* **14**: 1511–1520.

Hill J (2013) Intestinal Obstruction. In Williams NS, Bulstrode CJK and O'Connell PR (eds) *Bailey & Love's Short Practice of Surgery*, 26th ed. Kent, CRC Press, pp. 1181–1198.

Korner H, Nielsen HJ, Soreide JA, Nedrebo BS, Soreide K and Knapp JC (2009) Diagnostic Accuracy of C-Reactive Protein for Intraabdominal Infections after Colorectal Resections. *Journal of Gastrointestinal Surgery* **13** (9): 1599–1606.

Lunnis P and Nugent K (2013) The Anus and Anal Canal. In Williams NS, Bulstrode CJK and O'Connell PR (eds) *Bailey & Love's Short Practice of Surgery*, 26th ed. Kent, CRC Press, pp. 1236–1270.

Morneau M, Boulanger J, Charlebois P, Latulippe J-F, Lougnarath R, Thibault C and Gervais N (2013) Laparoscopic versus Open Surgery for the Treatment of Colorectal Cancer: A Literature Review. *Canadian Journal of Surgery* **56** (5): 297–310.

Tavakkolizadeh A, Whang EE, Ashley SW and Zinner MJ (2010) Small intestine. In Brunicardia FC, Andersen DK, Billiar TR, Dunn DL, Hunter JG, Matthews JB and Pollock RE (eds) *Schwartz's Principles of Surgery*, 9th ed. New York, McGraw-Hill, pp. 979–1012.

Further Reading

Phillips RKS and Clark S (2014) *Colorectal Surgery: A Companion to Specialist Surgical Practice*, 5th ed. London, Saunders Elsevier.

Smith CE (2011) Gastrointestinal Surgery. In Rothrock JC (ed) *Alexander's Care of the Patient in Surgery*, 14th ed. St. Louis, Elsevier Mosby, pp. 295–356.

Websites

Association of Coloproctology of Great Britain and Ireland: www.acpgbi.org.uk
British Hernia Society: www.britishherniasociety.org

38. Upper Gastrointestinal Surgery

References

Alderson D (2013) The Oesophagus. In Williams NS, Bulstrode CJK and O'Connell PR (eds) *Bailey & Love's Short Practice of Surgery*, 26th ed. Kent, CRC Press, pp. 987–1023.

Couper G (2014) Staging of Oesophageal and Gastric Cancer. In Griffin SM, Raimes SA and Shenfine J (eds) *Oesophagogastric Surgery*, 5th ed. London, Elsevier, pp. 38–62.

Findlay JM and Maynard ND (2014) Pathophysiology and Investigation of Gastro-oesophageal Reflux Disease. In Griffin SM, Raimes SA and Shenfine J (eds) *Oesophagogastric Surgery*, 5th ed. London, Elsevier, pp. 219–241.

Hardwick RH (2014) Other Oesophageal and Gastric Neoplasms. In Griffin SM, Raimes SA and Shenfine J (eds) *Oesophagogastric Surgery*, 5th ed. London, Elsevier, pp. 204–218.

Hardwick RH (2012) The Oesophagus, Stomach and Duodenum. In Garden OJ, Bradbury AW, Forsythe JLR and Parks RW (eds) *Principles and Practice of Surgery*, 6th ed. London, Elsevier, pp. 167–192.

Jobe BA, Hunter JG and Peters JH (2010) Esophagus and Diaphragmatic Hernia. In Brunicardia FC, Andersen DK, Billiar TR, Dunn DL, Hunter JG, Matthews JB and Pollock RE (eds) *Schwartz's Principles of Surgery*, 9th ed. New York, McGraw-Hill, pp. 803–889.

Primrose JN and Underwood TJ (2013) Stomach and Duodenum. In Williams NS, Bulstrode CJK and O'Connell PR (eds) *Bailey & Love's Short Practice of Surgery*, 26th ed. Kent, CRC Press, pp. 1023–1058.

Shenfine J and Griffin SM (2014) Oesophageal Emergencies. In Griffin SM, Raimes SA and Shenfine J (eds) *Oesophagogastric Surgery*, 5th ed. London, Elsevier, pp. 336–358.

Wayman J (2014) Benign Ulceration of the Stomach and Duodenum and the Complications of Previous Ulcer Surgery. In Griffin SM, Raimes SA and Shenfine J (eds) *Oesophagogastric Surgery*, 5th ed. London, Elsevier, pp. 317–336.

Further Reading

Burkitt HG, Quick CRG and Reed JB (2010) *Essential Surgery: Problems, Diagnosis and Management*, 4th ed. Philadelphia, Churchill Livingstone.

Scott-Conner CEH (2014) *Scott-Conner & Dawson Essential Operative Techniques and Anatomy*, 4th ed. Philadelphia, Lippincott Williams & Wilkins.

Websites

Association of Upper Gastrointestinal Surgeons of Great Britain and Ireland: www.augis.org
British Hernia Society: www.britishherniasociety.org

39. Hepato-Pancreato-Biliary Surgery

References

Bhattacharya S (2013) The Pancreas. In Williams NS, Bulstrode CJK and O'Connell PR (eds) *Bailey & Love's Short Practice of Surgery*, 26th ed. Kent, CRC Press, pp. 1118–1142.

Conlon K (2013) The Gallbladder and Bile Ducts. In Williams NS, Bulstrode CJK and O'Connell PR (eds) *Bailey & Love's Short Practice of Surgery*, 26th ed. Kent, CRC Press, pp. 1097–1117.

Fisher WE, Andersen DK, Bell RH, Saluja AK and Brunicardia FC (2010) Pancreas. In Brunicardia FC, Andersen DK, Billiar TR, Dunn DL, Hunter JG, Matthews JB and Pollock RE (eds) *Schwartz's Principles of Surgery*, 9th ed. New York, McGraw-Hill, pp. 1167–1244.

Garden OJ (2012) The Liver and Biliary Tract. In Garden OJ, Bradbury AW, Forsythe JLR and Parks RW (eds) *Principles and Practice of Surgery*, 6th ed. London, Elsevier, pp. 192–214.

Geller DA, Goss JA and Tsung A (2010) Liver. In Brunicardia FC, Andersen DK, Billiar TR, Dunn DL, Hunter JG, Matthews JB and Pollock RE (eds) *Schwartz's Principles of Surgery*, 9th ed. New York, McGraw-Hill, pp. 1093–1134.

Koti RS, Kanoria S and Davidson BR (2013) The liver. In Williams NS, Bulstrode CJK and O'Connell PR (eds) *Bailey & Love's Short Practice of Surgery*, 26th ed. Kent, CRC Press, pp. 1065–1086.

McKay CJ and Carter CR (2012) The pancreas and spleen. In Garden OJ, Bradbury AW, Forsythe JLR and Parks RW (eds) *Principles and Practice of Surgery*, 6th ed. London, Elsevier, pp. 215–232.

Oddsdottir M, Pham TH and Hunter JG (2010) Gallbladder and the Extrahepatic biliary system. In Brunicardia FC, Andersen DK, Billiar TR, Dunn DL, Hunter JG, Matthews JB and Pollock RE (eds) *Schwartz's Principles of Surgery*, 9th ed. New York, McGraw-Hill, pp. 1135–1166.

Further Reading

Garden OJ and Parks RW (2014) *Hepatobiliary and Pancreatic Surgery: A Companion to Specialist Surgical Practice*. London, Saunders Elsevier.

Neil JA (2011) Surgery of the Liver, Biliary Tract, Pancreas and Spleen. In Rothrock JC (ed) *Alexander's Care of the Patient in Surgery*, 14th ed. St. Louis, Elsevier Mosby, pp. 357–395.

Websites

Association of Upper Gastrointestinal Surgeons of Great Britain and Ireland: www.augis.org
British Association of Surgical Oncology – The Association for Cancer Surgery: www.baso.org.uk

SECTION 4

Surgical Scrub Skills

Sara Dalby

40 Basic Surgical Instrumentation

Introduction

Surgical instruments are precisely designed and manufactured tools which are used for single (disposable) or multiple use (non-disposable). They must resist physical and chemical effects, body fluids, secretions, cleaning agents and sterilisation in order to ensure they remain operational. For this reason, most of them are made of high-quality stainless steel; chromium and vanadium alloys ensure the durability of edges and springiness and provide resistance to corrosion.

It is important that the practitioners have a comprehensive knowledge of the uses of instruments as inappropriate use could lead to injury of the patient. Instrument types can be separated into six categories: sharps/cutting instruments, clamps, haemostatic forceps (artery forceps), grasping/holding instruments (close space), retractors and accessory instruments.

Sharps/cutting instruments

A broad spectrum of tissue formation in the human body highlights the need for appropriate choice of the most pertinent dissection technique (Guglielmi and Hunter 2011). These instruments are predominantly scissors and blades; they can be used for both sharp and blunt dissection.

Blade handles require the appropriately sized single-use sterile blade to be attached and removed using the appropriate instrument and to be handled in line with relevant sharp safety protocols. Smaller blades such as 11 and 15 may be more appropriate for finer dissection, port site dissection, and stab incisions for drain insertion. In contrast, larger blades such as 20 and 23 are utilised for initial skin incisions such as a laparotomy incision (Corley and Thomas 2011). For some procedures, the blade may need to be changed once the skin incision has been made before further dissection to reduce cross-infection of skin bacteria (Pirie 2010).

Scissors come in different shapes, sizes and angles depending on their purpose (Corley and Thomas 2011) (Photo 4). There are a number of surgical scissors, and it is important that they are used for their designed purpose; otherwise, there is a potential of damaging the instrument. For example, McIndoe scissors are for dissecting and should not be used for cutting ligatures or sutures, for which Mayo scissors are a more appropriate choice.

Clamps

There are several varieties of clamps which can be traumatic or atraumatic and are used for a number of specialities (Guglielmi and Hunter 2011). The two main types are:

- *Vascular and cardiac clamps*: These are used to occlude vessels without damaging the intimal layer. They allow for varying amounts of pressure and subsequent occlusion. They vary widely in size depending on their use and application (e.g. bulldog, De Bakey and

Rapid Perioperative Care, First Edition. Paul Wicker and Sara Dalby.

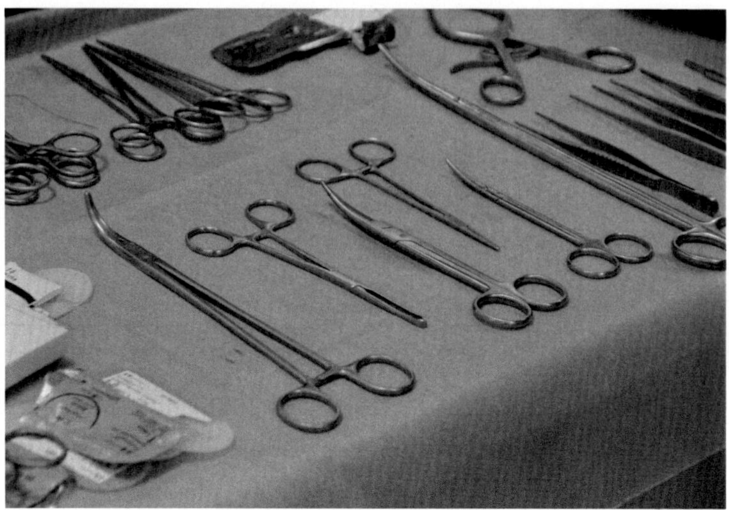

Photo 4 Basic instrumentation: scissors

Satinsky); they are curved in shape and allow partial or complete occlusion of the blood vessel.

- *Bowel clamps*: These clamps are grouped as crushing (Schoemaker) and non-crushing (Doyens). They are used to ensure that there is no spillage of bowel contents (Guglielmi and Hunter 2011). It is imperative that the practitioner has a good working knowledge of clamps as crushing clamps are used in the part of the bowel that is to be resected and can damage the integrity of the bowel tissue. Non-crushing clamps are applied to the proximal and distal part of the bowel which are to be used for an anastomosis.

Haemostatic forceps (Artery forceps)

They are used to occlude blood vessels to achieve haemostasis. As with other instruments, they vary in size and length depending on the type and depth of tissue for which they are appropriate (Corley and Thomas 2011, El-Sedfy and Chamberlain 2015). They are used for haemostasis, have ratcheted handles for varying pressure and are curved or straight. For example, Mosquitos are used for small superficial vessels compared to Roberts which are appropriate for deeper, larger vessels. They can also be used for blunt dissection or for holding sutures or swabs.

Grasping/holding instruments

This category includes tissue forceps, needle holders, dissecting forceps, sponge holders and towel clips (Pirie 2010).

- Tissue forceps are used to grasp tissue for retraction or dissection, with varying styles for different tissue types; but, if used inappropriately, they can tear through tissue. Babcock and Duval tissue forceps are for more friable tissue such as bowel, whereas Allis and Lanes tissue forceps have traumatic teeth and would tear through bowel tissue (Pirie 2010); Lanes and Allis tissue forceps are used to grasp denser tissue.

- Needle holders vary in size and weight. The selection of needle holder depends on the size of suture to be used. Some also have an integral scissors for independent suture cutting (e.g. Gillies and Foster Gillies).
- Dissecting forceps are in two categories: toothed (Gillies), which are used on tougher tissue and skin, and non-toothed (Debakey), which are used on more delicate tissue such as bowel and arteries (Corley and Thomas 2011).
- Sponge holders are used to prep patients, for absorption of fluid when used as 'a swab on a stick' and to retract, grip and handle tissue.
- Towel clips can be used to secure drapes and other items in the surgical field. They tend to be blunt these days due to risk of sharps injury.

Retraction

Retractors are used to optimise the surgeon's surgical vision by holding back wound edges, tissues or structures for the best exposure whilst causing the least damage possible to the tissue. They are either self-retaining or hand-held.

When selecting an appropriate retractor, the following needs to be considered:

- Stage of the procedure
- Type(s) of tissue to be retracted
- Availability of retractors
- Surgical preference
- Complexity of the operation
- Length and depth of the wound
- Time to perform operation
- Assistant experience and availability
- Amount of force needed to create exposure (Steele *et al.* 2013).

The assistant needs to be aware of the amount of force they are using as excessive force can compromise blood flow and cause tissue damage. The positioning of retractors is as important to consider as the force applied because misplacement can cause damage to tissue and structures such as nerves and vessels. Therefore, knowledge of anatomy is imperative, and placement of retractors is considered the role of a surgeon or a surgical care practitioner (Steele *et al.* 2013).

Handheld retraction has numerous advantages; it is easily placed, repositioned and removed. It allows the assistant to apply varying degrees of pressure as necessary, allowing perfusion of tissues. The assistant should not cause tissue distortion when pulling on the retractor. Excessive force may cause damage to the patient such as a laceration. If there is insufficient pull on the retractor, there may not be inadequate exposure. Self-retaining retractors should be placed only under direct vision with caution to prevent damage to body structures; once in place, they allow the assistant to carry out other surgical duties (Corley and Thomas 2011).

Accessory instruments

These are used to improve the basic instrumentation or assist the procedure. They include:

- Suction, such as pool suctions, which are reusable guarded suctions, to provide optimum surgical exposure by suctioning blood and fluid from the operative site.
- Dilators, such as oesophageal dilators and urethral dilators.
- Dissectors such as a McDonald dissector which can protect nerves, explore wounds or be used as a retractor (Pirie 2010).
- Probes/directors, which may be used to explore a tract such as pilonidal sinus.
- Mallets and screwdrivers (Guglielmi and Hunter 2011).

41 Surgical Positioning

Surgical positioning involves moving and securing the patient for the best exposure of the surgical site; access to the patient's airway, IV lines and monitoring devices; the patient's warmth and comfort; prevention of compromising of physiological functions; protection of body systems and protection of patient dignity (Beckett 2010).

Before positioning, it is important to evaluate:

- Patient factors
  - Age
  - Height and weight
  - Nutritional status
  - Skin condition
  - Pre-existing conditions (i.e. vascular, respiratory, circulatory, neurological or immunocompromised)
  - Physical/mobility limits (i.e. implants, range of motion and prosthesis)
- Intraoperative factors
  - Anaesthesia
  - Position required
  - Length of surgery
  - Surgical access.

The practitioner can identify any specific patient factors which may affect positioning if they undertake a preoperative visit or assessment.

Patients are susceptible to injury due to a loss of reflexes during general anaesthetics and muscle relaxants, resulting in a variety of potential nerve damage, compartment syndrome, deep vein thrombosis and pressure sores (Adedeji *et al.* 2010, Bale and Berrecloth 2010).

The mechanisms that contribute to perioperative positioning injuries are:

- Traction
- Stretch
- Compression
- Metabolic derangement (i.e. diabetes)
- Vascular compromise.

The specific predisposing factors associated with pressure sores are pressure, shear and friction (Pirie 2010). Prevention of injury is paramount, and it is essential to be able to identify the potential complications of each specific position.

Practitioners may also be injured during positioning. Adequate training, equipment and an appropriate number of staff may reduce the risk.

Supine

The supine position allows access to the abdominal cavities, head, neck and extremities. The patient's arms should be abducted less than 90° to prevent injury to the brachial plexus

Rapid Perioperative Care, First Edition. Paul Wicker and Sara Dalby.

and placed on padded arm boards, level to the padding of the surgical table. The preferred position for arms on arm boards is palms up, and elbows may need padding to prevent ulnar nerve compression between the ulnar groove and table apparatus (Adedeji *et al.* 2010). If the patient's arms are tucked in at the sides, attention should be taken to ensure that the patient's fingers will not be caught in the operating table, and wrists and fingers should be in a neutral position. The patient's arms may be across their chest with flexed elbows. In this instance, padding should be put proximal to the elbow to prevent cubital tunnel syndrome from resting on the operating table, protecting the ulnar nerve.

Emphasis must be placed on padding the patient's pressure areas in this position: the occiput, scapula, olecranon, thoracic vertebrae, sacrum, coccyx and calcaneus. Padding at the head prevents hyperextension or hyperflexion of the neck and alleviation of pressure on the occiput. The eyes should be protected by eye patches or taping the eyelids closed, ensuring a corneal lubricant is used to prevent corneal ulceration. Some patients may need a pillow under their knees which slightly flexes the hips and knees, improving comfort and taking stress off the knees as it is more physiologically neutral. As the heels are vulnerable to pressure areas, padding or heel supports should be used to prevent damage.

Cardiac output and workload are increased, especially if patients are obese. The weight of their chest increases intrathoracic pressure and further increases cardiac workload. In patients with cardiovascular deficiencies, it increases their risk of cardiac failure. Increased pressure on the inferior vena cava from abdominal viscera, abdominal masses or foetuses in pregnant women decreases blood return to the heart, thus lowering blood pressure. This can be overcome by tilting the patient to the left slightly by using a wedge (Pirie 2010). Respiratory function is compromised due to reduced tidal volume; in patients with severe pre-existing pulmonary disease, it may compromise oxygenation and ventilation.

Trendelenburg

The Trendelenburg position is used during abdominal surgery to improve visualisation of the pelvic organs in both open and laparoscopic surgery. It allows access for the placement of central lines and may be used to improve circulation to the cerebral cortex if the blood pressure suddenly lowers (Pirie 2010).

Pressure points are the same as in the supine position, and shearing risk is significant in this position. This position should only be maintained as long as necessary as blood pools in the upper torso, increasing blood pressure and intracranial pressure; it assists in drainage from the bases of the lungs and oesophagus, but the weight of the abdominal viscera hinders diaphragmatic movement, decreasing pulmonary compliance and tidal volume. Fluid moves into the alveoli, causing oedema, atelectasis and congestion. The patient should be moved slowly to Trendelenburg and back to supine to allow the patient's body to adjust to physiological changes.

Reverse trendelenburg

Reverse Trendelenburg is used to provide access to the neck and head and to move abdominal viscera from the diaphragm toward the feet. Venous circulation may be compromised if the patient is in this position for an extended amount of time (Bale and Berrecloth 2010). If used for laparoscopic surgery, it decreases venous return due to steep reverse Trendelenburg and increased intra-abdominal pressure due to pneumoperitoneum. Subsequently, the use of superficial venous return is recommended due to the increased risk of deep vein thrombosis. For patients having thyroid, neck or shoulder surgery, a soft roll may be placed horizontally under the shoulders to hyperextend the neck.

Lithotomy

The lithotomy position is used for gynaecological, urological and rectal procedures. The patient's anterior superior iliac spine is positioned at the break of the table, and the practitioner should ensure the patient's buttocks do not overhang the edge of the table (Pirie 2010). Stirrups should be securely attached to the operating table as slippage or dropping may cause hip dislocation, bone fractures and muscle or nerve damage. Both legs should be at the same height, and stirrups attached to the table at the same point. Hips should not be flexed more than 90°. A complication of this position is peripheral nerve injury; the sciatic nerve can be overstretched when flexion at the hip is exaggerated, combined with extension at the knees and external rotation. The femoral nerve and obturator nerve can be damaged by hyperflexion at the hip and strain the hip and joint muscles. The common peroneal nerve may be damaged (foot drop) due to compression against leg supports placed lateral to the knee. This is overcome by padding and distal placement of padded leg supports (Adedeji *et al.* 2010). The saphenous nerves are protected by adequate padding between the lower legs and leg braces. Lithotomy stirrups, which have thin ankle straps, put pressure on the distal sural and plantar nerves, resulting in neuropathies of the foot. Boot-type stirrups distribute the pressure fairly evenly, reducing the risk of localized pressure. Abduction should be limited to only what is necessary for surgery, and time in this position should be minimised.

This position significantly compromises both respiration and circulation, especially with extreme hip and knee flexion; it impairs respiratory function by increasing intra-abdominal pressure against the diaphragm and affects gravitational flow from the legs, causing pooling in the splanchnic region. Due to this pooling, blood loss may not immediately manifest, and when the legs are lowered the circulation will deplete and blood pressure drops. The effects of anaesthesia on the nervous system mean that normal compensatory mechanisms and haemodynamic adjustment are not achieved easily; volume repletion, vasoconstrictors and a slow change back to supine minimise these effects.

Prone

The patient is anaesthetised in the supine position with the airway secured and eyelids taped. The anaesthetist remains at the patient's head, whilst the rest of the team are positioned at the thorax, hips and legs. The patient is then turned in a controlled and coordinated manner. The first concern is the protection and patency of the airway (Adedeji *et al.* 2010).

If the patient's arms are to remain by their side, they are tucked in with a sheet, then elbows should face upwards to ensure less pressure on the ulnar nerve. Compression from the sheet being too tight or someone leaning on the arm may occur, but these can be minimised by padding the elbow. If the arms are being put on arm boards, then they are to be brought down and forwards with minimal abduction to prevent shoulder dislocation and brachial plexus injury. The arm boards are positioned to the same height as the operating table, and elbows should be flexed but not beyond 90° so as not to stretch the ulnar nerve, with padding of the elbow and arms ensuring the ulnar nerve is not in contact with the arm board.

The head is turned and positioned in alignment with the spine, the eyes are protected and padding is placed on the cheeks, ears, patellae and toes (Pirie 2010). Caution needs to be taken to ensure there is no pressure on the breasts or male genitalia. A pillow may be put under the pelvis to allow movement of the abdominal and anterior chest wall. The respiratory system is compromised as normal anterior lateral movement is restricted and the compressed abdominal wall and rib cage inhibit normal diaphragmatic movement (Bowers 2012). When the patient is returned to supine position, an inspection of pressure areas should be carried out.

Jack-knife

A small roll under each shoulder alleviates pressure on the brachial plexus from the clavicle. A pillow should be placed under the lower legs to eliminate pressure on the toes, and a restraint strap is placed over the thighs. Circulatory effects cause cephalad and caudad venous pooling, emphasising the need for assisted venous return. Breathing is severely compromised as anterior lateral chest movement is restricted, with pressure for the abdominal viscera and pressure from the flexed operating table. The bed should be straightened very slowly to enable the body to adjust haemodynamically.

Lateral

The patient's head should be supported with padding to prevent undue flexion, extension or side bending; the cervical spine should be aligned with the thoracic spine (Adedeji *et al.* 2010). The arms are placed at an angle of less than 90° anterior to the patient and flexed at the elbow, to prevent stretching which could lead to damage to the brachial plexus. The above arm may need to be supported by an arm support attached to the operating table; both must be well padded at the elbow to protect the skin and prevent nerve damage. The legs should be flexed at the knees, or the top leg may remain straight with the hips with a pillow between knees and ankles. Padding on the lateral side knee of the bottom leg prevents pressure on the peroneal nerve. The torso is supported at the hips or thighs with suitable restraints to ensure the patient is secure (Pirie 2010).

Systolic and diastolic pressures decrease. This is attributed to pharmacological processes depressing normal compensatory mechanisms. Respiratory function is compromised by the weight of the body on the lower chest, whereas the upper lung receives less blood flow.

Lateral chest

The lateral chest position allows surgical access to the highest part of the chest. The upper arm is flexed slightly at the elbow and raised above the head to elevate the scapula. The upper section of the bed is lowered, causing the mouth and trachea to be lower than the lungs; this means that secretions from the lungs leave via the mouth and don't drain into the unaffected side of the chest. Respiratory function is compromised as in the lateral position, with the upper lung less perfused but not compressed and the lower lung compressed but well perfused.

Lateral kidney

For the lateral kidney position, the iliac crest is positioned so that the lower iliac crest is just below the lumbar break. The toleration of this break depends on the patient's cardiovascular response to increased pressure to this area. It should be altered slowly with constant monitoring of blood pressure. Diaphragmatic movement is limited due to flexion of the lower limbs and the kidney bridge. Increases pooling in the legs causes decreased venous return to the heart which may reduce cardiac output, highlighting a need for superficial venous return.

Fowler

In the Fowler position, the upper body is raised 90° with flexed knees and lowered legs. A footrest prevents foot drop. Arms are either on padded arm boards or rested on a pillow flexed in the patient's lap. All sections of the spine should be in alignment. Main pressure areas include the scapulae, ischial tuberosities, calcanei and coccyx, with the need for padding at the lumbar area, under elbows and knees, and at the sacrum and heels. Blood pools in the lower extremities and torso, causing orthostatic hypotension and diminished perfusion to the brain. There is a potential for air embolism if a venous sinus is opened as the surgical site is above the heart. Additional monitoring in the form of a central venous catheter is utilised. In this position, there is the least effect on respirations, an acknowledgement that the arms in the lap don't restrict chest movement.

Semi-fowler

In this position, the upper section of the bed is flexed at a 45° angle and the leg section is lowered slightly, flexing the knees. The bed is tilted, reducing sliding and shearing and decreasing the haemodynamic effects. The positioning of the arms and feet is similar to that of the Fowler position.

Knee–chest

The patient is prone with the break at the hips, a safety strap is placed around the thighs and arms are placed on arm boards, flexed and lying next to the head (Pirie 2010). Pressure points include the anterior rib cage, anterior iliac crests, anterior tibial aspects of the calves, anterior tali, toes and knees, all of which need padding and support. Respiratory and circulatory compromises are the same as in the prone position, and venous return is compromised due to bended legs needing assisted venous return.

Documentation

Document any information gained from the preoperative assessment, the position of the patient, the types and location of equipment used and any specific actions taken to minimise injury (Spruce and Van Wicklin 2014).

Postoperative assessment

Following surgery, the theatre practitioners should assess the patient's pressure areas for the integrity of the skin and any potential musculoskeletal injuries. This should then be documented, and concerns highlighted to the recovery staff for monitoring (Spruce and Van Wicklin 2014).

42 Thermoregulation

It is important that the patient's temperature is monitored intraoperatively. The management of patient's temperature within the intraoperative phase is to prevent unplanned hypothermia. Patients can feel uncomfortable as a consequence of hypothermia but may also suffer additional detrimental health outcomes as a consequence. The patient's temperature should be monitored throughout the operative procedure and in the recovery phase to ensure normothermia is maintained. Inadvertent hypothermia is a common but preventable intraoperative complication which can be detrimental to patients. Recognition of the negative effects of hypothermia as a patient safety and quality-of-care issue has emphasised recommended practices, staff education and local guideline development (Wagner 2010).

Ways the body loses heat

- Radiation
  - 40% heat loss
  - Affected by room temperature and skin exposure
- Convection
  - 30% heat loss
  - Air temperature and draught (i.e. laminar air flow in theatres)
- Conduction
  - 5% heat loss
  - Cold theatre tables or cold fluids
- Evaporation
  - 8–15% percent heat loss
  - Skin prep, open wounds or respiratory loss
- Respiration
  - 8–10% heat loss
  - Anaesthetic gases (Anaesthesia UK 2016).

Assessment of patient's temperature

One of the main steps that practitioners can undertake to reduce the incidence of inadvertent intraoperative hypothermia is to regularly monitor the patient's temperature intraoperatively, identify if the patient's temperature is dropping and then take appropriate measures to maintain normothermia. A number of different thermometers can be utilised to monitor temperatures: rectal, bladder, forehead skin, oral or axillary (Hooper *et al.* 2009). The aim is to maintain the patient's temperature between 36.5 and 37.5 °C (Hamlin *et al.* 2010). Patients with temperatures below 36.5 °C may require active warming such as forced air

Rapid Perioperative Care, First Edition. Paul Wicker and Sara Dalby.

blankets or other warming systems. If the patient's temperature is above 37.5 °C, then there is a possibility of malignant hyperthermia, over-warming and sepsis, and it is necessary to seek advice.

Hypothermia is considered a core body temperature below 36 °C; however, hypothermia also can be categorised as mild, moderate and severe:

- Mild hypothermia is a core temperature between 32 and 35 °C.
- Moderate hypothermia is a core temperature between 30 and 32 °C.
- Severe hypothermia is a core temperature below 28 °C.

Inadvertent hypothermia

Hypothermia may be either deliberate or inadvertent; deliberate hypothermia may be necessary to reduce metabolic activity for cardiac surgery or neurosurgery to reduce oxygen consumption and therefore organ damage.

The development of a hypothermic state (a core temperature below 36 °C) occurs due to the effects of anaesthesia on metabolic rate and hypothalamic function, resulting in reduced functioning or non-functioning of normal physiological functions such as vasoconstriction and shivering, which normally preserve or increase temperature (AORN 2007, Kurtz 2008, NICE 2008, Greenberg *et al.* 2009, Hillier *et al.* 2009).

Additional factors which exasperate the development of hypothermia:

- Operating room temperature
- Length of operating procedure
- The use of cold IV fluids
- Cool abdominal wash-outs
- The use of cold anaesthetic gases
- Exposure of abdominal or thoracic organs.

Patients at increased risk of inadvertent hypothermia

Certain patients are more predisposed to hypothermia:

- Type of anaesthesia
- Type of surgery, such as patients with open abdominal cavities
- The elderly
- Neonates
- Burns patients
- Patients with a small body mass
- Patients with impaired metabolic rate
- Patients with circulatory failure
- Patients who have muscle atrophy
- Patients with hyperthyroidism or hypothyroidism (Berry *et al.* 2008, NICE 2008, Lynch *et al.* 2010).

Complications of inadvertent hypothermia

A number of adverse effects are suffered by patients whom have been hypothermic during surgery which results in an increased incidence of adverse outcomes and a potentially longer hospital stay (Berry *et al.* 2008).

A number of identified complications are consequences of inadvertent hypothermia:

- Metabolic acidosis
- Reduced tissue oxidation
- Increased postoperative anxiety and decreased patient satisfaction
- Oliguria
- Altered platelet and clotting function; therefore, increased risk of bleeding and needing a transfusion
- Increased risk of developing a pressure ulcer
- Decrease in cardiac output
- Reduced hepatic blood flow and slower drug metabolism
- Myocardial ischaemia
- Postoperative shivering and increased oxygen consumption
- Increased length of stay in recovery and a longer hospital stay
- Increased risk of postoperative infection due to suppressed immune system (Kurtz 2008, NICE 2008, Rajagopalan *et al.* 2008, Weirich 2008, Burger and Fitzpatrick 2009, Leeth *et al.* 2010, Carpenter and Baysinger 2012).

Despite the documented negative outcome of hypothermia, 70% of patients undergoing surgery have been found to experience some degree of hypothermia. However, if the patient is frequently monitored and appropriate warming techniques are utilised, inadvertent hypothermia is preventable (RCA 2012).

Preoperative management

The patient's temperature should be taken on admission and preoperatively; this is to be documented. Practitioners should be aware that patients who are given a pre-medication may need additional help to ensure they do not become hypothermic. Patients who are transferred from wards may become cold during their transfer or while waiting in reception; it is important to ask the patient if they feel warm and offer warm blankets as necessary (NICE 2008, AfPP 2011).

Anaesthetic care

The anaesthetic room should be warm, and the patient's temperature monitored and documented prior to induction. The induction of anaesthesia should not occur if the patient's temperature is below 36 °C unless delay is life or limb threatening. Once the patient is anaesthetised, the patient's temperature should be monitored and documented every 30 min (AfPP 2011).

Intraoperative management strategies

Perioperative thermal management techniques are safe, inexpensive and easy to use as long as practitioners have had the relevant training and follow local guidelines and policies. Only the operative site should be exposed; the rest of the patient should be covered. Theatre practitioners can take a number of steps to minimise the chance of hypothermia:

- Preoperative warming if necessary
- Active warming devices
- IV fluid-warming devices
- Warm irrigation fluids
- Blankets and head wrapping
- Increase the room temperature when possible (AfPP 2011, Roberson *et al.* 2013).

Postoperative management

The patient's temperature should be continually monitored postoperatively, preferably with the same technique as used intraoperatively (AfPP 2011).

Theatre practitioners should have knowledge of patients who are at the most risk and any additional compounding factors which should then help them make an informed decision for the most appropriate management strategies.

43 Skin Preparation

Rationale for skin preparation

Surgical site infections are distressing for patients and have financial implications for healthcare organisations. Preoperative skin preparation of the surgical site with an appropriate skin preparation solution is one of the most important steps a practitioner can take to reduce surgical site infections. Skin preparation methods all aim to reduce the risk of postoperative surgical site infections by removing dirt and transient microbes from the skin, reducing the microbial count in the shortest time possible whilst causing little irritation to the skin and preventing a rapid regrowth of microbes (Hemani and Lepor 2009, Alexander *et al.* 2011, AORN 2013).

General considerations

The general considerations for skin preparations include:

- Surgical site
- Numbers and conditions of contaminants
- Condition of site
- Skin characteristics
- The patient's overall condition
- The use of aseptic technique
- The selection of effective antimicrobial solutions
- Application techniques (Wanzer and Vane 2009).

Skin prep begins before the operating room by a preoperative shower, and patients having head and neck surgery are encouraged to wash their hair (NICE 2008). The site of incision and surrounding area should be cleaned by the patient showering or washing prior to surgery. As discussed in Chapter 47, 'Measures to Prevent Wound Infection', if deemed necessary hair removal should be undertaken immediately prior to surgery to reduce the incidence of infection.

Practitioners should consider the patient's condition prior to the choice of skin preparation, being aware that some patients are hypersensitive, that some antiseptics are absorbed and may become neurotoxic or oxytocic and that some are harmful to pregnant or breastfeeding women. The patient's skin should be checked for rashes, irritation, localized infection or abrasions. The practitioner should check if the patient has any allergies.

Antiseptic choices

There are three main choices for antiseptics:

1. Iodine/iodophor is a broad-spectrum bactericidal against both Gram-positive and Gram-negative organisms; it also has fungicidal, sporicidal, protocidal and viricidal properties. It maintains microbicidal activity for up to 8 h, and the brown staining makes the area

Rapid Perioperative Care, First Edition. Paul Wicker and Sara Dalby.

prepped easily identifiable. Iodine is inactivated by biomaterials. Pooling of betadine can cause skin irritation, and it can be a moderate eye irritant; it should not be used on areas such as the perineum, the genitalia or irritated or delicate skin, or on those with allergies to iodine. Contraindicated for use on pregnant or breastfeeding women. It should not be used on open wounds or dressings as it is toxic against fibroblasts and keratinocytes (Edwards *et al.* 2009, Zinn *et al.* 2010).

2. Alcohols are broad-spectrum, fast-acting antimicrobials. They are ineffective against bacterial spores but generally effective against fungal species and some viruses. They are fast acting in their antimicrobial action, but they are limited in their residual effect. Alcohol solutions cannot be used on open wounds or mucus membranes, as alcohol coagulates tissue protein; therefore, it is not indicated for use prior to transurethral or transvaginal surgery. Alcohol can be neurotoxic, so it should be avoided in use near brain or spinal tissue; it may also cause corneal damage to eyes and may affect the nerves of the inner ear. In neonates, alcohol can cause tissue trauma such as burns or necrosis. Alcohol can be combined with chlorhexidine gluconate or iodophors to optimise the activity of skin antisepsis. Caution must be taken when it is used due to its flammable properties, with special care taken to ensure there is no pooling. Avoid use when prepping areas with excessive body hair as it can delay the alcohol vaporising. Flammable solutions need to be allowed to dry prior to the application of the drapes to prevent a build-up of fumes underneath them (Hemani and Lepor 2009, Kehinde *et al.* 2009).
3. Chlorhexidine gluconate has a wide range of bactericidal activity against both Gram-positive and Gram-negative non-spore-forming bacteria; it also has some antiviral activity with good residual effect. It has a low incidence of patient reactions and lasts up to 6 h, it is not inactivated by blood or serum, and it is colourless, which may be preferable in aesthetic surgeries. Chlorhexidine gluconate has been identified as having persistent action but is inactivated by iodine. Prolonged skin contact may cause irritation, and rare severe hypersensitivity reactions have been reported. It should not be used on mucous membranes, may cause chemical burns in neonates, is ototoxic and is avoided for use near the eyes or brain and spinal tissue due to its neurotoxicity (Edmiston *et al.* 2010, Sivathasan *et al.* 2010, Zinn *et al.* 2010).

There are also combined preparations such as Tavasept, chlorhexidine gluconate and cetrimide which are used by urology and obstetrics and gynaecology for prepping genitals prior to scopes. It is also used for burns and occasionally washing out dirty trauma.

It is important for practitioners to acknowledge that chlorhexidine preps and povidine–iodine can be aqueous based or alcohol based; it is therefore important to double-check this before applying.

Optimum method of skin preparation

Both the application and choice of antiseptic have an impact on the effectiveness of the skin preparation.

In order to achieve the highest level of antisepsis, a combination of mechanical and chemical activity is required. The chemical process involves destroying microorganisms and also deterring their re-colonisation following cleansing; therefore, it is important to select the most appropriate antiseptic solution. The mechanical process requires an appropriate amount of friction to ensure all the cracks within the skin are sufficiently coated in antiseptic prep. Caution should be used in cases such as superficial malignancy and areas of carotid plaque, where friction should not be applied; gentle preparation techniques should be used when prepping patients with medical conditions such as diabetes and skin ulcerations.

Prior to prepping, the surgical site should be confirmed. The site of surgery influences skin preps because different preps target different endogenous flora; for example, genital skin flora are different to abdomen or oral flora. In the majority of instances when preparing the patient's skin, it is recommended to start with the incision site working outwards, and this is carried out by a person who is scrubbed using a swab on an instrument to maintain the sterility of the individual prepping; once soiled, the swab is discarded and never brought back over a scrubbed surface. Practitioners need to ensure that when prepping and draping, the area should be large enough for an extension of the incision and potential drain sites, as repositioning of the drapes and extending their area could cause contamination due to exposure of an unprepped site. Sufficient time needs to be allowed for the skin preps to be in contact with the skin prior to the application of the drapes (Wanzer and Vane 2009).

Caution needs to be used when prepping patients to prevent solutions from entering aural cavities. Practitioners must ensure that the solution doesn't 'pool' under the patient which may lead to irritation or electrocautery burns; to prevent this, it is suggested to have absorbent towels which can be removed after the patient is prepped. The causes of fire linked with alcoholic skin preparation are due to practitioners not allowing enough time for prep to dry or having prep-soaked swab in the operating field and near an ignition source (Rocos and Donaldson 2012). A number of considerations with regards to prepping: when preparing areas with a large amount of microbes (e.g. umbilicus, open wounds and pubis), these areas should be prepped last. Colostomies should be isolated by covering them, and burned, denatured or traumatised skin should be prepped with saline. No more than one antiseptic should be used to prep, as they may inactivate each other; bottles and sachets of prep should be single-patient use; and washing out cavities or soaking implants should be discouraged as not only are the products not licensed for this but also the solution may be contaminated, leading to infection (Wanzer and Vane 2009).

No single antiseptic solution is superior in all instances, so an assessment should be made taking into account patient factors, duration of surgery, type of procedure, area that is to be prepped and the product's efficacy. Differing operative sites have different endogenous flora, body contours and skin types, and the selection of skin prep must reflect these differences. Any allergies or sensitivities need to be taken into consideration. Finally, patient and environmental safety must be paramount and caution used when utilising alcohol-based surgical skin preparation.

44 Surgical Draping

The use of surgical draping for patients undergoing an operation is common practice and has been for decades. It is part of the steps taken to reduce the incidence of surgical site infections by providing a sterile environment surrounding the operative site and a barrier to potential contamination. If utilised appropriately, it has been shown to reduce surgical site infections and thus reduce the negative effects for patients and the financial implications associated (Gilmour 2010, Zinn *et al.* 2010).

Basic principles of draping

The practitioner must take into account a number of steps before, during and after draping the surgical patient:

- Check the patient's allergy status prior to applying the drapes.
- It is important to allow the skin preparation solution to dry prior to application of the drapes, especially if it is alcoholic to ensure fumes are not trapped under the drapes and reduce the incidence of fire.
- If using adhesive drapes, the surgical preparation solution will need to be left to dry before sticking the drapes to ensure sufficient contact is made.
- When placing the drapes, the practitioner should take into account the area needed, considering a need to extend the incision and insert drains.
- Consider the surgical procedure: is there going to be significant fluid loss or irrigation?
- Apply closest to the incision site first, and then apply peripheral drapes.
- If it has been appropriate to surgically mark the patient, this must still be visible once the patient is draped.
- Handle the drapes as little as possible.
- Once positioned, drapes should not be removed and repositioned.
- If the integrity of the drapes is compromised in any way (i.e. there is a hole), they must be discarded and an alternative utilised.
- When draping, the practitioner should not allow the drapes to go below their waist.
- Utilise gravity for the drapes to fall open, if required, to avoid the practitioner becoming contaminated.
- The practitioner must take into account their environment and ensure they do not accidently desterilise the drapes, thus compromising the sterile field.
- Best practice is for the practitioner to 'cuff' their hands with the drapes to reduce the chance of contamination.
- The drapes should not be in contact with the floor of the operating department.
- Practitioners should not reach across an unsterile area when draping.
- A minimum of two people is necessary to drape the surgical area effectively.
- Do not prematurely open out the drapes, as this may increase the incidence of contamination; stick the drapes in place, and then open in a controlled manner.
- It may be necessary to attach the drape at the head of the patient to metal poles (e.g. drip stands) to allow access for the anaesthetic team or to create a barrier if the patient is awake; it needs to be ensured that these are secure.

Rapid Perioperative Care, First Edition. Paul Wicker and Sara Dalby.

- When securing the quiver and diathermy cables and light leads, do not use anything that will penetrate the drapes.
- During long procedures, specifically those with bleeding or in which irrigation is necessary, the drapes may begin to lift, thus compromising the sterile field. An additional drape or tape should be utilised to reattach the drape as soon as this is identified.
- The drapes should remain in position until the dressing has been placed over the surgical wound to minimise surgical site infection.
- At the end of the procedure, the drapes should be disposed of appropriately; the recommended technique is to fold the contaminated side inwards to avoid spillage on the floor, and they are to be disposed in the appropriate bins for materials with contaminants and body fluids (Msaud *et al.* 2010, Nicolette 2011, Hamlin 2012, Kiernan 2012, Al-Hashemi 2013).

Considerations when selecting drapes

There are a number considerations which practitioners consider when selecting drapes:

- Absorbency and fluid control
- Barrier protection
- Strength
- Conformability
- Comfort and breathability
- Cost (both financial and environmental)
- Patient factors (i.e. allergies and skin integrity).

Reusable versus disposable drapes

Two types of drapes are available: reusable and disposable drapes.

Reusable drapes are said to be fluctuant in their quality; although some are waterproof, laundering this can diminish this effect, and it may be necessary to put a plastic sheet or a water-repellent paper sheet underneath the drapes to protect the patient (Gilmour 2010, Hamlin 2011). The use of towel clips may be needed to keep reusable drapes in position; these can be ballpoint which is preferable as the sharp towel clips have the potential to injure the patient and compromise the sterility of the surgical field. They may be an appropriate choice if the patient is allergic to the adhesive within the disposable drapes or if the patient has thin, fragile skin which could be damaged on removal of disposable drapes. They are also said to be more comfortable for the patient.

Disposable drapes have consistent quality and are designed to create an impermeable barrier between the patient and surgical field, but their effectiveness can be compromised by fluid or if they become torn (Humes and Lobo 2009, Rothrock 2011). Due to the malleability of the drapes, the practitioner can ensure that even the most difficult aspects of the patient are draped. They can be uncomfortable for the patient, and this needs to be considered for patients having surgery under local anaesthetic (Gilmour 2010).

Cost can have an influence when selecting which drapes to utilise, particularly in today's financial climate, and it has a direct effect on the availability within an individual's department. However, cost is not just outlay; there is also an environmental cost due to the disposal of disposable drapes, but there is an offset cost for the laundering of reusable drapes (Gilmour 2010). Due to strict standards of sterilisation of reusable drapes within Europe, there has been a shift to using disposable drapes (Gilmour 2010). An additional potential consideration for healthcare departments is that if the sterility of the drapes being utilised is questioned, the manufacturers of disposable drapes will carry some accountability and liability, especially if they are used within the manufacturer's recommendations.

45 Surgical Site Marking

An increased pressure on surgical throughput has led to the introduction and implementation of patient safety measures through checklists, time-outs and quality metrics. Perioperative practitioners need to ensure the perioperative environment meets safety standards to ensure optimal patient outcomes, including acting as an advocate in the instance of surgical site marking (Lee 2014).

Preoperative marking is essential to reduce the risk of wrong site surgery by identifying the correct site of surgery, particularly in instances of surgery where there are two sides (i.e. limbs). Operating on the wrong site is a 'never event' for any hospital but more importantly has serious implications for patients both physically and emotionally. Standardisation of practice and independent cross-checking by practitioners can minimise the risk (WHO 2008, Msaud *et al.* 2010).

With appropriate training and documentation in place, surgical site marking is well within the scope of practice of a surgical care practitioner. Although it is outside the scope of practice of the surgical first assistant or theatre practitioners, an understanding of the implications of wrong site surgery and legal issues of site marking is imperative for patient safety.

Wrong site surgery

The most common never events occurring in the National Health Service are from surgical specialities, including wrong site surgery which has significant negative outcomes for patients and financial implications for healthcare organisations (NHS England 2014).

Wrong site surgery includes:

- Removal of wrong organ
- Operating on the wrong patient
- Wrong procedure
- Wrong incision site
- Implanting a prosthesis incorrectly
- Administrating local anaesthetic to the wrong site (Mellinger 2014).

'Marking' practices used to be variable from individual surgeons and individual trusts, and it was identified that in order to reduce the incidence of wrong site surgery, it was necessary to unify practices and introduce a standard.

Steps to surgical site marking

The following steps should be taken to minimise the risk of wrong site surgery:

- The patient should be marked by the surgeon or a nominated deputy who will be present during the procedure prior to their arrival to theatre.
- Patient marking should involve the patient before sedation and possibly their relatives.
- The patient should verbally confirm the surgical site.

Rapid Perioperative Care, First Edition. Paul Wicker and Sara Dalby.

- The surgical site should be checked with the notes and images, and match the operation list.
- An arrow should point to the incision site or specific area (i.e. a digit), with an indelible marker.
- The mark should be in place after prepping.
- The mark should be visible after draping.
- Marking should be documented and should be confirmed throughout the patient's journey to the operation theatre, with a final verification from all the theatre team.

Standardisation of surgical site marking and cross-checking of the mark was introduced by the World Health Organization (WHO) in the form of a surgical checklist. The WHO Checklist provides the practitioners with a structured prompt to check the surgical site that should occur prior to the induction of anaesthetic and during the 'surgical pause' which should occur before commencing surgery, with a communication among all staff members ensuring the correct patient, site and procedure. This format of checking aims to minimise the risk of wrong site surgery by helping to avoid preventable surgical incidents (WHO 2008).

As an additional check, the surgical assistant should independently check the operating site even if it has been marked by the lead operating surgeon.

Surgical marking is within the remit of surgeons and Surgical Care Practitioners who have undergone training, as long as they will be present during the procedure and have been delegated the task by a consultant surgeon. It is outside the remit of a Surgical First Assistant (PCC 2012).

Factors which increase wrong site surgery

A number of factors increase the incidence of wrong site surgery:

- Time constraints
- Staffing problems
- Incomplete patient assessment
- Miscommunication between patient and surgeon
- Lack of protocols and procedures
- Poor preoperative planning
- Lack of verification in the operating room
- Distractions
- Failure of the surgeon to exercise due care
- Multiple procedures or surgeons at one time.

Theatre staff responsibility

Although the responsibility lies with the operating surgeon to perform surgical marking, it is important that checks are carried out throughout the patient's perioperative journey and that the surgical assistant should independently check and verify the correct site prior to the patient being anaesthetised (Shen *et al.* 2013).

To help reduce the risk of wrong site surgery, perioperative staff need to implement and adhere to proactive, evidence-based best practice. Effective communication and the confidence to speak up should there be any discrepancies are imperative (Mellinger 2014).

The responsibility can be delegated to a nominated deputy such as a junior surgeon or, if trained and covered by the healthcare institution within which they work, it can be within the remit of the Surgical Care Practitioner. Whichever individual has performed the marking, they must be present within theatre during surgery. If there is a potential that the junior surgeon or Surgical Care Practitioner will not be present, then they should not perform surgical site marking.

All perioperative staff have a shared responsibility to ensure surgery is performed on the correct site and appropriate safety checks have been undertaken. Staff are to act as patients' advocates to ensure that wrong site surgery is a thing of the past, with an increased awareness of not only patients who may have had sedation but also the elderly, those under stress and/or pain, and those confused or suffering from psychiatric problems or conditions which affect awareness (Msaud *et al.* 2010, Watson 2015).

It has been identified that, in an attempt to reduce the risk of surgical never events, education, training and standardisation of practices are key, encompassed with an environment of safety prevention. These principles can all be related to surgical site marking to minimise the risk of wrong site surgery (NHS England 2014, Watson 2015).

46 Swab Counts, Sharps and Instrument Checks

An integral part of being a theatre practitioner is maintaining the patient's safety. This can be manifested in a number of ways; one such way is the swab counts and instrument checks. The implications of a retained surgical item for a patient are pain, unnecessary additional procedures and a longer recovery. For staff, there is a reduction in morale and a risk of litigation. Each workplace has specific policies and procedures to follow to minimise the incidence of a retained item, and it is imperative that practitioners are familiar with them. The surgical count is a team process, and consistent methods of the counting process should be maintained to maximise patient safety (Woodhead 2009, Goodman and Spry 2014).

What should be checked?

Essentially, anything that is within the sterile field that the theatre practitioner should be able to account for should be checked. This includes:

- Swabs of all sizes (including swab ties)
- All instruments within the sterile field
- Sutures
- Hypodermic needles
- Blades
- Nylon tapes
- Sloops
- Scratch pads
- Pledglets (Hamlin *et al.* 2009).

When they should be checked

The initial count should be carried out prior to the commencement of surgery with all items being documented on the count board. Radiopaque swabs used during catheterisation should remain within theatre and be incorporated in the count. Checks should always be carried out before the closure of a cavity within a cavity, with a count prior to wound closure and a final count when the surgeon is closing skin (AfPP 2011).

When the checks are being carried out, it is imperative that the scrub practitioner ensures that the circulating practitioner can clearly see and verbally verify the items within the sterile field.

As such, swabs, which come in packs of five, should be counted in fives and marked on the board in fives. When checking swabs, the scrub practitioner and circulator should ensure the integrity (e.g. that the full nylon tape has been retrieved or the 'tail' on the swab is present) (AfPP 2011).

Rapid Perioperative Care, First Edition. Paul Wicker and Sara Dalby.

The scrub practitioner should provide the operating surgeon with a verbal confirmation that the counts have been carried out and if they are correct.

No items from within the operating theatre should be removed from the environment until the end of the procedure and all counts are carried out and accounted for (AfPP 2011).

Once within the sterile field, all countable items should be counted and noted on the count board. All countable items should be kept within packaging until counted (Hamlin *et al.* 2009).

Count board

All the counts should be clearly marked upon the count board and cross-checked during each count to minimise risk. Whenever the scrub practitioner is given additional items following the initial count, during the procedure the circulating practitioner should verbally state that they are adding an item to the count board. It is the scrub practitioner's responsibility (or the supervising registered practitioner's) to ensure that the item(s) is marked on the board appropriately (AfPP 2011). A verbal confirmation should also be carried out when an item is being marked off from the board following a count to remove items from the operating field. Items should never be rubbed off from the board but crossed out or circled to identify that they are no longer within the sterile field. Also, the circulating practitioner should never amend the board without confirming and communicating the changes with the scrub practitioner. The circulating practitioner who gave the scrub practitioner the item or counted an item down should be the person to mark it on or off the board.

Taking additional items

As when setting up, if the scrub practitioner requires additional items, this should be verbalised to the scrub practitioner. The circulating practitioner should never lean over the scrub table as they could contaminate the area, rendering it unsterile. The scrub practitioner should always lean out slightly to the circulating practitioner and take the item with a sponge forceps to minimise the incidence of contamination. For the same reason, the circulating practitioner should never 'drop' items into the sterile field. Also, if items are dropped onto the sterile field, the scrub practitioner may not be aware of the presence of the item which is dangerous from a count perspective. However, dropping of items may be deemed acceptable in an emergency (with the exception of blades); the circulating practitioner would ideally drop items into a bowl which allows the scrub nurse to identify the additional items and minimises contamination of the scrub trolley. As with the initial counts, all counts should be undertaken with the scrub practitioner and a circulator (one of whom must be a registered practitioner), verbalised out loud and recorded on the count board (Hamlin *et al.* 2010, Goodman and Spry 2014).

Swabs

It is necessary for the scrub practitioner to check that there is uniformity with the swabs and that there are five in a pack. It is important when checking swabs to ensure the radiopaque line is present within each individual swab and, if appropriate, the 'tail' is present and securely attached (Hamlin *et al.* 2010).

When soiled with blood, the scrub practitioner should replace the swab with a clean replacement and then should either lay them in a sterile bowl separated so they are easily distinguishable to be counted later into bags or place them into relevant plastic containers (AfPP 2011).

If the swabs become contaminated, such as being soiled with faecal matter, then they may be handed out of the sterile field and placed by the circulating staff within a 'dirty' bowl or swab container. This should be verbally confirmed with the scrub practitioner and carried out so the scrub practitioner can see the item.

Sharps and miscellaneous items

As with swabs, needles and blades have the potential to be retained during the operating procedure. The procedure for counting sharps is the same as for counting swabs. However, additional caution needs to be taken as there is a potential for a sharps injury. To minimise the chance of injury, it is recommended to keep needles in their packets until required. The scrub practitioner should have a designated area on their table for sharps (Goodman and Spry 2014).

Instruments

Instrument tray lists should be utilised to ensure that all items are present before, during and after the surgical procedure. Each instrument should be called out individually by name by the circulating practitioner, and the scrub practitioner should identify and separate the instrument to ensure the circulating practitioner has seen the identified item. The information identifying the theatre, patient ID and the names of the two practitioners who checked the tray should be documented on the tray list (Hamlin *et al.* 2009, AfPP 2011).

Who should carry out the checks?

If the scrub practitioner is a registered practitioner (i.e. registered nurse or operating department practitioner), they can carry out counts with any grade of circulating practitioner. However, if the scrub practitioner is a non-registered practitioner such as a student or a theatre assistant practitioner, then the circulating practitioner must be a registered practitioner (Hamlin *et al.* 2009).

Ideally, the same circulating practitioner should carry out all the checks during the procedure to minimise the risk of mistakes.

What happens if the count is wrong?

If the count is incorrect, the surgeon should be informed immediately (AfPP 2011).

If the swab count is incorrect with the board, then the practitioner has the additional check of the 'red tags' of which there should be one per five swabs. If the needle count is incorrect with the board, the packets are an additional check.

If the count is wrong and there is a swab missing, then the environment should be checked, including the patient, operating floor, bin bags and swabs which have been taken down to ensure an additional swab has not accidently been incorporated. This is the rationale for not removing any items, including disposal bins, from theatre until the end of surgery. The surgeon is asked to re-explore the wound to ensure a heavily blood-stained swab hasn't been missed within the wound cavity. Following this, an x-ray needs to be carried out to help locate the swab and ensure it is not inside the patient (AfPP 2011, Goodman and Spry 2014).

If a needle or blade is found to be missing, the scrub practitioner and circulating practitioner need to be careful when carrying out a search of the environment to minimise the risk of a sharps injury. Magnetic rollers can be utilised to try to find metallic sharps which may be on the operating floor. If a needle or blade breaks during the procedure, the scrub nurse should ensure all pieces are accounted for (AfPP 2011). X-ray can also be called to identify a retained needle and microvascular clamps too.

The closing stitch should never be given to the operating surgeon if the counts have not been carried out or if they are incorrect.

Documentation

Confirmation of the swab counts should be documented by the scrub practitioner in the perioperative document and the theatre register following the surgical procedure. Confirmation of the counts is signed by the circulating practitioner (Woodhead 2009).

If the count is incorrect and the appropriate policies and procedures adhered to but the item has still not been located, this needs to be documented in both the theatre register and perioperative document. In addition to this, an incident form needs to be completed by the scrub practitioner explaining the incident, including the item missing and steps taken to attempt to locate it (AfPP 2011).

47 Measures to Prevent Wound Infection

Infection is the most significant cause of interference with the process of wound healing. Infection delays healing, and there is potential for a localised wound infection to develop into a serious systemic infection. Surgical site infections (SSIs) can have serious implications to the health of patients and financial implications for healthcare organisations. The prevention of SSIs requires consideration of multiple contributing factors by perioperative practitioners (Korol *et al.* 2013).

Patient factors

A number of patient factors will increase the chance of SSIs (Reyes and Chang 2011). Patient factors resulting in a higher risk of infection include the following:

- Nutrition will influence wound healing. For example;
  - If a patient is obese or suffering from malnutrition
  - If a patient has protein deficiency, then wound healing is inhibited and the incidence of infection is increased due to a lower resistance.
  - Vitamin A deficiency negatively affects epithelialisation and collagen synthesis.
- Malignancies diminish nutrients and directly reduce wound healing.
- Vascular disease and cardiorespiratory disorders can inhibit wound healing due to a compromised blood supply, and sufficient oxygen levels are essential for fibroblast replication and collagen synthesis.
- The elderly, as they are more likely to have a degenerative disease and have changes in their skin structure that lead to slower healing
- Diabetics, as there is a delayed cellular response to injury, reduced cellular function at the wound and a defect in collagen production and wound strength with compromised microvascular circulation
- Immunodeficient patients whereby their immunodeficiency slows the cleansing of the wound bed and ability of the individual to fight infection
- Smoking due to its vasoconstricting effect
- Patients suffering from advanced cancer or major trauma, extensive burns, extensive surgery or chronic illnesses
- Areas which are heavily contaminated increase the chance of infection which will ultimately have a negative effect on local defence mechanisms, encroached by microorganisms, dead tissue, ischaemia, and anoxia and haematoma.
- Medications and treatments can also inhibit healing, such as:
  - Steroids reduce the normal inflammatory response and suppress collagen and fibroblast synthesis with long-term use, leading to tissue paper skin which can be easily damaged.
  - Cytotoxic drugs slow down the inflammatory response, suppress protein synthesis and inhibit the replication of cells.

Rapid Perioperative Care, First Edition. Paul Wicker and Sara Dalby.

- Anticoagulants, if they are not at the correct dose, cause excessive bleeding and an increased chance of haematoma.
- Immunosuppressive drugs increase the risk of infection by delaying the inflammatory response and radiation therapy.
- If the patient is known to have systemic infection prior to surgery, this increases their chance of contracting an SSI (Kirk 2010, Korol *et al.* 2013, Lobley 2013).

Preoperative practices to reduce surgical site infection

Certain preoperative procedures will reduce the incidence of SSIs.

Preoperative showering or bathing, especially with an antiseptic agent, is shown to decrease the incidence of SSIs. The site of incision and surrounding area should be cleaned by the patient by showering and washing prior to surgery, as well as by washing the site before arrival to the practice setting or immediately prior to application of antiseptic solution. Patients having head and neck surgery are encouraged to wash their hair (NICE 2014, AORN 2015).

Preoperative hair removal can increase the risk of SSIs. Factors influencing whether to remove hair encompass the amount of hair, the position of the surgical incision and the operation to be performed. Hair is removed as it may interfere with the exposure of the incision and wound, suturing of the wound, application of adhesive drapes and wound dressings. Best practice concludes that hair should only be removed if it is considered to get in the way of the surgical procedure; if deemed necessary, hair removal should be undertaken with clippers or depilatory cream (AfPP 2011, Jose and Dignon 2013, NICE 2014, AORN 2015).

There are three main hair removal methods:

- Shaving is deemed the cheapest, but during the process of shaving the skin it may cause small cuts and abrasions in which microorganisms can colonise, leading to SSIs.
- Clipper heads can be disposed of between patients to minimise cross-infection and are shown to be the least aggravating to skin, possibly as they don't come into contact with the patient's skin.
- Depilatory creams are a slower process as the cream has to remain in contact with the skin for between 2 and 20 minutes. There is a risk of skin irritation and allergic reaction, and patch tests should be carried out 24 h before use which would certainly not be feasible in emergency situations.

The patient should be shaved within the surgical suite, using clippers by someone proficient. The amount of time between shaving and the operation has a direct effect on the incidence of SSIs.

It is recommended to give antibiotic prophylaxis to patients who are to have surgery which will be contaminated, clean-contaminated or clean but involving the placement of a prosthesis or implant. Patients with a dirty or infected wound may need additional antibiotics. Antibiotics should not be used in instances where the surgery is clean and not involving prostheses. Adverse effects of the antibiotic should be taken into account before it is administered. It may be necessary for a single dose of antibiotic to be given prior to starting the anaesthetic, but it may need to be given earlier if the patient is to have a tourniquet during the procedure. Prior to the administration of antibiotic prophylaxis, the practitioner needs to take into consideration the timing, pharmacokinetics and infusion time of the specific antibiotic to be used. A repeat dose may be required if the operation is longer in duration than the half-life of the antibiotic. The optimum level of antibiotic should be in the tissue at the time of incision and therefore needs to be administered about 30 min prior to the commencement of surgery. It is important to tell the patient in advance that they will need antibiotics, if this is known. You should also inform them postoperatively that they were given antibiotics during their operation (Borchardt and Rolston 2012, NICE 2014).

Perioperative practices to reduce surgical site infection

During the procedure, there are steps which can be taken to minimise the chance of patients having a wound infection.

Hand hygiene is important to reduce skin flora, and sterile gloves and gowns provide a protective barrier and are utilised to prevent organisms from the hands contaminating the sterile area. Staff wear specific clothing and shoes within the perioperative environment; this reduces the risk of bringing potentially pathogenic organisms into the controlled environment (Rochon 2012).

Face masks are used to protect the patient from droplets from the nose and mouths of people within the surgical field. Sterile drapes provide a sterile field where the surgical team can operate without risk of contamination, and they also decrease the risk of desterilising instrumentation (Weaving *et al.* 2008).

Positive pressure ventilation directs bacteria from clean areas; ultra-clean laminar flow systems are used to reduce levels of microorganisms. Dispersion of microbes is increased with movement, most of which is derived from staff. Only necessary staff should be in theatre, restricting the number and movement of visitors.

Equipment used on tumours or 'dirty' areas, for example open bowel, should only be used on these areas and kept on either a separate trolley or a designated 'dirty' area on the sterile trolley. This is so they don't contaminate other areas, and they should not be used during wound closure. It is also necessary for the practitioner to be aware of using good surgical technique to ensure that microbes are not transferred to other areas of the body and don't contaminate the wound (Rochon 2012, Weston 2013, AORN 2015).

Preparation of trolleys is carried out using a sterile technique to ensure the sterility of items needed. Only sterile items are used within the sterile field; the circulating practitioner should ensure that the item is in date and packaging is intact, and check the sterilisation indicator. All instruments and consumables introduced to the sterile field should be sterilised, which removes all microbes (Weston 2013).

All skin preparation methods aim to reduce the risk of postoperative SSIs by removing dirt and transient microbes from the skin, reducing the microbial count in the shortest time possible whilst causing little irritation to the skin and preventing a rapid regrowth of microbes. Consider the patient's condition prior to the choice of skin preparation, being aware of patients with hypersensitivity and any contraindications of skin preparation (Alexander *et al.* 2011, AORN 2015).

Surgical skills are important to reduce the chance of SSIs, with prolonged procedures, haematoma, tissue damage and necrosis all increasing the risk. A collection of fluid and oedema increase the incidence of wound infection as they inhibit phagocytosis. The surgical team should ensure minimal blood loss, avoid shock and maintain blood volume leading to good tissue perfusion and oxygenation. Precise cutting and suturing techniques, along with efficient use of time to minimise the time exposure of the wound to air, eliminate dead spaces, and minimal pressure on retractors and other instruments which will minimise trauma all help reduce the risk of SSIs. Other considerations include avoiding excessive diathermy and appropriate use of drains, avoiding their use if unnecessary, along with unintended immunological effects.

It is important to handle the tissues gently, because if they are handled roughly they will become devitalised; and when using forceps during wound closure, do not to crush the tissues as the skin may die and scar postoperatively, subsequently increasing the incidence of wound infection (Kocker Fuller 2010, Nicolette 2011). The longer the operation, the higher the incidence of infection as the instruments are exposed for longer times; this increases the chance of contamination, and the wound site is exposed for longer.

The maintenance of homeostasis includes maintaining patient temperature; optimal oxygenation during the perioperative stage, which is particularly important during major surgery and the recovery period to ensure that patients have a saturation level above 95%; and maintenance of adequate perfusion. Also, it is vital not to administer insulin routinely to patients who aren't diabetic in order to optimise blood glucose postoperatively, aiming to minimise the incidence of SSIs. If the patient's temperature falls, it increases their susceptibility to infection; therefore, warming devices should be utilised. The chance of a patient contracting a wound infection is increased if they have operations in which there has been a lot of bleeding; therefore, it is essential for the practitioner to ensure that the operative field is dry, as stagnant blood is an ideal medium for microorganisms (Lobley 2013, NICE 2014, Peate and Glencross 2015).

Some surgical procedures have a higher risk of wound infection than others, such as if the procedure is 'dirty' or carried out on areas of the body which have a higher microbe level. In such cases, the practitioner closing the wound needs to acknowledge this risk and use interrupted stitches with a monofilament to lower the risk, and not to close under tension. It is important for wound healing that there is a good blood supply; therefore, the practitioner must ensure that the correct amount of tension is used as sutures pulled too tight will cut off the circulation.

The type of surgery also affects the incidence of infection. There is a higher risk of contamination in patients who have had abdominal surgery, as large numbers of endogenous bacteria are located in this region; therefore, there is an increased chance of cross-contamination. The presence of foreign bodies in the wound will affect healing and make the patient more susceptible to wound infections; therefore, it may be necessary to wash out the wound to eliminate the debris. Dead and ischaemic tissues should be removed as microorganisms require little or no oxygen to metabolise within this tissue. If the procedure requires the use of an implant, such as hernia mesh, patients have an increased risk of infection due to implants attracting and providing a supportive environment for the colonisation of microbes.

The theatre and equipment should be cleaned before the start of the day and between each procedure to minimise the incidence of cross-infection.

Methods to reduce SSIs are multifactorial, and a combination of the practices discussed in this chapter should minimise the incidence of infection for the patient.

48 Electrosurgery

Electrosurgery (diathermy) uses a high-frequency (2–3 MHz) alternating electrical current to heat tissues (Photo 5). High-frequency electrosurgical current does not stimulate muscles or nerves and therefore does not cause twitching, convulsions or fibrillation of the heart. Electrosurgery coagulates or cuts tissues quickly and easily. Practically every operating room in the world uses it. Therefore, most practitioners consider it as safe to use; however, human errors can still cause accidental harm to patients, evidencing a need for practitioner training (Feldman *et al.* 2012). Diathermy is commonly used for haemostasis and is divided into monopolar and bipolar.

Monopolar diathermy

A current is passed through the patient's body using a diathermy pencil or forceps which is then redirected to the diathermy machine via a return electrode (diathermy pad) which completes the circuit. The return electrode must be adequately sized and remain in contact throughout diathermy; if not, there will be a high concentration of energy and subsequent heat which leads to diathermy burns. The plate should be situated on a well-vascularised, muscular area to enhance conductivity and dissipation of heat near the site of diathermy and not where fluids will pool. The area may need to be shaved to enhance contact and should not be placed over bony prominences, an implanted prosthesis, scar tissue or areas below tourniquets where tissue perfusion is compromised. When securing the diathermy electrode to the drapes, a non-conductive material diathermy lead should be used, and diathermy leads should not be positioned round a metal clip to minimise injury from a stray current. The diathermy tip should also be cleaned frequently as build-up on the tip can hinder the current flow, causing the system to work less efficiently; such build-up also acts as a fuel source potentially leading to fires (Potty *et al.* 2010).

Monopolar settings

Several settings are available for monopolar diathermy: cutting, coagulation, blend (combining coagulation and cutting) and fulguration. Cutting uses a continuous wave form and is high frequency and low voltage; it focusses energy on a small area and results in intense heat and vaporising of intracellular fluid, bursting cells. When using the cutting mode, the electrode should be held a short distance from the tissue so the current arcs to the tissue. Coagulation uses an intermittent wave form, is lower current and lower voltage, and produces less heat, resulting in desiccation of the area through direct contact. Fulguration (spray) involves avoiding direct contact with tissues, uses high voltage and low current, and is used to spray over areas such as the gall bladder bed or the ends of bone, leading to coagulation and preventing bleeding. Blend is a combination of both cutting and coagulation that allows increased haemostasis when cutting.

Rapid Perioperative Care, First Edition. Paul Wicker and Sara Dalby.

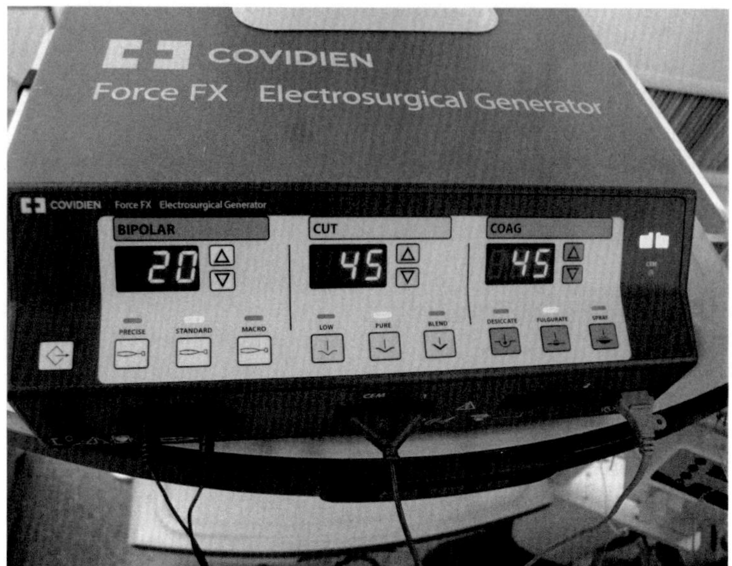

Photo 5 A diathermy machine

Bipolar diathermy

The electrical circuit is formed between two parallel tips, one positive and one negative, in close vicinity of each other with the current flowing only between the two, as they are so close to each other that only a low voltage is needed for the desired effect on the tissue. As the patient does not form part of the circuit, there is no need for a diathermy plate; subsequently, this should be the choice of diathermy for a patient with a pacemaker (as it avoids a current passing through the heart) and for patients with Cochlear implants in ENT (ear, nose and throat) surgery. Bipolar would be used in the following scenarios: when only coagulation is needed as, due to low voltage and power, it is incapable of cutting; when coagulation is needed for peripheral areas, as it reduces the risk of necrosis to peripheries which is caused by channelling current through narrow areas of tissue; and when pinpoint or micro coagulation is needed (O'Riley 2010).

Hazards of diathermy

A number of potential hazards are linked to the use of diathermy. Accidental burns can occur when the current is diverted away from the return electrode and causes a burn at the area where it departs the patient's body; other pathways may be through an electrocardiograph (ECG) electrode, or the patient being in contact with a metal part of the operating table or a table accessory. This can happen if the return electrode is not applied sufficiently (O'Riley 2010)

The chance of fire can be minimised by maintenance of the equipment, with checks of the machine for frayed wires, signs of moisture or loose plugs. Fluids should not be placed on the diathermy as spills can increase the incidence of fires. In order to reduce the risk of burns to patients, the electrodes should be stored in a holster or quiver when not in use in case the electrode is accidently activated; such activation could ignite drapes, and audible activation indicators and alarms should be able to be heard over the noise in theatre. Care should be taken when using surgical prep, in particular those which are alcohol based; sparks from an active electrode can ignite alcohol-based solutions, and chemical burns may occur around the diathermy pad due to pooling and trapped fluids; therefore, excess prep solution should be removed prior to diathermy use, and alcoholic solutions should be avoided whenever feasible (Spruce and Braswell 2012).

Healthcare professionals have been known to receive shocks from the diathermy, with holes in gloves being blamed. To avoid shocks, it is recommended not to lean on the patient as it would include the individual in the circuit, hold the diathermy pencil fully in hand to disperse the current over a larger surface area and touch the other instrument before activating diathermy. Use the diathermy briefly and sporadically, avoiding overheating of the tissues; once tissue is charred, the current will seek a more conductive path, shocking the individual.

It is preferable to use bipolar diathermy if the patient has a pacemaker, but if monopolar diathermy is used it is recommended to keep all diathermy cords and cables away from the pacemaker, use the lowest possible setting and ensure the distance between the electrode and pad is minimal and both are as far away from the pacemaker as possible. Pacemaker checks should be carried out pre- and post-operatively as per Trust protocols.

Smoke plume has been shown to be a biological and chemical hazard to both staff and patients; it has been found to incorporate toxic gases and vapours, blood fragments and viruses, and in high intensities it can cause ocular and respiratory tract infections (Bruske-Hohlfeld *et al.* 2008, Marsh 2012, Mowbray *et al.* 2013).

Laparoscopic diathermy hazards

Due to the number of instruments in a secluded space, and a limited visibility outside of direct surgical vision, minimal access surgery (MAS) provides healthcare professionals with a new set of challenges relating to electrosurgery. Complications from unintentional and unsuspected diathermy injuries include organ and vessel haemorrhage, contamination of the abdominal cavity, organ perforation and peritonitis. Electrosurgery injuries are due to direct coupling of current, insulation failure and capacitive coupling.

Insulation failure is said to be the most dangerous as the full strength of current can be reassigned to non-targeted tissue. Insulation damage occurs due to repeated use, the use of high voltages and rough handling; coagulation mode utilises higher voltages than cut mode, which is unfavourable as a weakened insulation can be converted to a break due to the increased force. Endoscopic instruments should be checked prior to use to ensure that insulation is intact. This ensures that the current only leaves the tip as intended and not at a point of the instrument which has suffered insulation damage, which could ultimately cause tissue damage by direct contact, an escaped current or arc to a metal trocar and serious patient injury, particularly if the patient is damaged internally and it is not detected instantaneously, as often this damage occurs outside of the vision of the surgical team. Small cracks in insulation are more dangerous as the current is more focussed and therefore more likely to cause significant damage (Spruce and Braswell 2012).

Direct coupling occurs when an active electrode touches or arcs to another instrument made of conductive material, such as a laparoscope or metal clip. The best prevention of direct coupling is to only activate the electrode when it is in direct contact with the intended site of diathermy. Three potential problems are necrosis of underlying tissue, frequency demodulation causing neuromuscular stimulation seen as muscular twitching and current flow to non-intended sites resulting in tissue damage. The surgeon must be continuously aware of the active part of the electrosurgical instrument, considering it as live, and the camera operator should ensure that all the metal area of the instrument is visible when activated. Sometimes surgeons use this technique intentionally by grasping tissue with one instrument and then touching it with a different active electrode; caution should be used as this could cause the current to be redirected to non-targeted structures (O'Riley 2010).

Capacitive coupling is two conductors separated by an insulator. For example, if a metal port was used and an insulated instrument was inserted into the port, the electrical current can move from the instrument through intact insulation to the metal port, which in turn can transfer the current to any bodily structures that it is in contact with; an adhesion or nearby organ can also be a conductor. The electrical charge will stay within the second conductor until a path to complete the circuit is found; this can usually be done safely through the abdominal wall from conductive ports, but if an insulator inhibits this, then a burn to any tissue in contact with the metal instrument will occur, such as a metal trocar sheath used with a plastic fixation sheath. Plastic ports can be equally dangerous, as the patient's own conductive tissue within the abdomen can act as the second conductor; omentum or bowel in contact with the plastic port may expel stored energy to nearby body structures; metal suction irrigations or laparoscopes can be conductors; and, if in plastic ports, the current can't escape safely to the abdominal wall, and subsequently it must return via non-targeted tissue. High voltages that are created when activating the electrode when not in contact with tissue or when an increase of power is needed for fulguration may produce capacitively coupled currents sufficiently intense to cause injury (Spruce and Braswell 2012).

The use of an active electrode monitoring system minimises the risk of capacitive coupling, direct coupling and insulation failure as it monitors and actively shields against stray currents and prevents electrosurgery burns.

49 Wound Healing and Dressings

Introduction

Any patient undergoing a surgical procedure is likely to need a dressing over the site of surgery. Surgical wounds vary and can include minor or major wounds, minimal access surgery, trauma, small incisional cuts or excision of large areas of tissue. The purpose of wound dressings is to reduce the risk of infection and also includes reducing pain, applying compression, immobilising injured areas, protecting the wound and promoting better healing. The wound needs assessing before applying the dressing to ensure use of the most appropriate dressing.

Physiology of wound healing

- *Haemostasis*: Blood cells are released to the wound, causing vasoconstriction, and coagulation factors are released.
- *Inflammation*: Vasodilation and increased capillary permeability, leakage of fluid and production of exudate and inflammatory phase begin which comprise a process of wound cleansing.
- *Proliferation*: Revascularisation and connective tissue formation which is weaker and less elasticated than in healthy tissue
- *Granulation*: Tissue formation
- *Epithelisation*: Wound closes its margins through cell migration, covering the wound with new skin.
- *Remodelling (maturation)*: Wound remodelling takes place within the scar (Beldon 2010, Wild *et al.* 2010, Flanagan 2013, Ward and Linden 2013, Peate and Glencross 2015).

Patient factors which inhibit wound healing

Patient factors which the practitioner should consider that affect wound healing include:

- Infection
- Dehiscence
- Effects of aging
- Obesity
- Nutrition state
- Pressure
- Desiccation
- Oedema
- Trauma
- Necrosis
- Incontinence leading to maceration

Rapid Perioperative Care, First Edition. Paul Wicker and Sara Dalby.

- Chronic illnesses
- Immunosuppressive and radiation therapy
- Vascular (arterial) insufficiency
- Environment of the wound
- Compliance
- Diabetes
- Smoking
- Steroids
- Stress response (Kotcher Fuller 2010, Sharp and Clark 2011, Ward and Linden 2013, Tickle 2014, Peate and Glencross 2015).

Environmental factors which inhibit healing

In conjunction with patient factors, there are also environmental factors that the practitioner should consider:

- Tissue handling
- Wound classification
- Improper choice of wound dressing
- Bleeding
- Infection
- Wound temperature (Kotcher and Fuller 2010, Zinn 2012, Peate and Glencross 2015).

Types of wound healing

- *Primary*: This is when skin edges are brought together by clips, sutures, glue or steristrips. Scar formation should be minimal, and it is considered the ideal; it can be seen in the majority of surgical wounds.
- *Secondary*: The skin edges are purposefully not put together as it isn't surgically practical (i.e. pressure sores and leg ulcers, or traumatic tissue loss); when the wound is encouraged to form granulation tissue from the base to fill the tissue deficit; is a common form of healing in chronic wounds.
- *Tertiary*: When a wound hasn't been primarily closed and is later sutured, or when the wound has broken down and is resutured later, two granulation surfaces are closed, which causes significant scaring (i.e. after wound debridement). Tertiary closure may be needed to allow topical treatment with antibiotics or in heavily contaminated or infected wounds (Dealey and Cameron 2009, Beldon 2010, Flanagan 2013, Peate and Glencross 2015).

Wound classifications

Wound Classifications

- Class I: clean
- Class II: clean-contaminated
- Class III: contaminated
- Class IV: dirty/infected (Simpson and Brooks 2008, Kotcher Fuller 2010, Zinn 2012, Zinn and Swofford 2014).

Things to consider when selecting dressings

Prior to selecting a dressing, a wound assessment must be performed. Things to consider include:

- How the wound occurred (i.e. surgical or chronic)
- Type of healing
- Amount of exudate
- Size and depth of wound
- Site
- Patient allergies
- Tissue perfusion
- Patient comfort and daily activities of living
- The type and state of skin around the wound
- Dressings available (Simpson and Brooks 2008, Kotcher Fuller 2010, Stephen-Haynes 2010, Broussard and Powers 2013, Tickle 2014, Peate and Glencross 2015).

Types of dressings

Hydrogels (IntraSite Gel, NU-Gel, Purilon Gel, GranuGel, ActiForm Cool, Curagel, Geliperm and Hydrosorb): These are non-adherent, non-absorbent, water and starch-based products which aid autolytic debridement in dry, necrotic or sloughy wounds. The gel should be put into the wound about 5 mm thick, with caution taken to ensure it doesn't seep onto surrounding skin which could cause maceration; or, if the dressing is used, it should be cut to the appropriate size wound, gently cover the wound or loosely fill the cavity to prevent moisture loss. A semi-permeable dressing should be used and removed after 3–5 days, depending on exudate levels (Benbow 2008, Tiaki 2012, Adis Medical Writers 2014).

Hydrocolloid (Granuflex, DuoDerm, Comfeel, Tegasorb, Hydrocoll and Aquacel): When they come into contact with the wound, the hydrocolloid component becomes a gel and creates a barrier to infection and microorganisms. They can handle light to very heavy exudate, can be used in a variety of wounds (e.g. pressure sores, surgical wounds and granulating, sloughy or necrotic wounds) and facilitate rehydration and debridement of dry, sloughy and necrotic wounds, but they can encourage growth of anaerobic bacteria on infected wounds. They may need an additional dressing on top and should overlap the wound and skin margins; they are ideally left in place for 3–5 days (Bennet- Marsden 2010, Tiaki 2012, Adis Medical Writers 2014).

Semipermeable films (Opsite, C-View, Hydrofilm and Mepore Film): These films are sterile, transparent, plastic sheets of polyurethane coated with an adhesive. A certain amount of air and water vapour can pass through, but the film is impermeable to fluids and bacteria. They aren't indicated for wet wounds and can't absorb exudate; if the moisture vapour transmission rate is low, there may be a build-up of moisture, wrinkling, skin maceration and dressing displacement. They may be used as primary or secondary dressings; it is important when applying the dressing that no traction is applied as this may result in blistering of the skin (Benbow 2008, Tiaki 2012).

Alginate (Aquacel, Kaltostat, Tegagen, Seasorb and Algosteril): Alginate absorbs 20–30 times its weight in exudate and therefore is useful in very moist wounds. As alginate absorbs, it converts totally or partially to gel; its sodium–calcium balance controls the amount of gel or residual dressing left in the wound. They come in ribbon or square form and are either put onto or into the wound; it promotes granulation and is comfortable for patients (Bennet-Marsden 2010, Tiaki 2012, Adis Medical Writers 2014).

Foam (Allevyn, Biatain, lyofoam, Mepilex and Tielle): Foam is manufactured as either polyurethane or silicone. Both transmit moisture vapour and oxygen, providing thermal insulation for the wound bed. Polyurethane is highly absorbent and prevents exterior leakage, and silicone has the facility to contain exudate and protects the area surrounding the wound from further damage (Tiaki 2012, Adis Medical Writers 2014).

Occlusive: This is said to increase cell proliferation and activity by maintaining an optimum level of wound exudate which contains vital proteins and cytokines, which facilitate autolytic debridement and promote healing.

Low-adherent, non-adherent and membrane (NA Ultra, Melonin, Tegapore, Tricotex, Release, Exu-Dry, Mepitel and Mesorb): These are used on lightly exudating wounds; some combine an absorbent layer which can be used in moderately to highly exudating wounds. Membrane dressings can be used for all levels of exudate, and they require a simple absorbent secondary dressing (Morris 2006).

Deodorising (CarboFlex, ActisorbSilver 200, Clinsorb, Lyofoam C and Carbonet): This is used for fungating and malodorous wounds; many dressings contain charcoal cloth which can absorb gas molecules, while others combine with other dressing materials such as foam, silver, absorbent pads and alginates (Morris 2006).

Honey (Activon range and Mesitran range): Honey has antibacterial, anti-inflammatory and debridement properties (Morris 2006).

Biologically based wound products: Hyaluronic acid (HYAFF) dressings re-stimulate the healing process, influencing quality tissue repair; enhance angiogenesis; and improve phagocytic response. They are used on neuropathic diabetic foot ulcers and venous leg ulcers (Collier 2006).

Antimicrobial: Cadexomer iodine (Iodoform and Iodosorb) contains 0.9% concentration of iodine, which is slowly released as the wound fluid is absorbed into the lattice. It is a moisture-retentive dressing which provides an antimicrobial environment as it absorbs exudate which promotes healing. Caution should be used when patients have thyroid disease, with all patients being monitored for thyroid function. Antimicrobial dressings impregnated with silver ions (Arglaes and Acticoat) are effective against antibiotic-resistant organisms; these may be used under compression wraps for venous stasis ulcers for seven days (Tiaki 2012, Broussard and Powers 2013).

Wound dressing contraindications

- Badly applied dressings can be painful and distressing to patients, and may in some cases lead to deterioration of the wound and surrounding skin.
- Maceration can occur when a dressing with low absorbency is used on a heavily exudating wound. If the dressing is highly absorptive, then more regular dressing changes are needed, and skin surrounding a heavily exudating wound may need additional protection from emollients or barrier films.
- A highly absorbent dressing used on a dry wound will cause disruption of healthy tissue and pain on removal.
- Both dressings and tapes used to secure dressings may cause allergic reactions; therefore, practitioners need to ensure they check the patient's allergy status beforehand.
- Dressings may need a secondary dressing; they should not be too tight, especially on patients with peripheral vascular disease (Benbow 2008).

50 Bladder Catheterisation

Bladder catheterisation increases the incidence of urinary tract infection (UTI). The longer a catheter is in situ, the higher that risk is. Indwelling urinary catheters should therefore only be used as a last resort after alternative items have been considered, such as a penile sheath or intermittent catheterisation, which have a lower rate of infection (NICE 2014). RCN (2012) states that nurses must assess whether the advantages of catheterising outweigh the disadvantages. Due to the risks involved, the assessment of the need for a catheter and the individual patient's medical status should be continually assessed, with removal as soon as possible. Informed consent should be obtained prior to catheterisation, with the patient understanding the reason, informed of other options and told of the consequences of not being catheterised (RCN 2012).

Steps of bladder catheterisation

Prior to bladder catheterisation, informed consent must be gained from the patient. The steps of the procedure should be explained, and the benefits and risks of the procedure discussed (Hughes and Patrick 2014). A clean environment should be sustained for both the procedure and the catheter equipment which maintains patient dignity and privacy. The equipment should be kept in a dry, cool and dark location which prevents damage and ensures sterility. Catheterisation must be carried out using an aseptic technique with sterile equipment. Hand hygiene is important, and sterile gloves must be used. When catheterising, plastic aprons should be worn to prevent bodily fluids from contaminating the health-care professional's clothing. The patient's dignity should be maintained at all times, and only essential staff should be present during the time when the patient is exposed to be catheterised.

Cleansing of the urethral meatus should be carried out prior to catheterisation with sterile saline away from the urethral opening. A single-use, sterile lubricating gel which contains local anaesthetic should be used as it reduces trauma and discomfort (EAUN 2012, RCN 2012).

When choosing a catheter, considerations may include:

- The duration of time it will remain in situ. Short-term catheters which are made of latex are suitable for four weeks. Long-term catheters which are made of silicone can be left in situ for up to three months.
- Patient allergies
- Gender of the patient, as recommendations vary for both circumference and length.
- Size of balloon required
- The purpose of catheterising (Hughes and Patrick 2014).

The narrowest and softest catheter that will be appropriate should be selected in order to avoid discomfort and decrease the chance of bypassing, and the smallest balloon appropriate should also be chosen as this will decrease mucosal and bladder irritation and prevent residual urine in the bladder.

Rapid Perioperative Care, First Edition. Paul Wicker and Sara Dalby.

The catheter should be advanced into the bladder with a sterile, non-touch technique. Prior to inflating the balloon, the healthcare professional should ensure that urine is draining from the catheter. The balloon should be filled as per the manufacturer's instructions as this maximises the drainage capacity of the catheter. The catheter should be attached to a closed drainage system to reduce the incidence of infection, and secured to avoid trauma. The drainage bag should be placed to prevent backflow of urine and elevated from the floor (EAUN 2012, RCN 2012).

Complications of bladder catheterisation

Complications from catheterisation include: blocked catheter, urinary stones, trauma to the urethra or bladder, urethral perforation, creation of a false passage, urethral stricture, bladder calculi, increased bladder cancer risk, chronic renal inflammation and introduction of infection, which in worst cases can lead to septicaemia and even death (Booth and Clarkson 2012, Hughes and Patrick 2014).

Documentation after bladder catheterisation

Following bladder catheterisation, the following should be documented: allergy status; whether consent was obtained; results of the risk assessment; if insertion was easy or difficult; if antibiotic cover was used; meatal or genital abnormalities, including discharge; any form of localised discomfort or pain shown by the patient; the patient's health status prior to catheterisation; indication for catheterising; residual urine amount, colour and smell; the details of the catheter used; the cleansing fluid used; if a specimen was taken and why; if lubricating gel was used and if the patient has a temperature or is taking antibiotics for a UTI (Geng *et al.* 2012, RCN 2012).

Indications for bladder catheterisation

- Urinary retention or to bypass an obstruction which may be due to a stricture, calculi or tumour
- For investigative purposes (i.e. retrograde pyelography)
- Intraoperatively to empty the bladder and increase the size of the pelvic cavity, allowing the surgeon a larger working area and reducing the risk of perforating the bladder, and to distinguish the ureters during pelvic or intestinal surgery
- Protection of a bladder anastomosis
- For bladder irrigation postoperatively to help with haemostasis
- Bladder dysfunction when alternatives were unsuccessful
- For women with persistent urinary retention which is causing incontinence, renal dysfunction or symptomatic infections which can't be managed alternatively
- For patients with urinary incontinence to improve comfort
- For terminally ill patients to minimise distress or disruption due to bed and clothing changes
- For monitoring renal function in critically ill patients
- Acute urinary retention and chronic urinary retention but only if symptomatic and/or renal compromise
- To introduce medication into the bladder
- Patients with neurological conditions which affect bladder function, such as multiple sclerosis and Parkinson's disease (Booth and Clarkson 2012, RCN 2012, NHS Choices 2013, NICE 2013, Hughes and Patrick 2014, Mangnall 2014).

Contraindications for bladder catheterisation

- If a patient refuses consent for catheterisation
- Where chronic wounds are present and there is likely to be cross-contamination to the urinary tract
- Catheterisation may increase the likelihood of pressure ulcers due to a reduction of patient interaction and subsequent movement.
- When a patient is unable to comprehend the need for a catheter and may try to remove it, causing damage to their bladder or urethra
- Patient allergies (e.g. latex, soap and medication)
- Urinary catheterisation, especially long term, increases the risk of wound infections.
- Increased risk of UTIs, which are associated with urinary tract stones and higher incidence of bladder cancer
- Certain patients are at an increased risk of infection from catheterisation, such as those with a debilitating or malignant disease, neonates and older patients, as they have a less proficient immune system; those having surgery, as the use of instruments and presence of foreign bodies increase the risk of infection; and those taking immunosuppressive drugs and broad-spectrum antimicrobials.
- Urethral stricture
- Urethral sepsis (RCN 2012).

51 Tourniquet Management

Having a bloodless field enables the surgeon to carry out complex surgeries in a safe and more effective manner. A tourniquet is a device placed around a limb or digit to prevent bleeding and isolate perfusion. Practitioners should have training and follow the policies and procedures within their local trusts for tourniquet management.

Types of tourniquet

There are two types of tourniquet in surgery:

1. *Simple tourniquet*: Used for the prevention of bleeding on a digit, such as a rubber tourniquet which comes in differing sizes depending on the digit to be operated on. They are used for procedures such as ingrowing toenail surgery.
2. *Limb tourniquet*: A pneumatic tourniquet is inflated, normally following limb exsanguination, to prevent bleeding during surgery.

Digit tourniquets

A digit tourniquet is usually made from brightly coloured rubber, usually with different colours corresponding to different sizes; there is also a tag attached. Both the tag and the colour are for safety to enhance visibility and prompt the practitioner to remove it postoperatively as one hazard is that it may be left in place post surgery. As an additional check, the removal of a tourniquet should be prompted during the swab check, with verbal confirmation of removal between circulating and scrub practitioner. The time of placement should be noted on the count board and documented postoperatively in the patient's notes. Practitioners should only utilise the specialised rubber tourniquets and should not create their own, such as with gloves and a clip. Postoperatively, the patient's digit should be checked for any signs of ischaemia (AfPP 2011).

Steps to tourniquet application for limb surgery

For orthopaedic limb surgery, tourniquets are used to reduce blood loss, maintain a clear operative field and also prevent the spread of local anaesthesia during IV regional anaesthesia (AfPP 2011).

It is important to pick a cuff that fits the extremity and evenly spreads the pressure. The practitioner should assess the patient and select a cuff which is of appropriate width and length depending on the shape and diameter of the extremity and the procedure. Wider cuffs are optimal as they occlude blood flow at lower pressure, and the length should be considered as excessive overlap of long cuffs increases the risk of wrinkling tissue and causing pressure (Karia 2011, AORN 2013).

The operative site should be confirmed, and appropriate surgical site safety practices should be complied with prior to the application of the tourniquet (AORN 2013).

Rapid Perioperative Care, First Edition. Paul Wicker and Sara Dalby.

To minimise the risk of 'pinching' and potential damage to the integrity of the patient's skin, it is necessary for the practitioner to wrap the area where the tourniquet will be placed with padding such as velband (Hamlin *et al.* 2009, AORN 2013).

Prior to the application of the tourniquet to the limb, it is necessary to exsanguinate the limb. This may be carried out by the practitioner by raising the limb or utilising a soft rubber exsanguinater (Angadi *et al.* 2010, AfPP 2011).

Another step the practitioner can undertake to minimise the risk of potential skin damage such as shearing is to apply a stockinette over the skin prior to using the exsanguinater.

The pressures for the tourniquet fluctuate depending on the limb, but the lowest pressure to achieve a bloodless field should be used:

- For an upper limb, the tourniquet pressure should exceed the systolic blood pressure by 50–75 mmHg (usually 200 mmHg in practice). The pressure should never be above 250 mmHg.
- For a lower limb, the tourniquet pressure should exceed the systolic blood pressure by 100–150 mmHg (usually 350 mmHg in practice). The pressure should never be above 450 mmHg (AfPP 2011, Karia 2011).

If the pressures are too high, the tourniquet may cause soft tissue damage, with thin patients being particularly at risk.

If the tourniquet accidently deflates or slips during the operative procedure, then there may be a partial or full return of blood flow to the limb which can compromise the surgeon's visualisation of the surgical field. Should this happen, the practitioner should deflate the cuff, reposition the tourniquet and elevate the limb prior to reflating the cuff. When carrying this out, the practitioner needs to ensure they communicate effectively with the surgical team and ensure they do not compromise the sterile field.

Depending on surgical preference, the surgeon may ask the practitioner to release the pressure in the tourniquet prior to wound closure to ensure haemostasis. However, some surgeons may prefer to close the wound and apply the dressing prior to releasing the pressure in the tourniquet. For this reason, it is imperative for the practitioner to confirm preference prior to releasing the pressure (Karia 2011).

Caution when exsanguinating a limb

The limb should not be exsanguinated in the following clinical situations:

- Suspected calf deep vein thrombosis
- Presence of distal infection
- Presence of foreign bodies
- Unstable fractures
- Malignancy (Angadi *et al.* 2010).

Caution also needs to be taken when exsanguinating a limb that is fractured or injured.

Caution and contraindications when using tourniquet

There is a need to exercise caution and not utilise tourniquets on patients with the following:

- Sickle cell disease
- Rheumatoid arthritis
- Regional infection
- History of deep vein thrombosis, thromboembolic disease or pulmonary emboli
- Known or suspected compartment syndrome
- Peripheral vascular disease

- Compromised blood flow to the intended limb
- Patients with an arterial venous access fistula
- Active malignancy
- If the patient has had vascular surgery on the limb (Afpp 2011).

Key points to remember when using a tourniquet on a limb

- There needs to be clear, visible documentation of the time of inflation and pressure to attempt to keep the duration to a minimum. This is usually documented on the count board in theatre and also in the patient's perioperative document postoperatively, as well as location and any changes to skin integrity.
- Care should be taken to ensure the cuff is not over bony prominences, as this can cause nerve damage and compression.
- Prophylactic antibiotics should be given about five minutes prior to the inflation of the tourniquet.
- Caution is necessary to ensure that alcoholic preps do not pool underneath the tourniquet.
- The considered safe time frame for application of tourniquet to an upper limb is an hour to an hour and a half.
- The considered acceptable time frame for application of a tourniquet to a lower limb is three hours, but this is not ideal.
- Theatre practitioners should make the surgeon aware of 60 min time intervals to ensure the tourniquet is not in situ over a safe time frame.
- For extended surgical times, it may be necessary to deflate the tourniquet and then re-inflate, but this is at the expense of a clear operative field (Hamlin *et al.* 2009, AfPP 2011, AORN 2013).

Complications of tourniquet use

- Haemorrhage once released
- Deep vein thrombosis or superficial venous thrombosis
- Ischaemic necrosis from prolonged use
- Pressure necrosis from insufficient padding or the tourniquet being too tight
- Distal ischaemia from arterial thrombosis
- Metabolic disturbances following release after prolonged use, such as lactic acidosis or hyperkalaemia
- Damage to skin, muscle or joints due to poor application or structures getting caught in the tourniquet, such as genitalia for a thigh tourniquet
- Damage to nerves causing nerve palsy (Smith and Hing 2010, Karia 2011).

Aftercare of limb following tourniquet use

Following surgery and the removal of the tourniquet, the circulation of the limb should be assessed to ensure perfusion and peripheral pulses. Skin integrity should also be assessed to ensure that no damage has occurred to the patient whilst the tourniquet has been in place (Hamlin *et al.* 2009).

Other information to be documented:

- Where the cuff was placed
- What was used to protect the skin (i.e. velband)
- Cuff inflation and deflation times

- The cuff pressure used
- If pressure was released at any point (AfPP 2011, AORN 2013).

The use of tourniquet helps with the surgical procedure by enabling a clearer operating field for the operative surgeon; it also helps to reduce the operative time. However, the use of tourniquets is not without hazards; it is important that practitioners have training and follow local policies and procedures. The patient should be assessed to ensure that the use of a tourniquet is appropriate, and the practitioner should take steps to reduce the risk if a tourniquet is to be used.

52 Haemostatic Techniques

Introduction

It is important as both a scrub practitioner and a surgical assistant to have a working knowledge of the potential haemostatic techniques. Knowledge of the methods to achieve haemostasis intraoperatively is majorly important to minimise bleeding (Paige 2009).

Contributing factors to surgical bleeding

Factors that contribute to surgical bleeding can be categorised as either patient factors or procedural factors.

Patient Factors

- Platelet dysfunction or deficiency
- Coagulation factor deficiencies
- Medical conditions (e.g. disseminated intravascular coagulation (DIC) secondary to sepsis, massive trauma)
- Fibrinolytic activity
- Nutritional status
- Specific anatomical considerations
- Medications (e.g. warfarin, novel oral anticoagulants (NOACs) and antiplatelet agents)
- Hypothermia (Gonzalez *et al.* 2010)

Procedural Factors

- Surgical incisions
- Tissues that cannot be sutured or low-pressure suture lines
- Exposed bone
- Large surfaces of exposed capillaries
- Unseen sources of bleeding
- Type of procedure
- Patient position
- Adhesional dissection (Samudrala 2008, cited in Moss 2013: 5)

Adverse effects of surgical bleeding

Intraoperative uncontrolled or diffuse bleeding can potentially result in a variety of adverse clinical and economic patient outcomes.

Clinical Effects

- Visual obstruction of the surgical field
- Thrombocytopenia

Rapid Perioperative Care, First Edition. Paul Wicker and Sara Dalby.

- Need for blood transfusions
- Hypovolemic shock (AORN 2013)

Economic Effects (Increased Incidence Of)

- Extended patient monitoring
- Longer procedure times and/or a return to theatre
- Extended length of hospital stay
- Further surgical intervention
- Postoperative intensive care unit stay
- Additional interventions (Schreiber and Neveleff 2011, cited in Moss 2013: 6)

Methods of haemostasis

As mentioned in this chapter, intraoperative haemostasis is important to ensure a clear operating field which reduces the overall operating time and reduces the incidence of blood transfusions. There are several methods of intraoperative haemostasis – mechanical techniques, chemical methods including haemostatic products and thermal/energy-based methods.

Mechanical methods

- *Haemostatic clips and staplers*: Clips allow quick and effective haemostasis when applied to arteries, veins, nerves and other small structures, decreasing the risk of foreign body reaction which can occur with sutures. They are ideal in small spaces where tying would be difficult and the use of diathermy may be hazardous as it may cause damage to adjacent structures. Prior to applying the clip, it is essential to visualise both tips to ensure that only the target tissue is within their grasp, with the applicator being fully released before removal to ensure that the clip is not dislodged; it is imperative that the correct size clip is selected for the structure. Staplers are used to provide haemostasis and closure of an organ; caution must be taken to ensure that the staples have enclosed all of the tissue for appropriate haemostasis and closure.
- *Vascular clamps*: Clamps are used to partially or completely occlude vessels whilst being atraumatic. Due to the range of clamp shapes and sizes, they can be used in numerous anatomical positions. It is essential to ensure the jaws are open prior to removal from the vessel to ensure that the vessel is not damaged.
- *Vascular tourniquets*: These are used by placing a tape or sloop around the vessel, tightening it until it occludes the blood flow and securing it with a clip.
- *Suturing and ligatures*: A ligature is a strand of material which is put round a vessel and tightened to occlude bleeding, close a structure or prevent leakage of substances. Sutures provide temporary or permanent haemostasis to tissues or vessel walls by approximating them during healing.
- *Direct pressure*: This is an effective method of haemostasis, and it may be considered the easiest and quickest and be less traumatic to vessels. A swab is normally used with digital pressure on the site of bleeding, but caution needs to be taken to ensure that once removed the swab doesn't dislodge clots; an instrument may be used to cover and compress bleeding. Indirect pressure may be placed above the bleeding with fingers or a 'swab on a stick', with packing of swabs used to apply pressure onto bleeding areas.
- *Pneumatic tourniquets*: These are used to provide a surgical field when operating on extremities with little or no bleeding which both aids with the visual field and reduces blood loss as it occludes both veins and arteries. However, they may cause vascular or neurological damage if not applied properly, and once deflated there is a need to control bleeding (Samudrala 2008, Paige 2009, Kotcher Fuller 2010, Guglielmi and Hunter 2011).

Chemical methods

Chemical methods can be divided into pharmacological agents and topical haemostatic agents.

PHARMACOLOGICAL AGENTS Pharmacological agents improve clot formation through mechanisms including increasing platelet function and reversing anticoagulation. They are used intraoperatively to control bleeding by boosting the patient's natural mechanisms of coagulation, such as epinephrine, vitamin K and tranexamic acid (Levy and Tanaka 2008, Samudrala 2008, Moss 2013, Camp 2014).

TOPICAL HAEMOSTATIC AGENTS A number of topical haemostatic agents are available within the theatre environment:

- Mechanical agents
  - Collagen-based products
  - Cellulose
  - Gelatine
  - Polysaccharide spheres
- Flowables
  - Flowseal
  - Surgiflo
- Adhesives
  - Skin sealants
  - Synthetic tissue sealants
- Active agents
  - Topical thrombins
- Sealants
  - Fibrin sealants
  - Polyethylene glycol (PEG) polymers
  - BioGlue
  - Cyanoacrylate (Samudrala 2008, Cheng *et al.* 2009, Gonzalez *et al.* 2010, Schreiber and Neveleff 2011, Sanjay *et al.* 2012, Moss 2013, Camp 2014).

Bonewax is used to stop bleeding from bone marrow. It should be applied to the exposed and bleeding area with only the smallest amount necessary, as foreign body reaction may occur from excessive use.

When selecting the appropriate selection of haemostatic agents, consider the size of the wound, the amount and type of bleeding and the properties of the haemostats available (Schreiber and Neveleff 2011).

Thermal-based methods

- *Monopolar diathermy*: A current is passed through the patient's body using a diathermy pencil or forceps which is then redirected to the diathermy machine via a return electrode (diathermy pad) which completes the circuit. The return electrode must be adequately sized and remain in contact throughout diathermy. If not, there will be a high concentration of energy and subsequent heat which leads to diathermy burns (Potty *et al.* 2010).
- *Bipolar diathermy*: The electrical circuit is formed between two parallel tips, one positive and one negative, in close vicinity of each other with the current flowing only between the two; they are so close to each other that only a low voltage is needed for the desired effect on the tissue (O'Riley 2010).

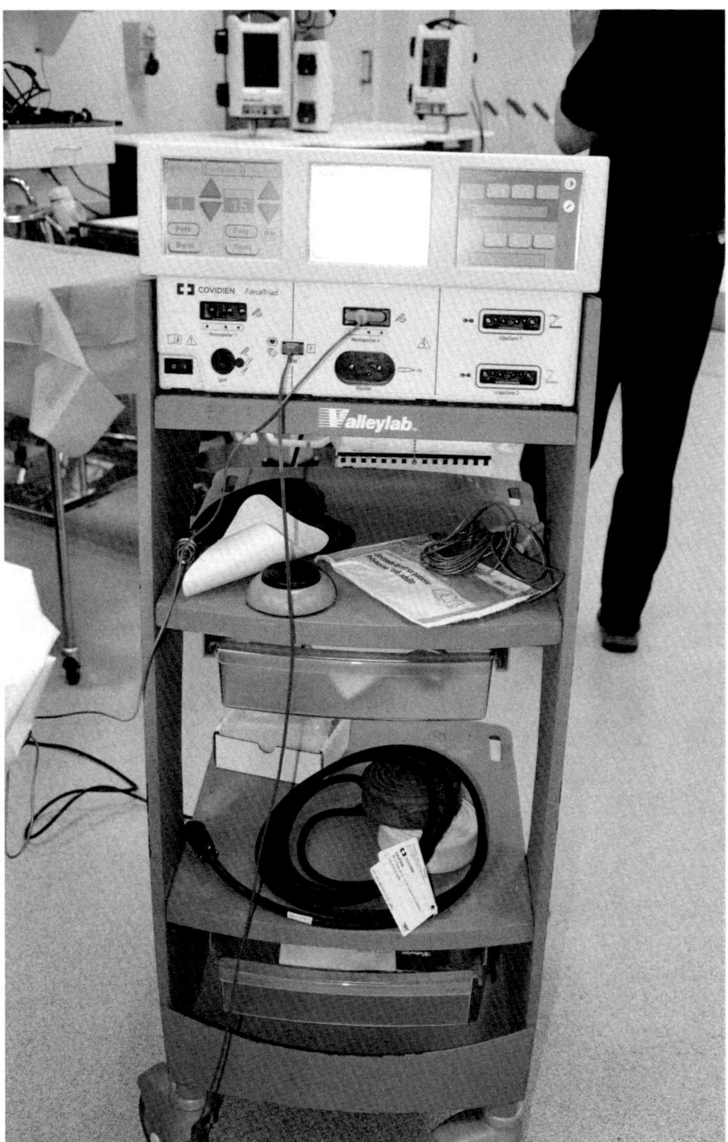

Photo 6 Ligature equipment

- *Ligature*: A ligature acts as a vessel sealant. It is a variant of biopolar electrosurgery which denatures the collagen and elastin in the vessel wall to create a seal (Janssen *et al.* 2012) (Photo 6).
- *Harmonic scalpel*: This scalpel cuts and coagulates simultaneously at a low temperature which means that it doesn't damage nearby tissue. It also causes less postoperative pain which may be due to its lack of electrical current and subsequent non-stimulation of nerves and muscles. It has been shown to reduce blood loss but has an increase in delayed bleeding. In laparoscopic surgery, it has numerous advantages, including improved wound healing, no stray currents or capacitive coupling, minimal smoke and char, and reduced heat damage to tissues; it is also said to make dissection of tissue planes easier (Earl 2012).

53 Surgical Drains

Wound drains are used commonly within most surgical specialities. With the implementation of enhanced recovery protocols, the use of wound drains is less common practice and at the discretion of the surgeon based on the surgical procedure.

Rationale for wound drains

For the renewal of tissue cells, wounds need to be free from a build-up of blood and serum, impaired circulation, mechanical injury and infection. Fluid collection and stasis predispose to infection; drainage reduces this and allows closer tissue apposition.

Drains enhance wound healing by:

- Obliterating dead space
- Preventing the formation of haematomas or seromas
- Preventing tissue devitalisation or wound margin necrosis
- Minimising a potential source of wound contamination
- Decreasing postoperative pain and minimising scarring (Findik *et al.* 2013).

A drain is used to allow the movement of fluid such as blood, pus, serum or air, which collect within a cavity in the body, to outside of the body. By removing the fluid from the spaces within the body, they reduce the risk of infection aiding wound healing and make the cavity smaller. They can aid in the monitoring of fluid balance, and if used subcutaneously, they prevent the formation of haematoma which would lift the tissue and compromise blood supply (Durai *et al.* 2009).

Drains are not, however, to be used as an alternative to good surgical technique or an alternative for the maintenance of haemostasis.

Drain uses

Drains may be used for therapeutic, prophylactic and decompressive drainage:

- *Therapeutic drainage*: To eliminate dead tissue bacteria, pus or other infected matter; drain air from the pleural cavity; drain ascites; reduce tissue damage; reduce dead space; and reduce the risk of abscess formation or recurrence.
- *Prophylactic drainage*: To deter infection; not recommended due to associated drain complications. There is little validation for using drains in this way, particularly as antibiotics can be used. Prophylactic drainage is chosen in instances where there will be fluid collection postoperatively, in postoperative cyst drainage (i.e. pancreatic cysts) as it will prevent cyst reformation, and to rest a new suture line. It can also be used to redirect natural body fluids via an alternative route for a certain amount of time such as T-tube drainage in the common bile duct or diversion of urine via a nephrostomy or suprapubic catheter. However, its main function is to stop haematoma formation and wound infection. A tube which will temporarily remain in situ in a hollow viscus, such as the bladder or common bile duct, may be fixed to the wall of an organ with an absorbable suture.

Rapid Perioperative Care, First Edition. Paul Wicker and Sara Dalby.

- *Decompressive drainage*: This prevents fluid accumulation in the wound or leakage around the wound, reducing the risk of haematoma or seroma; eliminates dead spaces; and prevents leakage of fluid such as urine, bile, and intestinal and pancreatic fluids (Durai *et al.* 2009, Durai and Ng 2010).

Disadvantages to surgical drains

There are several disadvantages to surgical drains:

- Drains may increase the risk of infection.
- Fragmentation of the drain in the abdomen
- May inhibit the tissue's resistance to the effects of local infection
- May cause foreign body response. This can cause pressure against vital structures which in turn can cause pressure necrosis.
- Pain and discomfort
- Decreased activity
- Loss of protein and fluids–electrolytes
- Loss of function due to obstruction
- Perforation of organs
- Potential problems with drain withdrawal
- Drains brought through the original incision may lead to incision hernias
- Maceration of the skin around the drain may occur if the fluid exudates (Durai *et al.* 2009, Durai and Ng 2010, Carlomangno *et al.* 2013, Ikeanyi *et al.* 2013).

Drains are said to provide the surgeon with an indication of the state of internal healing due to the fluid which is being evacuated; however, it cannot solely be relied upon to signal problems, and other indications should not be ignored if they point to a leak or bleed. This is because the holes of the drain may block with debris or blood clots, which may be falsely interpreted to mean that there is no further fluid to drain, leading to early removal of the drain.

If the drain is not secured properly, it may be accidentally pulled out by the patient or hospital staff; therefore, an understanding of the appropriate wound fixation is very important. With suction drains, it is important to be cautious when placing them as the suction tends to drag tissue to the holes, and this could cause damage to more delicate tissue (Kirk 2010).

Closed drainage systems

When possible, closed drainage systems should be selected as they minimise the incidence of infection and limit the amount of bodily fluid that healthcare providers will come into contact with. Closed drainage systems can be either active (including redivac, Jackson–Pratt drain, J-vac drain and vacuum-assisted closure devices) or passive (which include Robinson drainage system, Mallecot drain, pigtails, chest tube drains and T-tube drains) (Durai *et al.* 2009).

Passive or active drain selection

The selection of either a passive or active drain depends on patient activity, the area to be drained and overall healing capability.

Passive drains provide the path of least resistance. They are affected by pressure differentials and assisted by gravity; functioning by overflow and capillary action, they are usually used for the peritoneal cavity or skin wounds. Passive drains can be either open (and therefore drain into a dressing) or closed (and so drain into a collecting bottle or bag). As gravity is used for drainage of fluids in passive drains, the position of the drain needs to be carefully considered as does the patient's positioning (Durai *et al.* 2009, Phillips 2012).

'Sheet' drains such as penrose drains are often correlated to create spaces or may be made of a series of tubes. They work with gravity to drain cavities and body movement. They are secured by putting a safety pin through the end which is outside of the wound to ensure that it doesn't drop into the wound. It is advised to close the head of the safety pin with forceps to prevent it from opening and possibly stabbing the patient; for additional security, they are stitched to the skin, and an absorbent dressing is then put round the drain to catch excretions. It needs to be taken into account that if wound fluid has prolonged contact with the skin, it will cause irritation or erosion; these types of drains are used for abscess cavities in case there is any subsequent drainage (Wicker and O'Neil 2010, Phillips 2012).

For an active drainage system, the necessary drain needs to have a vacuum within a closed container. They are usually inserted near the incision through a stab wound. The tubing for these drains needs to be more unyielding as they need to be able to withstand the pressure caused by the vacuum without collapsing. They are usually secured by a loop suture attached to the skin, with orthopaedics as the exception if their patients may need to be removed from under plaster. Vacuum drains can only be used when they are put into closed wounds as they will only be able to work if a negative pressure gradient is sustained (Durai *et al.* 2009, Wicker and O'Neil 2010).

Vacuum-assisted closure

Vacuum-assisted closure (VAC) devices are used for open wounds such as the chest, abdomen and limbs. Abdominal VAC dressings are used when there is increased pressure in the abdominal cavity, and primary closure isn't an option due to a risk of abdominal compartment syndrome in primary closure or isn't possible. The abdominal viscera is protected by a nonadherent film, and the sponge and polyfilms are then applied. A vacuum pad is then used to create negative pressure (Durai *et al.* 2009).

Underwater drains

Underwater drains are closed drains. Their tubes are underwater, so air is not able to enter the tube, but they are not active. It is important to ensure that the bottle remains lower than the wound because if the bottle is higher the water may drain into the wound. Chest drains remove air and fluid from the pleural cavity. When the patient breathes, the fluid in the underwater tube swings due to the influence of pressure as a result of pleural cavity changes. Once the drain stops swinging, it is an indication that the drain can be removed as the lung has expanded, closing the pleural cavity and therefore stabilising the pressure (Wicker and O'Neil 2010).

Securing of wound drains

For tube drains, including passive or active, insert a stitch and tie loosely, then wrap the thread around the base of the drain, crisscrossing a few times. Tie a knot around the drain, ensuring not to occlude or puncture the tube. Cut the stitch, leaving the ends long. Drains are usually stitched with a non-absorbable monofilament suture, so it can neither slip into the wound nor fall out (Durai *et al.* 2009).

A purse string suture may be inserted around a drain. This is a continuous suture which, once the drain is removed, can be pulled tight to close the hole. Depending on the position of the drain, it may be taped into place as part of a dressing. In instances when it is necessary to bring the drain though the incision, the practitioner should ensure that the stitch used to secure the drain is different than those which close the wound.

To secure chest drains, it is recommended to insert a strong suture into the skin on either side of the tube, being careful not to put a stitch through the tube, tying it loosely to seal the hole and secure it to the skin, then wrapping it round the tube by crossing the threads over each other, tying a knot after each encirclement and ensuring that the tube is gripped but not piercing the tube. The other stitch should be left long and untied so that it can be used to close the hole once the drain is removed (Kirk 2010).

Other considerations

The number of holes in the drain and the size of the holes depend on the drain but need to be considered. Smaller drains have an increased chance of blockage, whereas larger tubes will cause more tissue erosion.

Prior to the insertion of drains, the practitioner needs to check that the patient doesn't have a latex allergy before choosing any of the drains made of latex.

By inserting the drain away from the main wound, the practitioner is inhibiting the chance of contamination.

Superficial wounds don't normally need to be drained. Having a drain in situ in such circumstances can increase the risk of infection, particularly as subcutaneous tissues are especially vulnerable to infection as they are fairly avascular. If a drain is necessary, then a suction closed system should be selected rather than a passive drain.

Different sites affect the choice of drain to be used, as subcutaneous tissues vary in depth and vascularity depending on the individual and areas of the body. Small collections can be drained using gauze wicks, corrugated sheet drains and gentle suction drains. A subfascial or intramuscular drain should be used when damaged muscle is trapped beneath as fluid collections may increase pressure, resulting in ischaemia and risking infection from anaerobic organisms. Intraperitoneal drains tend to be viewed by the body as a foreign body, and the discharge fluid may consist of reaction fluid. They can be used to draw attention to bleeding or an anastomotic leak.

Drain removal

The length of time that the drain will remain in situ depends on the amount of fluid which drains and the purpose of the drain. When the drain is to be removed, the patient should be informed about what is to happen and provided with analgesia. Drains should be removed using aseptic technique. The vacuum on suction drains should be released so there is less trauma to the tissues as it is removed. The suture is cut, and the drain is pulled steadily out. If there is any difficulty or disproportionate pain, there may be an adhesion and medical advice is needed. Wound drains should be disposed of as clinical waste.

Documentation

The following documentation is necessary, and any changes must be recorded and reported:

- Type of drain
- Position
- Recording the colour
- Amount
- Nature
- Viscosity
- Excessive drainage
- Changes in the type of fluid
- Stopping of drainage.

54 Handling of Specimens

The handling of specimens is an integral part of being a theatre practitioner. For the scrub practitioner, it is important to ensure that the specimen is in the correct medium, labelled appropriately and sent to the laboratory as these steps are essential for the patient's post-operative management. Practitioners should familiarise and follow the relevant trust policies and protocols for the handling of specimens as they are important for risk management and patient safety (Hamlin *et al.* 2009, Joint Commission 2015). The Human Tissue Act (2004) has the authority to 'regulate the removal, storage, use and disposal of human bodies, organs and tissue' and should be adhered to by practitioners and healthcare organisations.

Principles of specimens

During some surgeries, it may be appropriate to remove some of the patient's tissue as a specimen to be looked at in the laboratory; this helps with diagnosis, staging and postoperative management of the patient's condition. The discussion of specimen retrieval and the appropriate medium can be undertaken during the team brief but should be confirmed prior to placing the specimen in the container (AORN 2006).

Specimens should only contain organisms and tissue from the area which is being tested; therefore, sampling technique is important to avoid contamination. Utilisation of appropriate infection control techniques should also minimise cross-contamination. It is important at the operating table to handle specimens as little as possible if at all, particularly if they have cancer cells present, as there is the potential to shed cancer cells which could lead to spread.

Handling of the tissue could also cause damage to the cells, causing confusion and unconfirmed diagnosis due to the damaged cells. Small specimens should be handled very carefully as crushing with forceps or continually puncturing the biopsy with a needle to retrieve the specimen from punch forceps can also damage the cells. Swabs and instruments that come into contact with a cancerous specimen should be kept separate and not utilised on other tissues. Specimens should be removed prior to washout of cavities with an antiseptic solution and prior to antibiotics if possible, as antiseptics may affect diagnostic tests by killing organisms which were present. If used, it should be documented on the laboratory form.

When dealing with multiple specimens, it is important for the scrub practitioner, where possible, to label and place the specimens into the containers straight away, as this will minimise the chance of confusion and mislabelling.

The scrub practitioner must ensure that the specimen pot is big enough and contains enough preservative medium to adequately maintain the integrity of the specimen tissue (AORN 2006, Hamlin *et al.* 2009).

Specimens may be sent to:

- Pathology
- Microbiology
- Histology

Rapid Perioperative Care, First Edition. Paul Wicker and Sara Dalby.

- Cytology (AfPP 2011).

During the procedure, there may be a need to send a specimen for a frozen section. Where possible, the pathology department should be given advanced notice by the surgical team. Specimens for frozen section are sent immediately in a dry container. The results should then be relayed from the pathology department to the medical team (AfPP 2011, Murphy 2011).

Laparoscopic specimen removal

The site for removal of laparoscopic specimens should avoid contamination, cause minimal pain and consider cosmetic appearance.

Complications of laparoscopic specimen removal include:

- Losing the specimen internally
- Wound infection
- Port site tumour implantation, the risk of which can be reduced by using a specimen bag
- Visceral injury
- Incisional hernia
- Rupturing of the specimen which could lead to infection, dispersion of tumour cells and an insufficient pathological assessment.

Documentation

It is integral that the labelling of the specimen is carried out in a careful and concise manner from a patient safety issue as the result of the specimen findings can often alter the patient's postoperative care (Hamlin *et al.* 2009, Murphy 2011).

Two practitioners should confirm the patient specimen labelling and 'potting'. The scrub practitioner should always confirm with the surgeon what to label the specimen and ensure the correct medium. This should then be communicated to the circulator, who will complete the specimen label in black ball-tip pen (a fibre-tip pen can cause the ink to smear, causing difficulty in reading the label) including: patient information, date, name of consultant in charge of the patient's care and the specimen name and site. Once the operating surgeon has confirmed that the specimen can be 'potted', the specimen label should then be checked with the scrub practitioner. The circulating practitioner should then allow the scrub practitioner to place the specimen into the medium. The specimen should have two labels, one on the container and one on the lid, in case the lid is lost once removed in the laboratory (AORN 2006, Hamlin *et al.* 2009, Joint Commission 2015).

The correct identification and labelling of the specimen are imperative for correct diagnosis. The time frame in which the specimen is delivered to the laboratory may have an effect on the organism's survival depending on the specimen and what tests are required. A specimen container with the appropriate transport medium for the specimen should be selected (e.g. microbiology specimens are not to be put in formalin which is for histology) and the urgency of the specimen determined (AfPP 2011, Murphy 2011).

Placing a specimen into an unlabelled container is not good clinical practice, as it could result in a specimen of unknown origin arriving in the laboratory which could have negative consequences for the patient. Equally, a mislabelled specimen container could negatively affect patient management, potentially resulting in unnecessary additional surgery or interventions due to misdiagnosis or omission of treatment. Either of these actions could result in the patient suing the practitioner or healthcare organisation for negligence (Hamlin *et al.* 2009).

The specimen form should be filled in by a member of the surgical team and include:

- Patient's information
- Specimen site

- Type of tissue
- Clinical diagnosis
- Any additional pertinent clinical information (AORN 2006, Hamlin *et al.* 2009).

The scrub practitioner should ensure the specimen is removed from theatre prior to the next patient, and the information is documented in the patient's perioperative notes, the theatre register and the specimen book. Prior to the specimen leaving the theatre department, an additional cross-check is performed by a member of theatre staff to ensure all specimen forms are completed and correspond with the specimen labels. This safety procedure is documented, including the time and date of collection, and retained within theatre. Once the specimens are in the laboratory, a member of staff within the department will recheck the specimens. If there are any discrepancies, these are highlighted to the theatre department (Hamlin *et al.* 2009, AfPP 2011).

Safety issues

The integrity of the containers is important. They need to be leak-proof and impervious, have well-fitting lids and be rigid. Any specimen has the potential to carry hazardous microorganisms, and caution must be taken with their transportation to ensure that staff are not at risk of exposure. Containers must be securely sealed with contamination on the outside removed; it should be placed in an impervious bag and labelled as hazardous. Staff need to wear appropriate personal protective equipment to protect themselves from hazardous preservative media and adhere to the Control of Substances Hazardous to Health (COSHH) Regulations (COSHH 2002, AORN 2006, Hamlin *et al.* 2009, Murphy 2011).

The importance of specimen retrieval, labelling and appropriate preservative should not be trivialised as it has a significant impact on the postoperative management of patients.

References and Further Reading

40. Basic Surgical Instrumentation

References

Corley FG and Thomas R (2011) Basic Surgical Instruments and Their Use. *Operative Techniques in Sports Medicine* **19**: 200–225.

El-Sedfy A and Chamberlain RS (2015) Surgeons and Their Tools: A History of Surgical Instruments and Their Innovators – Part V: Pass Me the Hemostat/Clamp. *The American Surgeon* **81**: 232–238.

Guglielmi C and Hunter S (2011) Sutures, Needles and Instruments. In Rothrock JC (ed) *Alexander's Care of the Patient in Surgery*, 14th ed. St. Louis, Elsevier Mosby, pp. 174–203.

Pirie, S. (2010) Introduction to instruments. *The Journal of Perioperative Practice* **20**(1) 23–25

Steele PR, Curran JF and Mountain RE (2013) Current and Future Practices in Surgical Retraction. *Surgeon* **11** (6): 330–337.

Further Reading

El-Sedfy A and Chamberlain RS (2015) Surgeons and Their Tools: A History of Surgical Instruments and Their Innovators – Part I: Place the Scissors on the Mayo Stand. *The American Surgeon* **80**: 1089–1092.

El-Sedfy A and Chamberlain RS (2015) Surgeons and Their Tools: A History of Surgical Instruments and Their Innovators – Part II: The Surgeon's Wand – Evolution from Knife to Scalpel to Electrocautery. *The American Surgeon* **80**: 1196–1200.

El-Sedfy A and Chamberlain RS (2015) Surgeons and Their Tools: A History of Surgical Instruments and Their Innovators – Part III: The Medical Student's Best Friend – Retractors. *The American Surgeon* **81**: 16–18.

El-Sedfy A and Chamberlain RS (2015) Surgeons and Their Tools: A History of Surgical Instruments and Their Innovators – Part IV: Pass Me the Forceps. *The American Surgeon* **81**: 124–127.

41. Surgical Positioning

References

Adedeji R, Oragui E, Khan W and Maruthainar N (2010) The Importance of Correct Patient Positioning in Theatres and the Implications of Malpositioning. *Journal of Perioperative Practice* **20** (4): 143–147.

Bale E and Berrecloth R (2010) The Obese Patient: Anaesthetic Issues: Airway and Positioning. *Journal of Perioperative Practice* **20** (8): 294–299.

Beckett AE (2010) Are We Doing Enough to Prevent Injury Caused by Positioning for Surgery? *Journal of Perioperative Practice* **21** (1): 26–29.

Bowers M (2012) Prone Positioning for Surgery. *Journal of Perioperative Practice* **22** (5): 157–162.

Pirie S (2010) Patient Care in the Perioperative Environment. *Journal of Perioperative Practice* **20** (7): 245–248.

Spruce L and Van Wicklin SA (2014) Back to Basics: Positioning the Patient. *AORN Journal* **100** (3): 298–305.

Further Reading

Health and Safety Executive (2011) Getting to Grips with Manual Handling. Available at http://www.hse.gov.uk/pubns/indg143.pdf (accessed 26 January 2016)

Malik AA, Khan WS, Chaundry A, Ihsan M and Cullen NP (2009) Acute Compartment Syndrome – a Life and Limb Threatening Surgical Emergency. *Journal of Perioperative Practice* **19**: 137–142.

Rapid Perioperative Care, First Edition. Paul Wicker and Sara Dalby.

42. Thermoregulation

References

Anaesthesia UK (2016) Approximate Contribution to Heat Loss. Available at http://www.frca.co.uk/SearchRender.aspx?DocId=1529&Index=D%3a%5cdtSearch%5cUserData%5cAUK&HitCount=6&hits=6+7+11+12+2d+2e+ (accessed 15 February 2016)

Association for Perioperative Practice (AfPP) (2011) *Standards and Recommendations for Safe Perioperative Practice*, 3rd ed. Harrogate, Association for Perioperative Practice.

Association of Perioperative Registered Nurses (AORN) (2007) Recommended Practices for the Prevention of Unplanned Perioperative Hypothermia. *AORN Journal* **85** (5): 972–988.

Berry D, Wick C and Magons P (2008) A Clinical Evaluation of the Cost and Time Effectiveness of the ASPAN Hypothermia Guideline. *Journal of Perianaesthesia Nursing* **23** (1): 24–35.

Burger L and Fitzpatrick J (2009) Prevention of Inadvertent Perioperative Hypothermia. *British Journal of Nursing* **18** (18): 1114–1119.

Carpenter L and Baysinger CL (2012) Maintaining Perioperative Normothermia in the Patient Undergoing Caesarean Delivery. *Obstetrical and Gynaecological Survey* **67** (7): 436–446.

Greenberg SB, Murphy GS and Vender JS (2009) Standard Monitoring Techniques. In Barash PG, Cullen BF and Stoelting RK (eds) *Clinical Anaesthesia*, 6th ed. Philadelphia, Lippincott Williams and Wilkins, pp. 697–714.

Hamlin L, Richardson-Tench M and Davies M (2010) *Perioperative Nursing: An Introductory Text*. Sydney, Elsevier Australia.

Hillier SC and Mazurek MS (2009) Monitored Anaesthesia Care. In Barash PG, Cullen BF and Stoelting RK (eds) *Clinical Anaesthesia*, 6th ed. Philadelphia, Lippincott Williams and Wilkins, pp. 815–832.

Hooper VD, Chard R, Clifford T, Fetzer S, Fossum S, Godden B, *et al.* (2009) ASPAN's Evidence Based Clinical Practice Guideline for the Promotion of Perioperative Normothermia. *Journal of Perianaesthesia Nursing* **24** (5): 271–287.

Kurtz A (2008) Thermal Care in the Perioperative Period. *Best Practice and Research Clinical Anaesthesiology* **22** (1): 39–62.

Leeth D, Mamaril M, Oman KS and Krumbach B. (2010) Normothermia and Patient Comfort: A Comparative Study in an Outpatient Surgery Setting. *Journal of Perianaesthesia Nursing* **25** (3): 146–151.

Lynch S, Dixon J and Leary D (2010) Reducing the Risk of Unplanned Perioperative Hypothermia. *AORN Journal* **92** (5): 553–564.

National Institute for Health and Clinical Excellence (NICE) (2008) *The Management of Inadvertent Perioperative Hypothermia in Adults*. Clinical Guideline No. 65. London: NICE.

Rajagopalan S, Mascha E, Na J and Sessler DI (2008) The Effects of Mild Perioperative Hypothermia on Blood Loss and Transfusion Requirement. *Anesthesiology* **108** (1): 71–77.

Roberson MC, Dieckmann LS, Rodriguez RE and Austin PN (2013) A Review of the Evidence for Active Preoperative Warming of Adults Undergoing General Anaesthesia. *AANA Journal* **81** (5): 351–356.

Royal College of Anaesthetists (RCA) (2012) *Raising the Standard: A Compendium of Audit Recipes for Continuous Quality Improvement in Anaesthesia*, 3rd ed. London, RCA.

Wagner VD (2010) Patient Safety Chiller: Unplanned Perioperative Hypothermia. *AORN Journal* **92** (5): 567–571.

Weirich TL (2008) Hypothermia/Warming Protocols: Why Are They Not Widely Used in the OR? *AORN Journal* **87** (2): 333–344.

Further Reading

Journeaux M (2013) Peri-operative Hypothermia: Implications for Practice. *Nursing Standard* **27** (45): 33–38.

Llewellyn L (2013) Effect of pre-Warming on Reducing the Incidence of Inadvertent Peri-operative Hypothermia for Patients Undergoing General Anaesthesia: A Mini-review. *British Journal of Anaesthetic and Recovery Nursing* **14** (1–2): 3–10.

43. Skin Preparation

References

Alexander JW, Solomkin JS and Edwards MJ (2011) Updated recommendations for control of surgical site infection. *Annals of Surgery* **253** (6): 1082–1093.

Association of Perioperative Registered Nurses (AORN) (2013) Recommended Practices for Preoperative Patient Skin Antisepsis Standards, Recommended Practices and Guidelines. Available at http://www.hqinstitute.org/sites/main/files/file-attachments/skin_antisepsis_0.pdf (accessed 15 February 2016)

Edmiston CE, Okoli O, Graham MB, Sinski S and Seabrook GR (2010) Evidence for Using Chlorhexidine Gluconate Preoperative Cleansing to Reduce the Risk of Surgical Site Infection. *AORN Journal* **92**: 509–518.

Edwards P, Lipp A and Holmes A (2009) *Preoperative Skin Antisepsis for Preventing Surgical Wound Infections (Review) The Cochrane Library*. Oxford, John Wiley and Sons.

Hemani ML and Lepor H (2009) Skin Preparation for the Prevention of Surgical Site Infection: Which Agent Is Best? *Reviews in Urology* **11** (4): 190–195.

Kehinde E, Jamal W, Ali Y, Khodakhast F, Sahsah M and Rotimi VO (2009) Comparative Efficacy of Two Methods of Skin Preparation of the Perineal and Genital Skin of Male Urological Patients. *Kuwait Medical Journal* **41** (2): 103–107.

National Institute for Health and Clinical Excellence (NICE) (2008) Surgical Site Infection Prevention and Treatment of Surgical Site Infection. Available at http://www.nice.org.uk/guidance/cg74/chapter/1-recommendations (accessed 15 February 2016)

Rocos B and Donaldson LJ (2012) Alcohol Skin Preparation Causes Surgical Fires. *Annals of the Royal College of Surgeons of England* **94**: 87–89.

Sivathasan N, Sivathansan N and Vijayarajan L (2010) Chlorhexidine's Complications. *Journal of Perioperative Practice* **20** (8): 300–301.

Wanzer LJ and Vane EAP (2009) Prepping and Draping. In Rothrock JC and Seifert PC (eds) *Assisting in Surgery: Patient Centered Care*. Denver, Competency & Credentialing Institute, pp. 38–73.

Zinn J, Jenkins JB, Swofford V, Harrelson B and McCarter S (2010) Intraoperative Patient Skin Preparation Agents: Is There a Difference? *Association of Operating Room Nurses* (AORN) **92** (6): 662–674.

Further Reading

Al Maqbali MA (2013) Perioperative Antiseptic Skin Preparations and Reducing SSI. *British Journal of Nursing* **22** (21): 1227–1233.

Scowcroft T (2012) A Critical Review of the Literature Regarding the Use of Povidone Iodine and Chlorhexidine Gluconate for Preoperative Surgical Skin Preparation. *Journal of Perioperative Practice* **22** (3): 95–99.

Silva P (2013) An Evidence Based Protocol for Perioperative Skin Preparation. *Journal of Perioperative Practice* **23** (4): 87–90.

44. Surgical Draping

References

Al-Hashemi J (2013) Surgical Gowns and Drapes: Maximising Patient Safety. *Journal of Operating Department Practitioners* **1** (2): 69–73.

Gilmour D (2010) Considerations for Gown and Drape Selection in the United Kingdom. *AORN Journal* **92** (4): 461–465.

Hamlin L (2012) Operating Theatre Practice. In Hughes SJ and Mardell A (eds) *Oxford Handbook of Perioperative Practice*. Oxford, Oxford University Press, pp. 282–283.

Humes DJ and Lobo DN (2009) Antisepsis, Asepsis and Skin Preparation. *Surgery* **27** (10): 441–445.

Kiernan M (2012) Infection Prevention. In Woodhead K and Fudge L (eds) *Manual of Perioperative Care*. Chichester, Wiley-Blackwell, pp. 43–55.

Msaud D, Moore A and Massouh F (2010) Current Practice in Preoperative Correct Surgical Site Marking. *Journal of Perioperative Practice* **20** (6): 210–214.

Nicolette LH (2011) Infection Prevention and Control in the Perioperative Setting. In Rothrock JC (ed) *Alexander's Care of the Patient in Surgery*, 14th ed. St. Louis, Elsevier Mosby, pp. 48–110.

Zinn J, Jenkins JB, Swofford V, Harrelson B and McCarter S (2010) Intraoperative Patient Skin Preparation Agents: Is There a Difference? *Association of Operating Room Nurses* (AORN) **92** (6): 662–674.

Further Reading

Association of Perioperative Practitioners (AfPP) (2011) *Recommended Standards and Recommendations for Safe Perioperative Practice*, 2nd ed. Harrogate: AfPP.

Wanzer LJ and Vane EAP (2009) Prepping and Draping. In Rothrock JC and Seifert PC (eds) *Assisting in Surgery: Patient Centered Care*. Denver, Competency & Credentialing Institute, pp. 38–73.

45. Surgical Site Marking

References

Lee MJ (2014) Optimising the Safety of Surgery, before Surgery. *Clinical Orthopaedics and Related Research* **472**: 809–811.

Mellinger E (2014) Action Needed to Prevent Wrong-Site Surgery Events. *AORN Connections* **99** (5): C5–C6.

Msaud D, Moore A and Massouh F (2010) Current Practice on Preoperative Correct Site Surgical Marking. *Journal of Perioperative Practice* **20** (6): 210–214.

NHS England (2014) Standardise, Educate, Harmonise. Commissioning the Conditions for Safer Surgery. Available at https://www.england.nhs.uk/wp-content/uploads/2014/02/sur-nev-ev-tf-rep.pdf (accessed 27 January 2016)

Shen E, Porco T and Rutar T (2013) Errors in Strabismus Surgery. *JAMA Ophthalmology* **131** (1): 75–79.

Watson DS (2015) Concept Analysis: Wrong-Site Surgery. *AORN Journal* **101** (6): 650–656.

World Health Organization (WHO) (2008) *WHO Surgical Safety Checklist*. London, National Patient Safety Agency.

Further Reading

Khan IH, Jamil W, Lynn SM, Khan OH, Markland K and Giddins G (2012) Analysis of NHSLA Claims in Orthopaedic Surgery. *Orthopaedics* **35** (5): e726–e731.

Neily J, Mills PD, Paull DE, Mazzia LM, Turner JR, Hemphill RR and Gunnar W (2012) Sharing Lessons Learnt to Prevent Incorrect Surgery. *American Surgeon* **78**: 1276–1280.

46. Swab Counts, Sharps and Instrument Checks

References

Association for Perioperative Practice (AfPP) (2011) *Standards and Recommendations for Safe Perioperative Practice*, 3rd ed. Harrogate: AfPP.

Goodman T and Spry C (2014) *Essentials of Perioperative Nursing*, 5th ed. Burlington, Jones & Bartlett Learning.

Hamlin L, Jenkins M and Conlon L (2009) Patient Safety. In Hamlin L, Richardson-Tench M and Davies M (eds) *Perioperative Nursing: An Introductory Text*. Sydney, Elsevier Australia.

Hamlin L, Richardson-Tench M and Davies M (2010) *Perioperative Nursing: An Introductory Text*. Sydney, Elsevier Australia.

Woodhead K (2009) Safe Surgery: Reducing the Risk of Retained Items. *Journal of Perioperative Practice* **19** (10): 358–361.

Further Reading

Gilmour D (2012) Swab and Instrument Count. In Woodhead K and Fudge L (eds) *Manual of Perioperative Care: An Essential Guide*. Chichester, Wiley-Blackwell, pp. 177–183.

McClelland G (2012) Non-technical Skills for Scrub Practitioners. *Journal Perioperative Practice* **22** (12): 389–392.

Vats A, Nagpal K and Moorthy K (2009) Surgery: A Risky Business. *Journal Perioperative Practice* **19** (10): 330–334.

47. Measures to Prevent Wound Infection

References

Association of Perioperative Practice (AfPP) (2011) *Standards and Recommendations for Safe Perioperative Practice*, 3rd ed. Harrogate: AfPP.

Association of Operative Room Nurses (AORN) (2015) *Guidelines for Perioperative Practice*. Denver, AORN.
Borchardt RA and Rolston KVI (2012) Surgical Site Infection: Knowledge of the Likely Pathogens Is Key. *Journal of the American Academy of Physicians Assistants* **25** (5): 27–28.
Jose B and Dignon A (2013) Is There a Relationship between Preoperative Shaving and Surgical Site Infection? *Journal of Perioperative Practice* **23**: 22–25.
Kirk RM (2010) *Basic Surgical Techniques*, 6th ed. Edinburgh, Churchill Livingstone.
Kotcher Fuller J (2010) *Surgical Technology: Principles and Practice*, 5th ed. St Louis, Saunders Elsevier.
Korol E, Johnston K, Waser N, Sifakis F, Jafri HS, Lo M and Kyaw MH (2013) A Systematic Review of Risk Factors Associated with Surgical Site Infections among Surgical Patients. *PLoS One* **8** (12): 1–9.
Lobley SN (2013) Factors Affecting the Risk of Surgical Site Infection and Methods of Reducing It. *Journal of Perioperative Practice* **23** (4): 77–81.
National Institute for Clinical Excellence (NICE) (2014) Surgical Site Infection: Prevention and Treatment. Available at https://www.nice.org.uk/guidance/cg74 (accessed 27 January 2016)
Peate I and Glencross W (2015) *Wound Care at a Glance*. Chichester, Wiley-Blackwell.
Reyes GE and Chang PS (2011) Prevention of Surgical Site Infection: Being a Winner. *Operative Techniques in Sports Medicine* **19**: 238–244.
Rochon M (2012) Wound Healing and Surgical Site Infection. In Woodhead K and Fudge L (eds) *Manual of Perioperative Care*. Chichester, Wiley-Blackwell.
Nicolette LH (2011) Infection Prevention and Control in the Perioperative Setting. In Rothrock JC (ed) *Alexander's Care of the Patient in Surgery*, 14th ed. St. Louis, Elsevier Mosby, pp. 48–110.
Weaving P, Cox P and Milton S (2008) Infection Prevention and Control in the Operating Theatre: Reducing the Risk of Surgical Site Infections. *Journal of Perioperative Practice* **18** (5): 199–204.
Weston D (2013) *Fundamentals of Infection Prevention and Control: Theory and Practice*. Chichester, Wiley-Blackwell.

Further Reading

Eskicioglu C, Gagliardi AR, Fenech DS, Forbes SS, McKenzie M, McLeod RS and Nathens AB (2012) Surgical Site Infection Prevention: A Survey to Identify the Gap between Evidence and Practice in University of Toronto Teaching Hospitals. *Canadian Journal of Surgery* **55** (4): 233–238.

48. Electrosurgery

References

Bruske-Hohlfeld I, Preissler G, Jauch KW, Pitz M, Nowak D, Peters A and Wichmann HE (2008) Surgical Smoke and Ultrafine Particles. *Journal of Occupational Medicine and Toxicology* **3** (31). Available at http://occup-med.biomedcentral.com/articles/10.1186/1745-6673-3-31 (accessed 10 February 2016)
Feldman LS, Fuchshuber P, Jones DB, Mischna J and Schwaitzberg SD (2012) Surgeons Don't Know What They Don't Know about the Safe Use of Energy in Surgery. *Surgical Endoscopy* **26**: 2735–2739.
Marsh S (2012) The Smoke Factor: Things You Should Know. *Journal of Perioperative Practice* **22** (3): 91–94.
Mowbray N, Ansell J, Warren N, Wall P and Torkington J (2013) Is Surgical Smoke Harmful to Theatre Staff? A Systematic Review. *Surgical Endoscopy* **23** (2): 14–16.
O'Riley M (2010) Electrosurgery in Perioperative Practice. *Journal of Perioperative Practice* **20** (9): 329–333.
Potty AG, Khan W and Tailor HD (2010) Diathermy in Perioperative Practice. *Journal of Perioperative Practice* **20** (11): 402–405.
Spruce L and Braswell ML (2012) Implementing AORN Recommended Practices for Electrosurgery. *AORN Journal* **95** (3): 373–384.

Further Reading

Earl C (2012) Managing High-Risk Equipment. In Woodhead K and Fudge L (eds) *Manual of Perioperative Care: An Essential Guide*. Chichester, Wiley-Blackwell, pp. 190–202.
Neveleff DJ and Kraiss LW (2010) Implementing Methods to Improve Perioperative Haemostasis in the Surgical and Trauma Settings. *AORN Journal* **92** (5): S3–S15.

49. Wound Healing and Dressings

References

Adis Medical Writers (2014) Select Appropriate Wound Dressings by Matching the Properties of the Dressing to the Type of Wound. *Drugs and Therapy Perspectives* **30**: 213–217.

Beldon P (2010) Basic Science of Wound Healing. *Surgery* **28** (9): 409–412.

Benbow M (2008) Best Practice: Appliance of Dressing Products. *Journal of Community Nursing* **22** (3): 32–36.

Bennett-Marsden M (2010) How to Select a Wound Dressing. *The Pharmaceutical Journal* **2**: 363–366.

Broussard KC and Powers JG (2013) Wound Dressings: Selecting the Most Appropriate Type. *Journal of Clinical Dermatology* **14** (6): 449–459.

Collier M (2006) The Use of Advanced Biological and Tissue-Engineered Wound Products. *Nursing Standard* **21** (7): 68–76.

Dealey C and Cameron J (2009) *Wound Management*. Chichester, Wiley-Blackwell.

Flanagan M (2013) *Wound Healing and Skin Integrity: Principles and Practice*. Chichester, Wiley-Blackwell.

Kotcher Fuller J (2010) *Surgical Technology: Principles and Practice*. 5th ed. St. Louis, Saunders Elsevier.

Morris C (2006) Wound Management and Dressing Selection. *Wound Essentials* **1**: 178–183.

Peate I and Glencross W (2015) *Wound Care at a Glance*. Chichester, Wiley-Blackwell.

Sharp A and Clark J (2011) Diabetes and Its Effects on Wound Healing. *Nursing Standard* **25** (45): 41–44.

Simpson A and Brooks A (2008) Surgical Wounds. In Brooks A, Mahoney P and Rowlands B (eds) *ABC of Tubes, Drains, Lines and Frames*. Oxford: Blackwell.

Stephen-Hayes, J. (2010) Dressing Choice: A Practical Guide to Clinical Outcomes. *Practice Nurse* **40** (8): 27–31.

Tiaki K (2012) Modern Advances in Wound Care. *Nursing New Zealand* **18** (5): 20–24.

Tickle J (2014) Wound Care: Quality Dressing and Assessment. *Nursing and Residential Care* **16** (9): 486–488.

Ward JPT and Linden R (2013) *Physiology at a Glance*, 3rd ed. Chichester, Wiley-Blackwell.

Wild T, Rahbarnia A, Kellner M, Sobotka L and Eberlein T (2010) Basics in Nutrition and Wound Healing. *Nutrition* **26** (9): 862–866.

Zinn JL (2012) Surgical Wound Classification: Communication Is Needed for Accuracy. *AORN Journal* **95** (2): 274–278.

Zinn J and Swofford V (2014) Quality Improvement Initiative: Classifying and Documenting Surgical Wounds. *American Nurse Today* 9 (1). Available at http://www.americannursetoday.com/quality-improvement-initiative-classifying-and-documenting-surgical-wounds/ (accessed 1 February 2016)

Further Reading

Downie F, Edgdell S, Blelby A and Searle R (2010) Barrier Dressings in Surgical Site Infection Prevention Strategies. *British Journal of Nursing* **19** (20): S42–S46.

Naude I (2010) The Practice and Science of Wound Healing: History and Physiology of Wound Healing. *Professional Nursing Today* **14** (3): 17–21.

Nawaz Z and Bentley G (2011) Surgical Incisions and Principles of Wound Healing. *Surgery* **29** (2): 59–62.

50. Bladder Catheterisation

References

Booth F and Clarkson M (2012) Principles of Urinary Catheterisation. *Journal of Community Nursing* **26** (3): 37–41.

European Association of Urology Nurses (EAUN) (2012) *Catheterisation: Indwelling Catheters in Adults: Urethral and Suprapubic*. Evidence-based Guidelines for Best Practice in Urological Healthcare. Available at http://www.nursing.nl/PageFiles/11870/001_1391694991387.pdf (accessed 25 January 2016)

Hughes K and Patrick N (2014) Performing Urinary Catheterisation. *Journal of Operating Department Practitioners* **2** (2): 69–77.

Mangnall J (2014) Urinary Catheterisation: Reducing the Risk of Infection. *Nursing and Residential Care* **16** (6): 310–315.

NHS Choices (2013) Urinary Catheterisation. Available at http://www.nhs.uk/conditions/Urinary-catheterization/Pages/Introduction.aspx (accessed 25 January 2016)

National Institute for Health and Clinical Excellence (NICE) (2013) *Urinary Incontinence in Women*. Manchester, NICE.

National Institute for Health and Clinical Excellence (NICE) (2014) *Long Term Urinary Catheters: Prevention and Control of Healthcare Associated Infections in Primary and Community Care*. Manchester, NICE.

Royal College of Nursing (RCN) (2012) *Catheter Care: RCN Guidance for Nurses*. London, RCN.

Further Reading

Madeo, M. and Roodhouse AJ (2009) Reduced the Risks of Associated with Urinary Catheters. *Nursing Standard* **23** (29): 47–55.

Mangall J (2012) OptiLube Active. The Role of Lubricants in Urinary Catheterisation. *British Journal of Community Nursing* **17** (9): 414–420.

51. Tourniquet Management

References

Angadi DS, Blanco J, Garde A and West SC (2010) Lower Limb Elevation: Useful and Effective Technique of Exsanguination Prior to Knee Arthroscopy. *Knee Surgery Sports Traumatology Arthroscopy* **18**: 1559–1561.

Association of Perioperative Registered Nurses (AORN) (2013) Recommended Practices Summary: Recommended Practices for Care of Patients Undergoing Pneumatic Tourniquet-Assisted Procedures. *AORN Journal* **98** (4): 397–400.

Association for Perioperative Practice (AfPP) (2011) *Standards and Recommendations for Safe Perioperative Practice*, 3rd ed. Harrogate, Association for Perioperative Practice.

Hamlin L, Richardson-Tench M and Davies M (2010) *Perioperative Nursing: An Introductory Text*. Sydney, Elsevier Australia.

Karia RA (2011) Haemostasis and Tourniquet. *Operative Techniques in Sports Medicine* **19**: 224–230.

Smith TO and Hing CB (2010) Is a Tourniquet Beneficial in Total Knee Replacement Surgery? A Meta-analysis and Systemic Review. *The Knee* **17**: 141–147.

Further Reading

Earl C (2012) Managing High-Risk Equipment. In Woodhead K and Fudge L (eds) *Manual of Perioperative Care: An Essential Guide*. Chichester, Wiley-Blackwell, pp. 190–202.

Tai T-W, Lin C-J, Jou I-M, Chang C-W, Lai K-A and Yang C-Y (2011) Tourniquet Use in Total Knee Arthroplasty: A Meta-analysis. *Knee Surgery, Sports Traumatology Arthroscopy* **19**: 1121–1130.

Wall PL, Duevel DC, Hassan MB, Welander JD, Sahr SM and Buising CM (2013) Tourniquets and Occlusion: The Pressure of Design. *Military Medicine* **178** (5): 578–587.

52. Haemostatic Techniques

References

Camp MA (2014) Hemostatic Agents: A Guide to Safe Practice for Perioperative Nurses. *AORN Journal* **100** (2): 131–147.

Cheng CM, Meyer-Massetti C and Kayser SR (2009) A Review of Three Stand-Alone Topical Thrombins for Surgical Haemostasis. *Clinical Therapeutics* **31** (1): 32–41.

Earl C (2012) Managing High-Risk Equipment. In Woodhead K and Fudge L (eds) *Manual of Perioperative Care: An Essential Guide*. Chichester, Wiley-Blackwell, pp. 190–202.

Gonzalez EA, Jastrow KM, Holcomb JB and Kozar RA (2010) Haemostasis, surgical bleeding and transfusion. In Brunicardia FC, Andersen DK, Billiar TR, Dunn DL, Hunter JG, Matthews JB and Pollock RE (eds) *Schwartz's Principles of Surgery*, 9th ed. New York, McGraw-Hill, pp. 67–87.

Guglielmi C and Hunter S (2011) Sutures, Needles and Instruments. In Rothrock JC (ed) *Alexander's Care of the Patient in Surgery*, 14th ed. St. Louis, Elsevier Mosby, pp. 174–203.

Janssen PF, Brolmann HAM and Huirne JAF (2012) Effectiveness of Electrothermal Bipolar Sealing Devices versus Other Electrothermal and Ultrasonic Devices for Abdominal Surgical Haemostasis: A Systematic Review. *Surgical Endoscopy* **26**: 2892–2901.

Levy JH and Tanaka KA (2008) Management of Surgical Haemostasis: Systematic Agents. *Vascular* **16**: S14–S21.

Moss R (2013) *Management of Surgical Haemostasis: An Independent Study Guide*. Denver, Association of Perioperative Nurses.

O'Riley M (2010) Electrosurgery in Perioperative Practice. *Journal of Perioperative Practice* **20** (9): 329–333.

Paige JT (2009) Tissue Handling. In Rothrock JC and Seifert PC (eds) *Assisting In Surgery: Patient Centered Care*. Denver, Competency & Credentialing Institute, pp. 74–106.

Potty AG, Khan W and Tailor HD (2010) Diathermy in Perioperative Practice. *Journal of Perioperative Practice* **20** (11): 402–405.

Samudrala S (2008) Topical Haemostatic Agents in Surgery: A Surgeon's Perspective. *AORN Journal* **88** (3): S2–S11.

Sanjay P, Watt DG and Wigmore SJ (2013) Systematic Review and Meta-analysis of Haemostatic and Biliostatic Efficacy of Fibrin Sealants in Elective Liver Surgery. *Journal of Gastrointestinal Surgery* **17**: 829–836.

Schreiber MA and Neveleff DJ (2011) Achieving Haemostasis with Topical Haemostats: Making Clinically and Economically Appropriate Decisions in the Surgical and Trauma Settings. *AORN Journal* **94** (5): S1–S20.

Further Reading

Gruen RL, Brohi K, Schreiber M, Balogh ZJ, Pitt V, Narayan M and Maler RV (2012) Haemorrhage Control in Severely Injured Patients. *The Lancet* **380**: 1099–1108.

Spahn DR and Goodnough LT (2013) Alternatives to Blood Transfusion. *The Lancet* **381**: 1855–1865.

53. Surgical Drains

References

Carlomagno NI, Santangelo M, Grassia S, La Tessa C and Renda A (2013) Intraluminal Migration of a Surgical Drain: Report of a Rare Complication and Literature Review. *Annali Italiani di Chirurgia* **84**: 219–223.

Durai R, Mownah A and Ng PCH (2009) Use of Drains in Surgery: A Review. *Journal of Perioperative Practice* **19** (6): 180–186.

Durai R and Ng PC (2010) Surgical Vacuum Draining: Types, Uses, and Complications. *AORN Journal* **91**: 266–271.

Findik UY, Topcu SY and Vatansever O (2013) Effects of Drains on Pain, Comfort and Anxiety in Patients Undergone Surgery. *International Journal of Caring Sciences* **6** (3): 412–419.

Ikeanyi UO, Chukwuka CN, and Chukwuanukwu TO (2013) Risk Factors for Surgical Site Infections following Clean Orthopaedic Operations. *Nigerian Journal of Clinical Practice* **16**: 443–447.

Kirk RM (2010) *Basic Surgical Techniques*, 6th ed. London, Churchill Livingstone.

Phillips N (2012) *Berry & Kohns Operating Room Technique*, 12th ed. St. Louis, Elsevier.

Wicker P and O'Neil J (2010) *Caring for the Perioperative Patient*, 2nd ed. London, Wiley-Blackwell.

Further Reading

McEwen DR (2011) Wound Healing, Dressings and Drains. In Rothrock JC (ed) *Alexander's Care of the Patient in Surgery*, 14th ed. St. Louis, Elsevier Mosby, pp. 250–266.

Nanni M, Perna F, Calamelli C, Donati D, Ferrara O, Parlato A *et al.* (2013) Wound Drainages in Total Hip Arthroplasty: To Use or Not to Use? Review of the Literature in Current Practice. *Musculoskeletal Surgery* **97**: 101–107.

54. Handling of Specimens

References

Association of Operating Room Nurses (AORN) (2006) Recommended Practices for the Care and Handling of Specimens in the Perioperative Environment. *AORN Journal* **83**(3): 688–699.

Association for Perioperative Practice (AfPP) (2011) *Standards and Recommendations for Safe Perioperative Practice*, 3rd ed. Harrogate, Association for Perioperative Practice.

Control of Substances Hazardous to Health (COSHH) (2002) Regulations. Available at http://www.hse.gov.uk/nanotechnology/coshh.htm (accessed 15 February 2016)

Hamlin L, Jenkins M and Conlon L (2009) Patient Safety. In Hamlin L, Richardson-Tench M and Davies M (eds) *Perioperative Nursing: An Introductory Text*. Sydney, Elsevier Australia.

Human Tissue Act (2004) Available at http://www.legislation.gov.uk/ukpga/2004/30/contents (accessed 15 February 2016)

Joint Commission (2015) National Patient Safety Goals Effective January 1, 2015. Available at http://www.jointcommission.org/assets/1/6/2015_NPSG_LAB.pdf (accessed 15 February 2016)

Murphy EK (2011) Patient Safety and Risk Management. In Rothrock JC (ed) *Alexander's Care of the Patient in Surgery*, 14th ed. St. Louis, Elsevier Mosby, pp. 18–47.

Further Reading

Macqueen R (2012) Care of Specimens. In Woodhead K and Fudge L (eds) *Manual of Perioperative Care: An Essential Guide*. Chichester, Wiley-Blackwell, pp. 184–189.

SECTION 5

Surgical Assisting

Sara Dalby

55 Legal, Professional and Ethical Issues

Accountability and responsibility for practitioners in advanced roles

By performing a task within our working environment, we accept responsibility for it and its outcomes. As a professional, you are accountable for the results of your actions, especially if there is a negative result.

This accountability can be on a number of levels:

1. Towards patients due to a duty of care in common law
2. Legal responsibility through civil law
3. Professional responsibility as per code of conduct to your governing body
4. Employer due to contractual law and job description
5. Ultimately, the public (Dimond 2011).

The Perioperative Care Collaborative (PCC 2012) states that it must not be assumed that the surgeon is legally responsible for a qualified practitioner working as an Surgical First Assistant (SFA), as the law sees the person giving the care as responsible.

By taking on new roles and crossing traditional barriers, autonomous practice is becoming more commonplace. This is linked with increased responsibility, and therefore practitioners need to prove their competence and accountability. The NMC (2015) states that practitioners must work within our limitations. The PCC (2012) provides SFAs with a specification incorporating all the tasks which are deemed within the remit of their role. It is recommended not to undertake the role of SFA unless the organisation within which you work has a policy which supports practice, with the individual having an extended role in their job description and contract of employment; it is important to confirm that the SFA has vicarious liability (PCC 2012).

Delegating responsibility

When delegating responsibility, the NMC Code of Conduct (2015: 10) states that as a professional you must be accountable for your decisions to delegate tasks and duties to other people, and this is achieved by the following guidelines: 'only delegate tasks and duties that are within the other person's scope of competence, making sure that they fully understand your instructions', 'make sure that everyone you delegate tasks to is adequately supervised and supported so they can provide safe and compassionate care' and 'confirm that the outcome of any task you have delegated to someone else meets the required standard'.

Record keeping

Record keeping is an important aspect of patient care and is considered an indication of a competent and safe professional. Practitioners should use clinical judgement to decide

Rapid Perioperative Care, First Edition. Paul Wicker and Sara Dalby.

which content is pertinent, documenting in an accurate, consistent and precise way which is both legible and comprehensible (NMC 2012). In a society in which there is an increasing rate of litigation, it is important for professionals to keep accurate records as those documents may be used in their defence in a court of law if liable action is taken. Record keeping is considered an aspect of duty of care owed to patients; therefore, if documentation is not maintained and of a reasonable standard, it could be interpreted as professional misconduct (Dimond 2011). Record keeping should include terms which patients can understand; avoid jargon, abbreviations, irrelevant speculation, and distasteful or subjective accounts; and ensure that any record is easily identifiable and recorded in a manner which cannot be tampered with (NMC 2012). There has been the introduction of a legislation which regulates documentation. The Data Protection Act 2000 controls the rights of people to their health records. The Freedom of Information Act 2000 allows anyone access to information which is not protected by the Data Protection Act 2000. The Computer Misuse Act 1990 secures computer programmes and data from unauthorised alteration or access. The Access to Health Records Act administrates access to the health records of the deceased.

A responsibility to maintain patients' privacy and deal with information confidentially is a crucial part of all healthcare professionals' ethics, which are important components in ensuring trust within professional–patient relationships; if trust is diminished, patients may not disclose sensitive information to professionals, which may be detrimental to their health. An individual who believes their confidence has been broken can sue through civil law, and a breach of confidentiality which cannot be justified can lead to disciplinary action. Nurses who choose to disclose confidential information must be able to justify their actions, and disclosure without consent must be carried out only in the public interest to protect individuals, groups or society from the risk of harm (e.g. child abuse or serious crime) (NMC 2012).

Informed consent

Healthcare professionals need to uphold the interests and rights of patients by acting as advocates as they have a moral, professional and legal responsibility towards them with regards to consent. Consent is important at every level of care, from basic personal care to major surgery, as patients are entitled to predetermine what happens to them and should be empowered to do so by healthcare staff (DH 2009). In order for consent to be valid, it needs to meet certain criteria; it must be given voluntarily and uncoerced, by a competent adult who has been provided with the information to make an informed judgement (Dimond 2011). An important aspect of consent which is commonly disregarded is the patient's right to refuse consent or withdraw their consent which can take place at any time and should be documented (DH 2009). Adequate information needs to be provided to the patient so they can make a decision whether to consent. If a patient feels they received insufficient information, they may take legal action. If healthcare professionals don't gain valid consent or go against a patient's wishes, they may find themselves liable for charges of assault and battery (Dimond 2011).

Children under 16 may be able to consent for treatment if deemed to be able to comprehend the implications (Gillick competence). If not, a parent may consent for them. A child in this instance may be able to accept treatment, but their refusal of treatment needs to be examined in context of the severity of their decision. Children who are 16 or 17 are considered competent to consent for themselves, but as good practice parental involvement should be encouraged. It should be noted that if a child up to the age of 18 refused treatment, parents may overrule the child. On occasion, depending on the circumstances, a court order may be necessary (Carey 2009, DH 2009).

It is best practice that the person carrying out the procedure should gain consent; however, colleagues may gain consent on your behalf if they are trained to seek consent for that procedure or can carry out the procedure (DH 2009). Consent can be given in three ways; verbal, implied and written. All are legally equal, although written consent is often deemed as preferable as this can act as evidence of the event, particularly if the treatment is hazardous, difficult or extensive. Verbal consent should be used with caution, especially when no witnesses are present. It is important to understand that a signature on a consent form doesn't necessarily prove the patient has been consented. It is merely evidence of the patient's choice (DH 2009). It is suggested that in procedures considered to carry large or serious risks, it is recommended to use a two-stage process; the first stage is covering the information and discussion of options and obtaining verbal consent, and the second is obtaining the signature which confirms the patient's decision to continue with the proposed treatment. In instances when there is a language barrier, translators should be utilised to enable the patient to consent.

When considering if patients are competent to give consent, practitioners should always assume adults have competence unless they demonstrate otherwise. Patients may be incompetent temporarily due to sedation or long-term due to unconsciousness or mental illness. If patients do not meet one of the following three criteria, then they are deemed as lacking capacity:

- Unable to take in or retain information provided about their treatment or care
- Unable to understand the information provided
- Unable to weigh up the information as part of the decision-making process (Dimond 2011).

No one is able to give consent on behalf of an adult who lacks capacity for medical treatment, unless they have been authorised under a Lasting Power of Attorney or they have been made a court-appointed deputy and have the authority to make treatment decisions (DH 2009). Therefore, in most circumstances, a family member cannot make decisions on behalf of another adult. In instances when a patient is deemed incompetent to give consent, healthcare professionals are expected to act in the patient's best interests, whilst keeping relatives informed. It does not affect the legitimacy and legality of the consent. It is important to note that just because a patient has a mental disorder, it doesn't mean that they necessarily lack the capacity to consent.

In emergency situations when patients may be temporarily unable to give consent (i.e. if they are unconscious), healthcare professionals should act in the patient's best interests. Any treatment which can be delayed until the patient can consent should be given once the patient can consent, but life-preserving treatment can be given without consent. Living wills or advanced directives enable patients to determine what treatment they would receive in an instance when they are incapable of making decisions. They are not automatically legally binding, but they give an insight into the wishes of the patient and in instances where healthcare professionals are brought to court to explain their treatment of patients they can be used as a defence (Dimond 2011).

Risk assessment

Risk assessments are important for protecting employees, patients and organisations as well as complying with the law; it is not feasible to eliminate risk but to acknowledge the potential and minimise that risk (HSE 2014). Therefore, risk assessment and management are key to the role of any practitioners within an advanced capacity. There is a legal requirement under the Management of Health and Safety at Work Regulations 1999 (Management Regulations) to carry out risk assessment and guidance published by the Health and Safety Executive (HSE 2014). It explains that the five steps to a risk assessment are:

- Identify the hazards.
- Decide who might be harmed and how.
- Evaluate the risks and decide on precautions.
- Record your findings and implement them.
- Review your assessment and update if necessary.

A hazard is considered as something that could cause harm, and risk is the chance of the harm occurring and the degree of severity. Also considered is the number of people who could potentially be harmed. The PCC (2012) explains that individuals practising as SFAs and their management department require explanations regarding the expectations, limitations and implications both legally and ethically of the role. Working in a theatre presents its own risks, as surgery is technically complex and requires a range of people with different skills collaborating. Risk can be reduced by the practitioner being competent in the role by having the correct training and qualifications.

Guidelines, policies and protocols

It is important to acknowledge that in court procedures, guidelines, policies and protocols have no hierarchy, with the same principles applicable to them all equally (Dimond 2011). Guidance issued by an employer, professional association or governing body should be followed, but there may be instances when following the guidelines may not be appropriate, in which case the practitioner should modify their actions accordingly. The practitioner may need to seek advice as to whether flexibility to the recommendations would be apt, and documentation of the rationale for the decision is imperative (Dimond 2011). Clinical guidelines provide a structure and evidence-based approach to specific conditions. Local implementation is imperative as these are normally based on national guidelines. Once guidelines are introduced at a local level, they are considered protocols. Protocol-based care is considered evidence based, provides care collaboratively, and integrates and enhances patient-centred care.

As healthcare professionals take on advanced practice, these come with increased autonomy and independence which in turn may lead to liability issues. Therefore, it is important that they work within their scope of practice, maintain registration and incorporate continual educational and liability coverage be it vicarious liability or independent indemnity insurance. In order to achieve vicarious liability, an SFA must work within set protocols and must show that they are practicing in the best interests of patients.

56 Surgical First Assistant

The Surgical First Assistant (SFA), formerly known as Advanced Scrub Practitioner (ASP), is a predominantly intraoperative role with set skills which can be transferred to any surgical speciality. Unlike the Surgical Care Practitioner role, in which the practitioner specialises within a surgical speciality, an SFA can perform set skills for across a number of specialities and they are generically trained.

Background to role

Due to the introduction of the European Working Time Regulation (DH 2007), stricter immigration rules and the potential introduction of Seven Day Working, there is a potential for gaps in the care for patients. This includes within the intraoperative setting, where acting as an assistant was previously the role of a junior doctor.

Traditionally, it has become custom and practice that theatre practitioners will surgically assist within the operating theatre. Due to this, it is now the expectation of some surgical staff that it is within the remit of perioperative practitioners. This may be as an additional person or in a dual-role capacity. If a practitioner performs a *dual role*, this means they are acting as a scrub practitioner and a surgical assistant, which is generally considered as bad practice as the practitioner is unable to perform either role safely (Sutton 2003, Mardell 2004, Timpany and McAleavy 2010).

In addition, perioperative practitioners would historically undertake this additional role without any additional formalised training or education. This can put patients at risk due to the potential of compromised care, and practitioners may be found negligent should damage to the patient occur. Due to increased awareness and litigation, there is currently a shift within the perioperative environment and theatre staff are requesting a surgical assistant, which may result in staff feeling undervalued. However, when undertaking the additional training required, it becomes apparent to even experienced staff that the knowledge they had was superficial. However, this can sometimes leave perioperative staff in the uncomfortable position of either assisting or performing a dual role in the absence of an assistant (Brame 2011, Halliwell 2012).

Role definition

The scope of the Surgical First Assistant role has to be clarified and is defined as a:

> Role undertaken by a registered practitioner who provides continuous competent and dedicated assistance under the direct supervision of the operating surgeon throughout the procedure, whilst not performing any form of surgical intervention (PCC 2012: 1).

The SFA must have advanced knowledge and skills to ensure they can provide competent and safe assistance during surgical procedures. They work as an additional member of the team. SFAs may work ad hoc as an assistant, but the ideal would be for the SFA to be pre-scheduled for necessary operating lists where necessary.

Scope of practice

The scope of the role includes:

- Pre and postoperative visits
- Urinary catheterisation
- Positioning
- Skin preparation
- Draping
- Assisting with haemostasis
- Indirect diathermisation
- Camera holding
- Cutting of sutures
- Retraction
- Assisting with wound closure
- Application of dressing (PCC 2012).

The SFA has a clinical supervisor who is a Consultant Surgeon and either a more experienced SFA, a surgical care practitioner or a senior member of the perioperative staff for support and to help facilitate their role.

Experiences of the role

Practitioners who undertake the role underestimate the differences between the scrub role and being utilised as an assistant. The interactions can differ with the surgeons, who may expect a different level of anatomy knowledge (Deighton 2007). Being in an assisting role provides the practitioner with a different perspective and improves and enhances their scrub ability. This is similar to the knowledge and skills of a good circulator making the individual better within the scrub role.

Often practitioners who are new to the role find it a challenge to not step back into the role of team leader or scrub practitioner, particularly when they still have these aspects within their role when not working in the SFA capacity (Deighton 2007). If the practitioner was acting as an assistant and also acting as a team leader. that could be considered another form of 'dual' role.

The two skills which the majority of perioperative practitioners find challenging are camera holding and pre and postoperative visits. Pre and postoperative visits can be challenging due to shortage of staff and time constraints but also due to practitioners being outside of their comfort zones and unsure what the patients may ask (Brame 2011). However, the benefits to the patients, particularly allaying their fears and being 'a friendly face', add to the practitioner's job satisfaction. Camera holding is challenging, both mentally as the assistant needs to maintain the correct horizon and orientation and physically due to the position needed to maintain a safe view.

Expanding into an enhanced or advanced role allows senior practitioners to have an alternative clinical role and further develop in an alternative pathway to management.

Professional and legal considerations

The registered practitioners maintain accountability for their own actions. They must always act within the parameters of their respective Code of Conduct. The practitioner should have the SFA role reflected in their job description/job contract, and the role should have been risk assessed. Necessary Trust policies should be established to support the SFA role. It is recommended that SFAs consider private indemnity insurance, in particular if they work within the private sector (PCC 2012).

57 Surgical Care Practitioner

A Surgical Care Practitioner (SCP) works within a surgical speciality providing pre, peri and postoperative care for surgical patients, unlike the Surgical First Assistant role which is an intraoperative role.

Background to role

As with the Surgical First Assistant role, due to the impact of national drivers such as European Working Time Regulation (DH 2007), stricter immigration rules and the potential introduction of Seven Day Working, there is a potential for gaps in care for patients. The gaps in care are not purely interoperative; other care previously delivered by a junior doctor needs to be supported. These areas are across the patient journey and include elective and emergency services.

An SCP can provide care along all aspects of the patient journey and may work in clinics or preoperative assessment, provide ward-based care, assist in theatre, perform independent surgery, provide postoperative care and follow-up and provide out-of-hours support services.

Benefits and challenges of the surgical care practitioner role

There are identified benefits of advanced roles for the patient, practitioner and organisation. The benefits of the SCP role are the continuity and consistency of care. They are a permanent member of the surgical team along with the Consultant Surgeons and other specialist or advanced roles.

As a consequence, they:

- Provide skilled surgical assistance and can subsequently reduce operative time.
- Provide holistic care for the patient as they follow the patient pathway.
- Improve patient experience.
- Provide continuity of care.
- Provide consistency of care and have a familiarity with the organisation.
- Can provide specialist advice and information to the patient and other staff.
- Enhance patient safety.
- Improve quality of care.
- Reduce waiting times.
- Increase patient satisfaction.
- Promote self-development and improve self-confidence for the practitioner.
- Create new challenges and offer an alternative career pathway for practitioners other than management (Lowe *et al.* 2011, Christiansen *et al.* 2012, Quick 2013).

Rapid Perioperative Care, First Edition. Paul Wicker and Sara Dalby.

However, there are some identified challenges to being in an advanced role such as an SCP:

- Challenging to gain acceptance of the role by healthcare practitioners and patients
- Inadequate management support
- Lack of role standardisation
- Confusion surrounding titles
- Lack of appropriate education
- Excessive protocols
- It can be difficult to motivate doctors to change from a traditional model.
- Crossing of traditional professional boundaries is challenging.
- Development may be inhibited due to embedded resistance to change within a clinical setting (Lowe *et al.* 2011, Christiansen *et al.* 2012, Quick 2013).

Definition of role

A Surgical Care Practitioner is defined as:

> A registered non-medical practitioner who has completed a Royal College of Surgeons accredited programme (or other previously recognised course), working in clinical practice as a member of the extended surgical team, who performs surgical intervention, pre-operative care and post-operative care under the direction and supervision of a Consultant surgeon (RCS, 2014: 13).

The SCP must have extensive advanced skills and knowledge to competently and safely be able to perform their advanced role.

Practitioner background

SCPs can come from a variety of registered backgrounds, such as nursing, operating department practitioners and physiotherapists, but it is a requirement that they have a background in caring for surgical patients.

Scope of practice

The scope of the role can fluctuate depending on a number of factors: the individual surgical care practitioner and their education and what they wish to undertake, the surgical team within which they work, the departmental needs and the level of trust support.

Under the direction of a Consultant Surgeon and in conjunction with local guidelines and where applicable taking additional qualifications, the RCS (2014: 12–13) outline the scope of practice of the SCP as:

- (In clinics) Seeing specific preoperative patients and listing them for surgical procedures
- Assessment, including clinical examination and enhanced recovery education
- Arrangement of appropriate pre and postoperative investigations
- The consent process, following guidelines from the GMC and local trust
- Liaison with medical, theatre, ward and clerical staff to support coherent service provision
- The World Health Organization Safe Surgery checklist
- Preparation of patients for surgery
- Surgical procedures in the operating theatre as part of the multidisciplinary team for the surgical speciality under the supervision and direction of the operating surgeon
- Acting as first or second assistant as directed by the supervising surgeon
- Performing some technical and operative procedures
- Facilitating continuity of patient care

- Daily ward rounds, making assessments and formulating plans for patients' postoperative care
- Writing of operation notes and ward round note taking
- Postoperative care, including wound assessment, initial treatment and identification of surgical problems and complications
- Identifying acute deterioration of patients and having knowledge of national early warning scores
- Provision of support to on-call and emergency services
- The evaluation of care, including the discharge process and follow-up care arrangements for surgical patients
- A variety of outpatient activities
- Facilitation of the training of trainee surgeons
- Research, development, education and audit within their surgical department
- The prescription of medications appropriate to their individual speciality.

Educational requirements

The National Curriculum outlines a two-year master's-level course in which SCP students are required to spend a minimum of 2200 hours gaining clinical learning, with half of those hours in theatre. This emphasises that SCPs are not just intraoperative practitioners, and in order to fulfil the programme requirements they need to be involved in the surgical patient's complete journey (RCS 2014).

The courses include both generic and specialist aspects of caring for surgical patients. However, the student Surgical Care Practitioner has to identify a specific surgical pathway (listed below) prior to commencing their course. Generic aspects include research, leadership skills and the intraoperative skills of assisting, history taking, clinical examination and diagnostics, interpretation of common tests (i.e. blood tests, chest and abdominal x-rays and electrocardiographs (ECGs)) and ward management of patients, including the identification of common postoperative complications such as haemorrhage and sepsis. The speciality-specific components of the course include educational and technical aspects that are relevant to the surgical speciality, and they are outlined in the National Curriculum. They include specific presentations of both elective and emergency patients, intraoperative tasks, interpretation of specialist tests and scans and specific postoperative complications.

As discussed, SCPs perform aspects of a junior doctor's role and as a consequence should be educated and assessed similarly. As per the National Curriculum, the methods of clinical assessment have been brought in line with those of junior doctors and are similar to the assessments set out by the Intercollegiate Surgical Curriculum Programme. This has an added benefit of ensuring familiarity and consistency of assessment for the Surgical Consultants who are assessing the SCP students. Along with these assessments, the students are also assessed with a variety of methods; exams, assignments and an objective structured clinical examination (OSCE) (RCS 2014).

Surgical speciality pathways

There are generic aspects of surgical patient management but also 11 possible surgical speciality pathways:

- Trauma and orthopaedic
- General surgery
- Urology
- Gynaecology
- Neurosurgery
- Cardiothoracic surgery
- Vascular

- Paediatric surgery
- Otorhinolaryngology
- Maxillofacial surgery
- Plastic and reconstructive surgery (RCS 2014).

Professional and legal considerations

As discussed in this chapter, the scope of practice of an SCP is extensive, and they are expected to perform at an advanced level with the required clinical decision making and level of autonomy. Although they work under the direction of a Consultant Surgeon to whom they are clinically responsible (RCS 2014), they are registered practitioners and subsequently accountable for their actions and omissions. The SCP must always stay within their scope of practice, follow guidelines and protocols, work within their outlined job description and within a predetermined level of supervision.

Although it can be a challenging role, the benefits for the patient, practitioner and healthcare organisation are well documented. With increasing pressures on the National Health Service to provide high standards of patient care whilst offsetting financial limitations, the need for such roles is increasing.

58 Pre and Postoperative Visiting

Introduction

The value of pre and postoperative visits can often be underestimated. For the patient, it is comforting to have a 'familiar face' when they arrive at theatre having met the practitioner earlier, thus reducing stress and anxiety. For the practitioner, it enhances job satisfaction by having additional knowledge of the patient and seeing them during the recovery period. Preoperative visits help with the smooth running of the list as potential problems can be identified and solved in a timely manner. During the postoperative visit, the patient may feed back to the practitioner suggestions which will enhance the patient perioperative journey. Nowadays, due to on-the-day admissions and same-day discharges, it becomes more difficult for practitioners to see the patients.

Preoperative visits

It must be emphasised that a preoperative visit differs from a preoperative assessment.

The preoperative visit consists of:

- Evaluating the patient's intraoperative needs specifically from a theatre practitioner's perspective
- Informing the patient of the intraoperative process and clarifying expectations
- Allaying any concerns the patient may have (Hurley and McAleavy 2006).

When carrying out a preoperative visit, it is important that as a practitioner you do not make promises as nothing can be completely guaranteed. It can be difficult if the patients ask questions regarding the surgical or anaesthetic procedures. It is important to remember that it should be members of the respective medical teams who have those specific conversations. However, this is an opportunity for the practitioner to ensure the patient has completed the consent process and facilitate discussions with the medical teams if necessary in advance to sending for the patient, thus resulting in smooth running of the list. Preoperative visits may also allow the practitioner to identify any health problems or conditions which may not have been identified which may affect the intraoperative phase, such as allergies, organisation of additional equipment or minimal range of movement which may affect positioning. The practitioner may also be able to reduce waste of resources by being a communication link between the ward, medical teams and theatre as they may gain additional information which the theatre team are not privy to (Hurley and McAleavy 2006).

Rapid Perioperative Care, First Edition. Paul Wicker and Sara Dalby.

Postoperative visits

Postoperative visits are often deemed less important; however, for the patient, it provides a continuity of care following the immediate intraoperative phase and an opportunity to discuss any positive experiences or things which could be improved upon. For the theatre practitioner, it allows an insight into the patient's recovery and an opportunity for feedback which could positively change practice. As with the preoperative visit, it may be preferable for the practitioner to redirect certain questions from the patient to the medical team and ensure that they stay within their professional limitations.

Patient-centred communication

A patient-centred approach should start with the patient's perspective and aims to meet their individual needs. The practitioner should listen, help the patient to reflect on and clarify significant aspects and provide professional insights which the patient may not have thought about.

The environment for discussion needs to be considered. Privacy should be maintained, with the patient being consulted as to whether they would like to talk in a separate room (if available) or at the bedside. Interruption and disruption should be minimal; aim to ensure the patient feels comfortable to disclose information. The room should be well lit and well ventilated; the 'set up' of the environment should encourage conversation, taking into account a comfortable distance (Arnold and Underman Boggs 2011).

When we communicate with another person, we begin to build a relationship with them, and it is up to us to determine that type of relationship. Relationships are developed through self-disclosure in which the people involved divulge information, feelings and attitudes. To develop a good relationship, positive social and perception skills are necessary with emphasis placed on the qualities of empathy, respect, trust and confidentiality. The therapeutic relationship that is formed enables nurses to provide all aspects of nursing care from physical care to emotional support and health education. A patient's feelings of anxiety and stress need to be considered as they may hinder communication (Berry 2006, Arnold and Underman Boggs 2011).

It is best to ask 'open' questions which encourage people to talk and expand on their responses as 'closed' questions are only answered with a short response. During the conversation, it is useful to utilise reinforcement which encourages the communicator to continue or repeat what they have said. To assure the patient that you are actively listening, it is important to maintain attention through eye contact and appropriate facial expressions and delay evaluation of the conversation until you fully comprehend. Patients seldom ask questions, but instead provide cues to concerns which they may repeat until either they are picked up on or the patient feels that the professional feels the cues are unacceptable. Medical terminology should be avoided (Berry 2006).

As the conversation is ending, it is important to summarise the conversation so the patient knows that the healthcare professional has understood and any misunderstandings can be corrected. Screening questions can ensure that all important issues have been addressed as it enables the patient to feel they have had the opportunity to talk about all major concerns.

It is also important to document the visit and any specific findings relevant to the patient's intraoperative management (Holmes 2005).

Things to consider

- *Non-verbal communication*: These can either enhance what is said verbally or contradict verbal expression. There are three main categories; body language, paralanguage and dress. Body language is the conscious or unconscious body movements or actions when communicating. The emotional status of the individual can be interpreted from body language, taking into account posture, gesturing and rhythm of movement. Facial expression reveals a lot about our mood and emotion, with our eyes and mouths being the most dominant features. Individuals tend to evaluate us by our facial expression. Paralinguistic features include rhythm, pace, pitch, emphasis, tone of voice and intonation. They help with the interpretation of the person's mood and are particularly useful in instances when the people communicating can't see each other (e.g. telephone conversations). Our personal appearance and presentation affect non-verbal communication. Some we can alter; others are outside of our control. These include body shape, skin colour and facial features. Clothing, jewellery and hairstyle can affect perceptions of our intelligence, social confidence, warmth and friendliness, emphasising the importance to present ourselves appropriately for each situation (Ellis *et al.* 2003, Berry 2006, Arnold and Underman Boggs 2011).

- *Language and speech characteristics*: Verbal language is the primary form of communication and can be spoken and written. Reflecting feeling happens when the listener is able to identify the speaker's feelings by sensing the underlying emotion and reading between the lines (Berry 2006).
- *Spatial factors*: Body space and proximity are something we need to be conscious of when communicating with people, as everyone needs their personal space to feel comfortable. This varies with factors such as culture, age, gender and the familiarity of the people interacting. Acknowledgement of this is particularly pertinent in a healthcare setting, where patients' personal space is frequently invaded, possibly causing the patient to feel a loss of dignity and vulnerable (Berry 2006).
- *Location*: The physical setting of the interaction needs to be taken into account. Factors such as the type, layout and decoration of the room; noise levels; and types of sound can affect the person's behaviour and interpersonal communication (Berry 2006).
- *Listening*: This can be divided into active and passive listening. In active listening, it is made obvious that the content of the conversation is being heard and responded to, which encourages disclosure; with passive listening, the recipient shows no signs of registering what they are being told. Listening barriers include external distractions; lack of interest; verbal battling, where we debate ideas from the conversation in our own heads instead of listening and subsequently lose focus of the other person's points; and fact hunting, where we focus on the detailed facts, overlooking the main theme of the conversation. Also consider preoccupation, personal insecurity, unusual speech or behavioural patterns, physical discomfort, psychological discomfort and information overload as barriers to active listening (Arnold and Underman Boggs 2011).

Barriers to pre and postoperative visits

Factors which impinge upon effective communication are labelled as barriers and include:

- Physical barriers such as noise, a physical problem like deafness, a lisp which affects the formation of speech or a breakdown of equipment necessary for communication.
- Semantic barriers are caused by the careless use of words. If words are used which are not understood, such as slang terminology or (more pertinent to our job) medical terminology, they may be incomprehensible to the public.
- Interpreters may need to be arranged if there is a language barrier between the patient and the practitioner.
- Psychological barriers are caused by attitudes, beliefs and values. They affect how we express ourselves and how we interpret others. We must ensure we do not make assumptions or speak before first thinking about how we may be perceived.
- It is important to consider the patient's cognitive state as they may be in pain or anxious which may inhibit the receptiveness of information.
- Time is a barrier, as patients are more frequently admitted on the day of surgery and may be discharged on the day of surgery.
- Short staffing may make it difficult for staff to be released to perform the visits.

- Practitioners may feel anxious due to being in an alternative department and not having specific training for pre and postoperative visits.
- Patients may not wish to have a preoperative visit as they may not want any additional information. The practitioner should always confirm with the patient first (Hurley and McAleavy 2006).

Although there are many barriers to pre and postoperative visits, the benefits outweigh the difficulties, specifically with relieving patient anxiety and helping the smooth running of the intraoperative phase by identifying potential issues which may not be considered by medical teams.

59 Retraction

Retraction and tissue manipulation are important for the surgical assistant as ineffective performance of these tasks negatively affects the operating surgeon by not providing them with a clear operating field.

Handling of tissues

Whilst it is important for the safety of the patient that the operating field is exposed appropriately for the surgeon, the assistant must also remember the effect retraction has when handling tissues. When tissues are handled, an inflammatory response ensues, creating swelling and a release of serosanguinous fluid. This is a natural response; however, rough handling can cause an exacerbation of this response. This results in having a negative effect by providing an environment suited to increased infective microorganisms (Paige 2009, Kotcher Fuller 2010). If the practitioner uses too much pressure, they may cause damage to tissue and organs, potentially leading to swelling and tissue bruising. When assisting with wound closure, it is particularly important for the practitioner to not apply excess force on the wound edges, as this may lead to poor wound healing and an increased risk of infection (Kotcher Fuller 2010). Rough handling could also cause excessive bleeding due to damaging blood vessels; this could result in a haematoma which can result in wound breakdown. Practitioners also have a potential to cause damage to nerves if the retractor is placed incorrectly or too much force used.

Considerations when retracting

Retractors can be divided into self-retaining retractors such as Golligers and Travers or handheld retractors such as Morris and Langenbeck (Photo 7). The benefits of self-retaining retractors are that the assistant is free to assist in other manners, and also they are not at risk of causing musculoskeletal damage. However, handheld retractors are easier to position and reduce the tension, even for the short term, to allow perfusion of the tissues. Self-retaining retractors can also be bulky and be obstructive to the operator (Paige 2009).

The practitioner needs to consider the following:

- Select the correct size retractor to minimise potential damage to tissue due to correct distribution of pressure.
- It may be beneficial to protect the wound edges with swabs, particularly with self-retaining retractor blades as they will be in situ for extended periods.
- Skin hooks and some 'teeth' on self-retainers can be sharp and have the potential to cause sharps injuries to the practitioners.
- Retraction, particularly during long cases, can be physically demanding for surgical assistants; to avoid or minimise the risk of musculoskeletal injury, the practitioner needs to be aware of their posture and the appropriate use of the retractor.

Rapid Perioperative Care, First Edition. Paul Wicker and Sara Dalby.

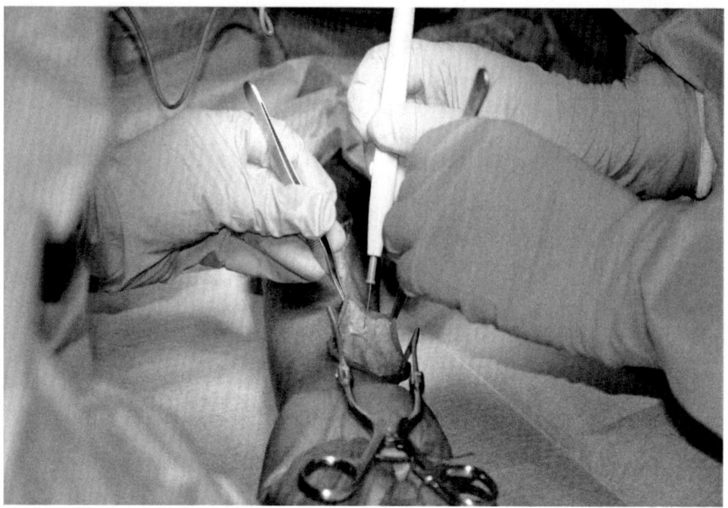

Photo 2 Self-retaining retractor

Choice of retractor

The basic principle of retraction is that an appropriate retractor is placed (in most instances by the lead operating surgeon) on the tissue surrounding the operating field whilst taking into account the surrounding structures to minimise potential damage. The retractor is then to remain in both positions and has equal tension as when it is first positioned.

The choice of retractor is based on a number of factors:

- The procedural requirements
- Surgeon's preference
- Availability
- Cost
- Availability of an assistant
- Assistant's experience (Steele *et al.* 2013).

Alternative methods of retraction

Although retraction has always been a basic necessity for adequate surgical exposure, new techniques have developed due to different specialities, techniques and procedural requirements. In Chapter 40 on surgical instruments, the use of retractors was discussed; however, aside from the use of retractors, there are numerous alternative methods of retraction.

- *Positioning*: During laparoscopic procedures, the table will be tilted to manipulate the movement of internal organs to move from the operating site. For example, for a laparoscopic anterior resection, the patient is positioned 'head down and left side up' to remove the small bowel from the operating field and thus minimise incidence of damaging the small bowel.
- *Stay sutures*: These allow the practitioner to apply tension on tissue; they may be used to stabilise structures or temporarily retract tissue.
- *Sloops*: These are used primarily in vascular surgery to isolate, manipulate and retract vessels.

- *Hands*: A practitioner's hands can be utilised; this technique can be particularly good for delicate and friable tissue and organs. However, the assistant is potentially put at increased risk of a sharps injury and can get in the way due to a lack of space in the operating field.
- *Swabs*: Whether to 'pack' the small bowel away from the operating field or to use a 'swab on a stick' to keep tissue from occluding the surgeon's view.
- *Pneumoperitoneum*: During laparoscopic surgery, the creation of a pneumoperitoneum separates the abdominal wall from the abdominal content.
- *Graspers*: In both open and laparoscopic surgery, graspers can be placed on tissue to manipulate it from the operating field. Graspers can be traumatic and atraumatic, and caution needs to be utilised by the practitioner to ensure that the appropriate grasper is used on the correct tissue. If an incorrect selection is made, the grasper can tear through and damage tissue.
- *Tape*: Tape can be used in cases such as the bottom end of an extra-levator abdoperineal resection when the patient is positioned jack-knife to aid with the exposure of the perineum, allowing the assistant to retract deeper tissues.
- *Haemostats*: These can be used to retract tissue layers (Paige 2009, Kotcher Fuller 2010, Spera *et al.* 2011, Steele *et al.* 2013).

Placement of the retractor

Placing of the retractor is the responsibility of the lead operating surgeon and is deemed outside the Surgical First Assistant's scope of practice; however, Surgical Care Practitioners are allowed to place retractors as part of their scope of practice (PCC 2012). The rationale of the operating surgeon positioning the retractor is that they have an advanced level of knowledge of anatomy and thus have a smaller chance of causing damage. They also have a better visualisation of the surgical field, and therefore it is safer for them to position the retractor to minimise the risk of damage.

Retraction is an important aspect of surgery and can significantly affect the efficiency and safety of the operative field. However, there are numerous potential hazards, including nerve and tissue damage, which the practitioner must take into consideration.

60 Cutting of Sutures

The cutting of sutures is another assisting skill outlined by the PCC (2014) Position Statement for Surgical First Assistants. It can be an underestimated and undervalued skill; however, it is an important skill and particularly difficult when cutting a suture or tie deep in the pelvis.

Communication with the surgeon

Effective communication with the operating surgeon is vital at all times during the surgical procedure to ensure patient safety (Wicker and O'Neill 2010). It is important during the task of cutting sutures too. It allows the surgeon to confirm if the suture or ligature is to be cut rather than clipped as a 'stay suture'. The number of 'throws' can fluctuate depending on the type of knot and suture material, and effective communication ensures confirmation that the stitch is ready to be cut. There may also be a dialogue regarding the required length the surgeon would like the suture strands to be (Guglielmi and Hunter 2011).

If the practitioner has been asked to cut a suture or ligature and they are unable to see the tip of the scissors, then they should communicate to the operating surgeon that they are unable to cut the suture safely.

Importance of having the right tools

It is important that the suture-cutting scissors are sharp, as blunt scissors would fray the suture material.

The length of the suture-cutting scissors needs to be appropriate for the specific part of the operation. If operating in the pelvis, Nelson scissors are more appropriate than Mayo scissors. If a practitioner used scissors which were too short to cut a suture in the pelvis, they risk needing to lean in and advance their hands into the operating field, thus potentially occluding vision. Equally, if Nelson scissors were used to cut a stitch at the skin level due to the positioning, the practitioner would have less control over the cutting of the stitch as the scissors are too long and could accidently cause damage to the patient (Kirk 2010).

Dissecting scissors should not be used to cut sutures as cutting causes blunting to the blades.

Handling the scissors

The practitioner should use their thumb and ring finger in the handles of the scissors; the index finger on the same hand should be placed on the shaft of the scissors to stabilise. With their other hand, the practitioner should use their index and middle fingers under the jaws of the scissors to stabilise them. It is important when cutting sutures to use the tip of the scissors, and the tips should be visualised at all times (Kirk 2010).

Rapid Perioperative Care, First Edition. Paul Wicker and Sara Dalby.

Knowledge needed

It is important for a surgical assistant to have a working knowledge of suture materials and their indications. Suture materials can be categorised into multifilament (braided) or monofilament (single strand). Monofilament sutures are much more friable, and the practitioner needs to ensure when handling them that they are not crushed. Monofilament sutures also retain a memory which affects the handling and knot security.

The benefits of the multifilament in this context are that it is easy to handle and has better knot security. Due to the increased knot security, the strands on multifilaments can usually be shorter than those of monofilaments as the risk of them unravelling is less (Kotcher Fuller 2010).

A knowledge of whether a suture is absorbable or non-absorbable is also important, particularly when the surgeon performing superficial wound closure. The type of wound closure method will give the practitioner an indication on how long the strands of the suture need to be too. For example, if the surgeon chooses to use a simple interrupted method with an nylon suture, the stitches will require removal, and therefore the practitioner will need to leave the strands fairly long to make it easier for removal. However, if the surgeon chooses a subcuticular stitch with a Monocryl suture, then the stitch will normally be tied with an Aberdeen knot and buried, so the assistant needs to cut the suture just above skin.

A knowledge of the stages of the procedure is important for the assistant so they can pre-empt and proactively assist. This is true for all aspects of assisting, but in the context of cutting sutures there may be a part of the procedure where the sutures may be required to be cut long, for example on a tissue specimen to aid the identification of lymph nodes or orientation (Whalan 2006). There may also be instances where the surgeon only wants one strand long and the other clipped.

Potential risks

If a stitch or ligature is cut too short, then it has the potential to unravel which could have severe implications if it was on a vessel or part of an anastomosis. If the suture unravelled, the following could occur: wound separation, haemorrhage and wound dehiscence (Muffly *et al.* 2009).

If the stitch is cut too long, then it has the potential to cause a stitch sinus which can be uncomfortable for patients and may even require further surgery to remove. Also an inflammatory suture material can cause an inflammatory response, so the less left in situ, the less tissue reaction.

If the suture or ligature was not cut effectively and the practitioner withdraws their hand, they may pull on the suture which will pull on the vessel, potentially tearing the vessel and thus causing bleeding (Whelan 2006).

If the practitioner slips, does not utilise the tip of the scissors to cut the suture or has limited vision of the suture when they intend to cut it, there is a risk that they may cut tissue or structures adjacent to the intended suture (Phillips 2013).

Cutting sutures poses an increased risk of a sharps injury for practitioners; a sharps injury could also happen when passing the scissors.

For the safe cutting of sutures, it is important that the practitioner uses the right tools appropriately, has good visualisation and communicates effectively with the operating surgeon.

61 Suture Materials

Suturing is a method of wound closure which promotes healing by eliminating dead space, realigning tissue, and apposing and holding together the skin edges until they have healed and no longer require support.

Selecting suture materials

A number of features need to be considered prior to the selection of suture material, including:

- Absorbable or non-absorbable
- Monofilament or multifilament
- Natural or synthetic
- Tensile strength
- Tissue reactivity
- How the suture knots (Hamlin *et al.* 2010, Goodman and Spry 2014).

Patient factors

Patient factors such as infection, obesity, respiratory problems, presence of malignancies or debilitating injuries, immunodeficiency, blood loss, fluid and electrolyte imbalances, inadequate nutrition, debility and chronic disease influence the rate of healing and must be considered when selecting wound closure. The age of the patient is an important consideration; paediatric patients need a smaller suture than adults, and the child's age will influence the decision of removal, with absorbable sutures being favoured when appropriate. Older patients have a decrease of elasticity in their skin tissue and an increased likelihood of bruising or injury. Their skin is more thin and fragile due to disease, age and medication (Davis 2009).

Wound support

Wound support fluctuates depending on the type of tissue; several days for muscle, skin and subcutaneous tissue; weeks or months for fascia or tendon; and long term in the instance of vascular prosthesis. Fascia and skin have a longer healing period than visceral tissues. Subsequently, when choosing sutures for skin and fascial closure, a suture material which sustains its tensile strength should be selected. When choosing suture materials for tissue that heals quickly, a suture should be selected so that it loses its tensile strength at the same rate as the tissue gains its strength, which then dissolves, leaving no foreign material in the healed wound. Tensile strength is measured by the amount of tension or pull that the thread will endure before it breaks when knotted (Davis 2009, Phillips 2012, Goodman and Spry 2014).

Rapid Perioperative Care, First Edition. Paul Wicker and Sara Dalby.

The 'perfect' suture

The 'perfect' suture should be made of a material which can be used in every operation, altering only in tensile strength and diameter; it should be easily manipulated when used, with nominal tissue reaction; not be prone to bacterial growth; and preferably, in the majority of situations, should be absorbed after achieving its objective in supporting wound healing. Unfortunately, there is no such 'perfect' suture; the practitioner must use decision making based on numerous factors to select the optimum wound closure method. Suture materials should be strong and reliable, and have a minimal inflammatory or allergic response. The three main points to consider are material properties, how it handles and tissue reaction. The aim is to choose a suture which causes the least reactivity, whilst providing optimum strength during wound healing (Davis 2009, Hamlin *et al.* 2010, Kirk 2010, Goodman and Spry 2014).

Disadvantages of suturing

There are a number of disadvantages to consider before selecting suturing as the wound closure method. Suturing requires someone with the knowledge and skill to carry it out. There is a risk of needle stick injury, and it can be time consuming; damage may occur to the tissues from, for example, crushing the wound edges with forceps or injecting with local anaesthetic. Suture material increases the risk of infection, and the suture thread can act as a path for bacteria to enter the wound (Davis 2009).

Absorbable and non-absorbable

Suture materials can be distinguished into two categories, depending on what happens to them inside the body: absorbable and non-absorbable.

Absorbable sutures can be either natural or synthetic and are used to provide short-term wound support until the wound is healed enough to endure stress; they lose their tensile strength within 60 days. The regularly used absorbable sutures are catgut, polyglycolic acid (Dexon), polydioxanone (PDS), polyglactic acid (Vicryl) and polyglyconate (Maxon). Natural absorbable sutures are slowly digested by tissue enzymes, whereas synthetic absorbable sutures are primarily destroyed by hydrolysis which occurs naturally as part of the healing process. A rise in temperature or change of pH can increase the rate of hydrolysis. The absorption rate of suture material is significant when considering delayed suture complications such as suture granuloma and sinus formation. The rate at which the material loses its strength is important in the selection to ensure that the wound is supported; catgut strength remains for about a week; Dexon, polysorb and Vicryl for two weeks; and PDS, Monocryl and Maxon for up to three months. PDS, Maxon and Monocryl, due to their prolonged support for wound healing, are selected for fascial closure or elderly patients as they have the benefits of prolonged wound support and absorbability. Absorbable sutures should not be placed in fluids as moisture lessens their tensile strength. It is important to note that in the presence of infection, the strength of catgut decreases significantly, but this isn't commonly the same for synthetic absorbable sutures (Price and Sinclair 2008, Davis 2009, Hamlin *et al.* 2010, Kirk 2010, Hussey and Bagg 2011, Goodman and Spry 2014).

Non-absorbable sutures can be divided into *natural*, which include silk and cotton, and *synthetic*, which incorporate Dacron, prolene, nylon, ethibond and wire. Synthetic sutures are able to retain their tensile strength for longer than absorbable sutures; however, they do lose some of their strength, but it is so minimal that it is of little significance. When silk is concealed in tissue, it loses strength quickly in comparison with other non-absorbable materials. Silk loses its strength after 60 days, nylon loses only 16% of its tensile strength after 70 days and prolene keeps its strength for up to two years. Non-absorbable sutures stay in situ within the wound until they are deliberately removed; unlike absorbable sutures, they are capable of withstanding the process of enzymatic digestion. They tend to be utilised in areas which have slow-healing tissues such as skin, fascia and tendons. When they are to remain permanently within the body, such as abdominal wound closure and the suturing of vascular grafts, they become encapsulated or walled off by the body's fibroblasts. For skin closure, they provide the best cosmetic result as they cause minimal tissue reaction and are effortlessly and painlessly removed. For best results, they are to be removed when the wound has healed before there is scarring from the suture tracts. Non-absorbable sutures are chosen for percutaneous skin closure, which in healthy patients is anything from 5 to 8 days; however, the site of the wound and the amount of tension that the wound is under also affect the amount of time that they need to remain in situ. The wound may be reliant on the strength of the fascial or subcutaneous sutures to support it. Silk is a braided suture which increases its tensile strength and improves its handling qualities; silk is pliable and provides safe, fixed knots. It is treated to eradicate its capillarity properties; if untreated, bodily fluids may track infection along the suture; therefore, it needs to be kept dry. Silk can form tracts due to the suture moving to the surface of the wound and can occur up to a year after it is used. Silk sutures may cause an extreme tissue reaction and are no longer recommended due to suture sinus formation and a higher risk of excessive scarring (Andrews and Cascarini 2008, Price and Sinclair 2008, Davis 2009, Hamlin *et al.* 2010, Kirk 2010, Hussey and Bagg 2011, Goodman and Spry 2014).

Natural versus synthetic

Natural sutures are obtained from animals such as catgut or plants such as linen and cotton. Synthetic materials are made from polymers and are more consistent in their functioning and more predictable in their absorption rates than natural materials. Synthetic non-absorbable sutures last longer than natural non-absorbable suture materials. Sutures can be classed as a foreign material which is implanted into the body; as with all foreign material, they will cause the body to have an inflammatory reaction. Usually, this reaction is fairly mild; however, it is important to be aware that synthetic materials are less reactive and are less irritating to tissue than natural suture materials. Natural materials are cheaper than synthetic ones, but synthetic materials are designed to meet specific requirements of duration of strength, handling and absorbability (Kirk 2010).

Monofilament versus multifilament

Monofilament materials are robust, but they do not provide strong knots due to them retaining a 'memory' of what shape they were when they were packaged, making them rigid and springy and subsequently less easy to handle. In contrast, multifilament sutures are easier to manipulate into knots and form more reliable knots which are less likely to unravel. Monofilaments are made of a single strand, which means they run smoothly through the tissues as they expose a smaller amount of surface area. Therefore they are easy to use, produce less reaction, cause only moderate trauma to tissues and, as they have a smooth surface, do not provide cavities in which bacteria can harbour, so they are preferable when the wound is infected or has the potential to become infected. They are, however, easily weakened if damaged when handled poorly (Hamlin *et al.* 2010, Kirk 2010, Goodman and Spry 2014).

Multifilament material is twisted or braided, resulting in increased tensile strength. They provide good handling due to increased flexibility and tying qualities. It is important to note that there may be some inconsistency in knot strength which results from the braiding or twisting process. Multifilament sutures have an increased probability of infection when compared to monofilament as bacteria can become ensnared within the weaves of the material. Our bodies' natural defence mechanisms are unable to terminate them, leading to replication of the bacteria and infection. The choice of whether to use a multifilament or monofilament suture needs to be carefully considered when a wound is infected or has the potential to become infected. Braided materials pass less easily through the tissue, causing trauma and leading to increased tissue reaction. This can be lessened by suture materials having coatings with substances such as silicone, Teflon or a variety of polymers to reduce capillarity and friction when passing through tissue (Hamlin *et al.* 2010, Kirk 2010, Goodman and Spry 2014).

An understanding of the rationale for suture selection and the advantages and disadvantages of different categories of suture materials allows the practitioner to select the most appropriate for the wound closure method to provide the patient with optimum wound closure.

62 Surgical Needles

It is important for all theatre practitioners and surgical assistants to have a working knowledge of needle types, as it is a daily consideration during surgical procedures and pertinent to all surgical procedures.

Needle selection

When selecting an appropriate needle, it is necessary to choose one which brings the suture through the tissue, causing minimal tissue damage:

- They should not break easily.
- Should be sharp enough to go through tissue with minimal pressure but not too strong for the tissue.
- Be of a similar size as the suture thread to reduce tissue trauma.
- Be rigid enough so that there isn't disproportionate bending but pliable enough so it doesn't break after bending (Davis 2015).

The shape and size of the needle need to be appropriate for the tissue variety, for ease of access and without decomposition or burrs subsequently, avoiding infection and tissue trauma (Phillips 2012).

Needle classification

Needle classification is by needle type. The selection of needle shape is due to the accessibility of the area to be sutured, with more restricting operating areas requiring greater curve on the needle.

The majority of needles are curved; half needles are able to be utilised for many different purposes, quarter circles are used in microvascular anastomoses and three-quarter circles for hand closure of the abdominal wall. Straight needles are also available and are usually used for securing drains or skin closure. The needle length differs depending on the depth required to suture and the delicacy of the surgery (Kirk 2010, Goodman and Spry 2014).

The shape of the needle may be determined by the area which is to be sutured; particularly if it is restricted (i.e. for limited spaces), a five-eighths circle or J-shaped needle is selected. The needle type also needs to be contemplated; round-bodied needles divide through tissues rather than cutting them, cutting needles are utilised in dense tissue and spatulate needles (broad or rounded) are used in ophthalmic surgery (Hamlin *et al.* 2010, Davis 2015).

Handheld needles

Handheld needles are less frequently used due to their risk of needle stick injury, and the majority of needles are used with needle holders. Needle holders should be chosen to match the size and strength of the needle. A needle holder which is too big may damage the needle

Rapid Perioperative Care, First Edition. Paul Wicker and Sara Dalby.

and distort the curvature. The needle holder should be in good condition as any defects can cause damage to the needle, leading to a loss of strength, unnecessary force being applied and even breakage. Needles should be mounted on the needle holders securely at the tip and on the flattened area not too near the shaft or tip. Needles without a flattened area should be placed about one-third down from the eye of the needle. To pass the needle through the tissue, it should follow the curvature of the needle. If for any reason you need to reposition the needle, it shouldn't be manoeuvred within the tissue and should be removed and readjusted (Ethicon 2005b, Kirk 2010).

The main aspects of a surgical needle

Surgical needles can be divided into three main aspects:

1. The point is the end which breaks through the tissue first, the design of which varies depending on the tissue. The basic categories are cutting, blunt and taper.
2. The shaft influences the shape, size and diameter of the needle. It is the place where the needle holder is positioned, and may be flat or ribbed to reduce the incidence of slippage of the needle holder.
3. The body of the needle may be round, oval, triangular, side-flattened rectangular or trapezoidal; they are measured in chord length, needle radius and length. When selecting a needle, it is important to consider shape, thickness and size which may be dependent on the position and ease of access to the tissue to be sutured. The thickness of the needle is influenced by the tissue and size of suture to be used (Hamlin *et al.* 2010, Phillips 2012, Goodman and Spry 2014, Davis 2015).

Most needles are now eyeless. They are attached to the thread during manufacture by either swaging or crimping the needle onto the thread or by drilling a hole into the needle and introducing the thread into the needle after applying an adhesive to the tip. This means that the needle is only a little larger than the thread (Kirk 2010, Goodman and Spry 2014).

Different types of needles

- Cutting needles are triangular in the cutting section with edges laterally and on the inside of the curvature. They are capable of piercing through resilient tissue such as tendons, skin, pharynx, ligaments, nasal cavity, oral cavity and aponeuroses; if they carry through thread under tension, they may tear towards the edge of the tissue (Andrews and Cascarini 2008, Kirk 2010, Davis 2015).
- Reverse cutting needles have a third cutting edge on the outside of the curvature to avoid tearing through the tissue, as with cutting needles; they are used on heavy muscle, fascia, ligament, nasal cavity, oral mucosa, tendon sheath, pharynx and skin (Andrews and Cascarini 2008, Hamlin *et al.* 2010, Kirk 2010).
- Tapercut needles combine the sharpness of the tip of a cutting needle with the minimised trauma of a round-bodied needle as the sharp tip fuses into a smooth round cross-section. Tapercut needles are used to stitch abdominal tissues except skin. They are capable of going through fascia and muscles, but it is very difficult to break the skin with them which minimises the incidence of needle stick injury. They can be used on an extensive list of tissues: bronchus, calcified tissue, fascia, ligament, nasal cavity, oral cavity, ovary, perichondrium, periosteum, pharynx, tendon, trachea, uterus and vessels (sclerotic) (Hamlin *et al.* 2010, Davis 2015).
- Round-bodied needles go through soft tissues which are opened by the movement of the needle, but the tissues then seal around the thread, creating a leak-free stitch. They are ideal for use with intestinal and cardiovascular sutures. They are selected for tissue which is fragile or tissue which is in strands and can be displaced as round-bodied sutures cause minimal damage (Kirk 2010).

- Taperpoint needles are used for closing delicate tissue, providing easy penetration of selected tissues. They have a flat part along the needle for placement of the needle holder to achieve additional stability, leading to a more exact positioning of sutures. They are used on aponeurosis, biliary tract, dura, fascia, gastrointestinal tract, muscle, myocardium, nerve, peritoneum, pleura, subcutaneous fat and urogenital tract vessels. A 'taperpoint plus' needle has been designed so that the tapered cross-section behind the tip is flattened into an oval shape rather than round. This improves the separation of the tissue layers (Andrews and Cascarini 2008, Hamlin *et al.* 2010, Kirk 2010, Goodman and Spry 2014).
- Blunt taperpoint needles have been designed to be sharp enough to go through fascia and muscle but not skin, thus minimising the chance of needle stick injury. They can also be used on fragile and easily torn tissue such as liver. A blunt-point needle is used to suture fragile tissue such as the liver, fascia, intestine, muscle, spleen, uterine cervix (for ligating incompetent cervix) and kidney. As the blunt points don't cut through tissue, they are less likely to puncture a vessel (Andrews and Cascarini 2008, Phillips 2012, Davis 2015).

Damage can be caused to the patient if an inappropriate needle selection is made; therefore, a knowledge of different needles and their uses is imperative to minimise the risk.

63 Wound Closure

Rationale for wound closure

Wound closure removes dead space, thereby reducing the risk of infection and haematoma formation; brings together and everts skin edges; supports the wound whilst the tissue heals; evenly distributes tension along the wound; and realigns tissues for the optimum cosmetic appearance (Davis 2015).

The following factors are important to establish optimum healing of wound edges, an aesthetically pleasing scar and a wound that is secure, robust and healed without infection or dehiscence:

- A good blood supply
- Accurately opposed edges with no tension or trauma
- No infection
- Foreign material kept to a minimum
- Good surgical technique
- Maintenance of the sterile field
- Selection of appropriate incision
- Technique and choice of wound closure materials (Kirk 2010).

There are various types of wound closure which all have specific indications and advantages and disadvantages; these include sutures, tapes, staples and adhesives. Before selecting the appropriate suturing technique, the location and size of the wound, along with the tissue type, need to be considered (Davis 2015).

If there is infection present or wound contamination, it is better to have less suture material. The practitioner should be aware that in infected wounds, absorbable sutures dissolve quicker; therefore, they should not be used. Monofilament nylon and prolene are ideal for closing infected wounds.

Patient factors for consideration

Prior to the selection of wound closure, it is important to make a patient assessment for factors which will increase the incidence of infection and inhibit wound healing, such as diabetes mellitus, chronic renal failure, obesity, malnutrition and the use of immunosuppressive medications such as steroids and chemotherapy. Suturing as a form of wound closure is selected in instances when the wound is long or large, for oily or hairy areas, for areas under tension, or where there is a lot of mobility around the wound or it is in need of frequent washing. Suturing is not the best choice when the patient has thin, friable skin as the sutures will tear through the tissue. Poor suturing technique leads to unpleasant scarring, tissue ischaemia and tissue oedema. Traumatised or crushed skin shows little damage at the time as it is not until later that the skin may die and scar; therefore, practitioners must be careful not to roughly handle tissue and to be conscious of this when using forceps on the tissue (Kirk 2010, Davis 2015).

Rapid Perioperative Care, First Edition. Paul Wicker and Sara Dalby.

Selection of wound closure materials

The selection of the gauge of the suture depends on the size and location of the wound; more often than not, the suture with the smallest gauge that will adequately support the healing wound edges will be selected (Kirk 2010). The aim of wound closure is to ensure that the suture selected should provide support to the wound edges until the tissue has enough strength to remain closed itself.

Selection of closure materials should take into consideration:

- The condition and position of the wound
- The healing characteristics of the tissue to be sutured
- The patient's condition
- The properties of the closure material
- The consequences of local and systematic factors on wound healing whilst taking into account the principles of delayed healing (Davis 2015).

Consideration of different wound closure methods

Sutures are classed as foreign material. Selection of the type of suture is due to the wound characteristics and suture material traits: non-absorbable sutures cause less tissue reaction than absorbable ones, but absorbable ones are preferential if there is infection or a potential for infection, as non-absorbable sutures can cause sinus tract development or lead to extrusion. Monofilament and coated sutures are preferable if the wound is infected or may become infected, as multifilament fragments allow sinus formation. The wound strength is linked to the tissue condition and number of stitches in the edges; the minimum amount of stitches necessary should be used, taking into consideration that the amount of tissue within each suture directly affects healing rates by influencing the adequacy of blood supply to the tissue or causing swelling. It is important as a practitioner not to use excessive force when handling any type of thread as you may break the thread or weaken it which could result in breakage later. Particularly when utilising monofilament sutures, the practitioner needs to be careful not to damage the material by handling it roughly as it weakens the thread (Kirk 2010, Phillips 2012).

One cause of wound dehiscence is poor technique. Closing muscle with fascia makes the wound stronger than just closing fascia alone, but taking muscle can lead to tissue ischaemia.

Fascia should be closed by placing the stitches 1 to 1.5 cm back from the wound edge and 1 cm across. Knots should not be tied too tightly. The practitioner needs to take into account the 30% postoperative wound expansion, and if sutures are too tight it will cause ischaemia of the tissue, leading to suture pull through and dehiscence; continuous sutures are equally as strong as intermittent sutures. If sutures are too loose, the wound will gape and not heal by first intention. The practitioner needs to be cautious that the knots aren't too tight. The practitioner also needs to consider that, during the inflammation process, the tissue will swell and if the knot is too tight it may result in tissue necrosis. It is recommended to tie the sutures tight enough that the edges just meet.

64 Suturing Methods

The practitioner should have knowledge of the different types of suturing methods that can be used to close skin. The indication may differ depending on the type of wound, site of the wound and practitioner's preference.

Simple interrupted

A number of individual sutures are used to close the wound. Stitches are placed at right angles to the wound, and each is tied and cut individually, providing increased security because if one were to break, this will have no impact on the other sutures which will all stay intact. Therefore, the wound will remain approximated (Guglielmi and Hunter 2011).

The practitioner must be careful not to use excessive tension and leave enough length of suture on either side of the wound for knot tying. Interrupted sutures are used extensively on vessels and tissues; they are deemed the strongest and most secure, and also assist in wound healing as less sutures are used. They are usually used on skin and underlying tissue layers. Skin edges should be slightly everted; this flattens as healing occurs, and if the edges are inverted the end result will be a depressed scar (Guglielmi and Hunter 2011).

There are a number of advantages to using interrupted sutures:

- Removal is generally easy and less painful.
- They are technically straightforward to put in compared to continuous sutures.
- If one is misplaced, it is simple to replace without disturbing the other sutures.
- Alternate sutures may be removed; this is invaluable for facial wounds which require a good cosmetic result or when wounds have become infected.
- It is easier to precisely bring together the wound edges; this is because each suture can be placed independently at premeditated positions of the wound.
- Interrupted sutures are used when the wound will be under tension, particularly when sutures may break due to tension or tissue weakness. This enables more particular approximation of tissues which is therefore desirable for use in plastic surgery.
- It is important if the wound is infected or has the potential to become infected, as it would be less likely for microorganisms to spread through interrupted sutures.
- Interrupted sutures create a more robust incision line and prevent devascularisation of the wound edges (Davis 2015).

Disadvantages of interrupted sutures:

- The practitioner must be careful not to tie the knots too tight, as if it is under too much tension, the thread will either snap or tear through the tissue.
- A possible weakness of interrupted sutures is the need for so many knots; a knot which is perfectly thrown and tightened significantly increases the strength of the thread, whereas a badly tied knot which has been roughly handled, snatched or not tightened adequately may reduce the strength of the thread by over half.

Rapid Perioperative Care, First Edition. Paul Wicker and Sara Dalby.

- Tension for all the stitches must be equal; if not, the tightest stitch will be under the greatest strain and may give way, possibly leading to other stitches following suit. Also, over-tightened stitches will lead to tissue strangulation and pulling out through the tissue.
- Interrupted sutures take longer to close the wound than continuous ones (Kirk 2010, Davis 2015).

Horizontal mattress

Mattress stitches are used for wounds which are under tension. Horizontal mattress stitches are placed parallel to the wound edge, with each bite being used instead of two interrupted stitches; in comparison, vertical mattress stitches take deep and superficial bites across the wound vertically at right angles to the incision. These are ideal for deep wounds; their results have good wound edge approximation. Start on one side of the wound, taking a bite of tissue, then take a bite from the other side of the tissue, followed by another bite of the same side a little further distance from the previous stitch, and then stitch across to the initial side, tying a knot with the two thread lengths. Mattress stitches may cross the wound parallel to each other or in the same line (horizontal mattress and vertical mattress), and they are to be removed at varying times; in the face, they should be removed after 5–7 days to avoid leaving tram line scars, but for abdominal wounds they may be left for approximately 10 days. Both horizontal and vertical mattress stitches have a section of suture above the surface, pulling the surface away from the edge and subsequently everting the edge (Price and Sinclair 2008, Kirk 2010, Phillips 2012).

If the skin edges start to invert, then a mattress stitch can be used to evert the edges which will ensure that the wound will be able to heal as inverted skin brings together the dead keratinized layers. Mattress stitches are far less likely to pull through the tissue as they have a portion of tissue between its threads, especially when used on tissues in which their fibres run at right angles to the wound edge. They aid wound approximation when there is an irregularity of depth or disposition. Mattress stitches provide the best eversion of skin edges whilst apposing deeper tissue, thereby reducing the incidence of haematoma or seroma (Kirk 2010, Thomas 2013).

Subcuticular

Subcuticular stitches avoid the chance of patients being scarred by suture marks as they are placed under the epidermal layer of the skin. When using an absorbable suture, a bite of tissue from both sides near one end of the wound should be taken with a knot tied and then buried; then, starting at the apex of one side, the suture is taken in and out of the wound at either side along the whole incision, ensuring there are no gaps in the suture line until the end of the wound is reached. With the last stitch catching both sides, a knot is then made and buried. When using a subcuticular technique, the practitioner must ensure that there are no gaps in the suture line by placing the sutures close together; maintaining an adequate amount of tension to keep the wound together whilst not strangulating the tissue or pulling the suture out of the tissue is imperative. Horizontal sutures should be avoided as they can compromise the blood supply to the skin (Price and Sinclair 2008, Kirk 2010, Thomas 2013).

It is important that stitches are placed at the same depth on each side; otherwise, the wound will be uneven. It is crucial not to put the needle too deeply into the skin as this may risk piercing the skin, as this exposes the suture thread to the outside of the skin which supplies an opportunity for bacteria to access the wound, subsequently leading to infection. Subcuticular sutures should be used when there is no tension in the wound or if there is support in lower levels due to deeper sutures. If the patient's dermis is thin, then a subcuticular suturing method should be avoided. A non-absorbable subcuticular stitch is usually a monofilament, withdrawn from the wound by removing the anchoring suture from one end and then pulling the thread through. Subcuticular stitches can be either continuous or interrupted, and they are placed in the dermis under the epithelial layer. This gives the best cosmetic result, producing a very fine scar (Guglielmi and Hunter 2011, Davis 2015).

Continuous

Continuous sutures, also known as running stitches, are a series of stitches made with the same thread of suture, and only the first and last are tied. The tension along the wound is equal along the wound; a downside of this type of suture is that if one suture breaks, it will cause disturbance to the whole suture line. This risk can be minimised by avoiding instrument damage and over-tensioning; it is selected for the closure of wound layers where there is some tension but a tight closure is needed (i.e. the peritoneum to avoid intestinal loops protruding, or blood vessels to avoid leakage). A continuous suture may be either knotted at the end normally using an Aberdeen knot, or the thread from the beginning and end of the suture may be tied together. The knots for this type of suture are critical, because if one were to come undone, the stitches which are under tension will unravel. Practitioners may choose to use beads or clips on continuous sutures as an alternative for surgical knots (Kirk 2010, Guglielmi and Hunter 2011).

The strength of a continuous stitch is from evenly distributed tension along the wound, but the practitioner must be careful not to pull the suture through too tight as this may lead to tissue strangulation and subsequent necrosis, or it may result in the suture thread pulling through the skin edges. For this type of suture, it is recommended that a monofilament is chosen, as they have no areas to harbour bacteria and this type of stitch may allow the spread of infection along the whole wound. When using a continuous stitch on a long wound, the practitioner may encounter a problem: the suture may loosen in one area, causing gaping along the wound edge, whilst another area is being tightened; this can be overcome by using a locking stick every couple of centimetres along the wound or asking an assistant to follow the suture, catching the last stitch to hold the sutures in place. When inserting continuous sutures, in order to ensure that they are lying correctly, use a closed forceps or your finger to place the thread appropriately prior to its tightening. Also, as continuous suturing tends to twist the thread, it is advised to run your finger and thumb along the thread to unwind the twists. If the thread is not long enough for the wound, then tie a knot in the end of the first thread, leaving the end loose; and start with a second length of thread, inserting and tying it, then tie the loose end of the first thread to the second. A benefit of this type of suturing is that it is a quick method of wound closure and leaves less foreign body material within the wound. The cosmetic results of continuous sutures are not as good as those of interrupted sutures (Price and Sinclair 2008, Thomas 2013, Davis 2015).

As discussed in this chapter, each of the different suturing techniques has advantages and disadvantages. It is important for the practitioner to consider these when selecting the suturing technique which is most appropriate for each patient.

65 Alternative Methods of Wound Closure

Alternative methods of wound closure to suturing are skin clips and skin glue.

Skin clips

Skin stapling uses an applicator that, when squeezed, an open staple is forced against an anvil within the tip of the stapler which bends the staple. This results in the staple piercing the everted skin edges, leading to the staple's final rectangular shape. When applied properly, skin clips effectively evert the edges of wound. They need to be removed within a few days, usually between 5 and 10 days depending on the location, to ensure that the staple marks are not permanent. Clips are perhaps not as versatile as sutures, and although they can be inserted quickly, the time it takes to ensure the edges are brought together correctly can take as long as it does to stitch (Kirk 2010, Goodman and Spry 2014, Davis 2015).

Benefits of skin staples include:

- The reduction of use of sutures which reduces the risk of needle stick injury.
- Less inflammatory reaction compared with sutures, as the materials in staples are non-reactive.
- Enhanced wound healing due to the correct level of tension.
- No tissue strangulation if the staples are applied correctly.
- Decreased incidence of wound infection associated with skin staples when compared with sutures when closing contaminated wounds.
- Better cosmetic results.
- Staples can achieve haemostasis without causing tissue necrosis.
- Easy and quick to insert.
- Stapling needs little skin penetration; as a result, fewer microorganisms are carried into the lower skin, thus lessening the incidence of secondary infection.
- Quick and straightforward to remove (Vuolo 2006, Hochberg *et al.* 2009, Hussey and Bagg 2011, Dignon and Arnett 2013, Davis 2015).

The disadvantages of clips:

- Less elastic and therefore weaker than sutures
- Can cause pain on removal
- Can leave permanent track marks
- More expensive than sutures (DeBoard *et al.* 2007, Lloyd *et al.* 2007, Dignon and Arnett 2013).

Rapid Perioperative Care, First Edition. Paul Wicker and Sara Dalby.

Surgical glue

Wound edges are brought together after being cleaned, and glue is applied to the outside of the wound and left to dry. Wound edges should be clean and dry, with haemostasis achieved prior to application, as the adhesive will not work if there is excessive moisture. The glue is not to be put in the wound itself as this causes pain and excessive scarring and increases risk of infection, but instead it is applied to opposing edges. Once sealed, a dressing is not required but may be preferred by some. In this instance, it is necessary to wait several minutes before application of the dressing so the glue doesn't adhere to it. The glue will naturally slough off after 7–14 days (Reynolds and Cole 2006).

With skin glue, wound closure time is said to be 20–50% shorter than with suturing. Skin glue has an equal tensile strength to that of 5–0 sutures, but the first day of strength is much less than that of sutures. As a result, surgical glue tends to be restricted to wounds on the face, extremities (apart from over joints) and certain areas of the torso (Dowson 2006, Reynolds and Cole 2006).

Prior to the application of glue, an assessment of the patient for infection should be undertaken, and symptoms such as redness, warmth, swelling and erythema should be eliminated.

Benefits are:

- No need for anaesthesia.
- Nothing to remove postoperatively, eliminating the need for early postoperative follow-up.
- Can be used on its own to close superficial wounds or combined with subcutaneous sutures if the wound is deeper.
- Gluing is relatively painless; however, it is important to be aware that polymerisation releases heat and may be uncomfortable.
- Does not leave track marks.
- Quicker than suturing and no need for local anaesthetic, the combination of which means there is no concern regarding sharps injury.
- Glue imparts a waterproof seal which acts as a barrier to dirt and bacteria.
- Use of glue diminishes some of the problems identified with sutures, in particular unpredictable absorption rates or reactivity.
- Shown to enhance the aesthetic appearance of wounds.
- Cross-infection is not perceived as problematic because of single-use applicators and because glue doesn't encourage the growth of bacteria.

There are situations in clinical practice where the use of skin glue is ideal. One example is wounds on the face or scalp, where sutures and staples would be difficult to use. Glue is also useful in children and patients with learning difficulties, as there is no need for removal, although the glue can be picked off (Coulthard *et al.* 2009, Sajid *et al.* 2009, Goodman and Spry 2014).

Disadvantages:

- Glue is not suitable for wound closure of incisions that are over joints or in positions where they are under a lot of tension, or for areas where frequent washing is required.
- It is not appropriate for extensive or complex wounds, and it may crack over long wounds or when used over skin creases which may then harbour bacteria.
- Glue can be removed and reapplied, but this is not ideal.
- When gluing wounds on the face, it is imperative to ensure that the glue does not get into the patient's eyes.
- Should not be used on patients who are at high risk for poor wound healing (Reynolds and Cole 2006, Davis 2015).

Contraindications include:

- Avoid use on wounds with evidence of infection.
- Avoid use on wounds near the eyes or mouth.
- Avoid on patients with a hypersensitivity to cyanoacrylate or formaldehyde.
- Liquid or ointment medications should not be applied to the wound after closure (Ethicon 2008, Davis 2015).

It is important to note that the adhesive has not been studied on patients who have peripheral vascular disease, are insulin-dependent diabetics, have blood-clotting disorders or have a personal or family history of keloid formation, hypertrophy or wounds from animal or human bites, puncture or stab wounds or burst stellate lacerations (Ethicon 2008).

66 Injection of Local Anaesthetic for Wound Infiltration

Local anaesthetics work by reversibly inhibiting nerve transmission; this is done mainly by inactivating sodium channels and stopping electrical depolarisation. Smaller, thinner nerves are more sensitive than thicker ones, so larger doses are needed to block fibres which transmit sympathetic pain, temperature, proprioception and motor impulses; this process is known as *differential conduction blockade*. It is why patients can feel pushing, pulling or more movement but nothing sharp, and why nerve blocks should be tested prior to initiating the surgical procedure by testing for pain or temperature.

Ideal local anaesthetic

The 'ideal' local anaesthetic should be rapid and reliable with regards to its onset; have a low toxicity; be effective for the duration of time necessary, with no sympathetic fibre blockade and minimal motor block, preferably having a selective pain fibre block; be non-addictive, non-antigenic and non-irritating to tissues; and subsequently should not negatively affect wound healing. Although not essential, they also should be as effective when used topically as when injected, and should be soluble and stable in solution.

The length of time which the anaesthetic works for is affected by not only the pharmacological properties of the drug but also the volume and concentration used, local blood flow, drug additives, protein binding and local metabolism (Phillips 2013).

Delivery of local anaesthetic

Local anaesthesia can be divided into four categories:

1. Topical (e.g. use of EMLA cream before cannulation)
2. Wound infiltration for analgesia or procedural
3. Regional blocks used either prior to surgery to numb the area or postoperatively for analgesia
4. Central blocks such as spinal and epidural anaesthesia (Cox and Bhudia 2009, Culp and Culp 2011).

Types of local anaesthetic

Local anaesthetics have a tertiary amine group related to an aromatic group. They are categorised as either esters which include cocaine, procaine, amethocaine and benzocaine or amides which include prilocaine, lignocaine, bupivicaine and ropivacaine. Their organisation

Rapid Perioperative Care, First Edition. Paul Wicker and Sara Dalby.

depends on the connection between them; the liver metabolises amides, whereas esters are broken down by plasma cholinesterases. Amides cause fewer allergic reactions than esters but have greater systemic toxicity (Clark 2008, Parry 2011).

Local anaesthetics can be divided into three groups determined by their potency and duration of action:

1. *Low potency and short duration*: procaine, chloroprocaine
2. *Moderate potency and intermediate duration*: lidocaine, mepivacaine, prilocaine
3. *High potency and long duration*: tetracaine, bupivicane, etidocaine.

The local anaesthetics which can be utilised will vary in their potency, duration of action, toxicity, solubility in water, stability and ability to infiltrate mucus membranes; these differences will determine their appropriateness of use, such as infiltration, topical application, intravenous regional anaesthesia, epidural block, spinal block or peripheral nerve block (BNF 2016).

The more commonly used local anaesthetics are as follows:

- *Lignocaine (lidocaine)*: It is often the drug of choice when the operation will have no additional anaesthetics. Starting its effects quickly, it lasts between 60 and 120 min, producing a high-quality block as it is able to pass through the tissues easily. For the injection of lidocaine, the patient's weight and the procedure need to be considered with regards to the dosage.
- *Bupivacaine*: This has a slow onset which can take up to 30 min for the full effect to occur but a prolonged action. Bupivacaine is used for nerve and plexus blockade, local infiltration and spinal and epidural anaesthesia; however, it is known to be particularly cardiotoxic, and it is now available as a single enantiomer called levobupivicaine (Chirocaine) which is safer with respect to cardiac side effects.
- *Ropivicane*: This is the newest local anaesthetic and has similar properties to bupivicane in potency and length of duration, but it is less toxic and has less motor block.
- *Prilocane*: This is as potent as lignocaine, having a similar onset but shorter duration; it is used during IV regional anaesthesia, and it can cause methaemoglobinaemia.
- *Cocaine*: This is one of the few ester local anaesthetics still used. Cocaine is a vasoconstrictor which is why it is used frequently in ear, nose and throat (ENT) surgery, but it has a large systematic side effect profile, including myocardial ischaemia, tachycardia and cerebral vascular accident.
- *Benzocaine*: This is used only as a topical agent and has low toxicity.
- *Procaine*: This is rarely used due to it being very short acting, but it is only a quarter as toxic as cocaine and doesn't have a topical effect. It has a vasodilatory affect; therefore, it can be used intraoperatively on small vessels to combat arteriospasm (Cox and Bhudia 2009, Anaesthesia UK 2016, BNF 2016).

The practitioner needs to calculate the maximum safe dose when considering this. It is crucial to take into account a number of factors: absorption rate; rate of excretion; patient factors such as age, physique, pre-existing disease and clinical condition; duration of administration; the vascularity of the area where the local anaesthetic is to be administered; and other factors which affect the rate of absorption (Parry 2011, BNF 2016; Table of Local Anaesthetic Drug Information taken from Anaesthesia UK 2016).

1% solution of any drug contains 1 gram (i.e. 1000 mg) of drug per 100 ml of solution.

If a healthy 50 kg woman comes for a procedure requiring local anaesthesia, the drug of choice is bupivacaine without epinephrine. As bupivacaine without epinephrine is 2 mg/kg, when considering her weight, 50 kg = 100 mg bupivacaine (1% bupivacaine = 10 mg/ml). Therefore, a safe dose for a woman who weighs 50 kg is either 10 ml 1% bupivacaine or 5 ml 2% bupivacaine.

Drug	Lidocaine	Prilocaine	Bupi-vacaine	Levobupi-vacaine	Ropi-vacaine
Description	Amide	Amide	Amide	Amide	Amide
Relative potency	2	2	8	8	6
Onset	5–10 min	5–10 min	10–15 min	10–15 min	10–15 mins
Duration without epinephrine	1–2 h	1–2 h	3–12 h	3–12 h	3–12 h
Duration with epinephrine	2–4 h	2–4 h	4–12 h	4–12 h	4–12 h
Maximum dose without epinephrine	3 mg/kg	6 mg/kg	2 mg/kg	2.5 mg/kg*	3 mg/kg*
Maximum dose with epinephrine	7 mg/kg	9 mg/kg	2.5 mg/kg	3 mg/kg*	4 mg/kg*

*INDICATES PROBABLE SAFE MAXIMUM DOSE (INSUFFICIENT DATA).

Local anaesthetic additives

A number of additives may be incorporated into local anaesthetic, including epinephrine, felypressin, clonidine and sodium bicarbonate. They reduce toxicity risk and extend the intensity and length of the block. With the exception of cocaine, most local anaesthetics cause vasodilatation. Epinephrine can be used alongside a local anaesthetic for its vasoconstricting properties, resulting in a slower rate of absorption for the local anaesthetic, lower incidence of toxicity and a longer duration of action as there is reduced blood flow to the area; but it should be used with caution in patients with diabetes, heart disease or hypertension. The adrenaline must be a low concentration, for example 1 in 200,000. Local anaesthetics with adrenaline should not be injected into areas of the body where the blood supply, distally from the injection site, is marginal (e.g. toes, nose, fingers or external ears), as it may cause ischaemic necrosis (Anaesthesia UK 2016, BNF 2016).

Communicating with the patient

The practitioner should discuss with the patient that although they will feel touch, they should not feel pain and should inform the practitioner if they do so. There should be extra local anaesthetic kept available to increase the dose if necessary, and the patient should also be told to say if they have any unusual feelings which may be signs of toxicity (AORN 2007, Kirk 2010).

The monitoring of the patient should include blood pressure, heart rate and rhythm, respiratory rate, oxygen saturation with pulse oximeter, temperature, skin condition and colour, mental status and level of consciousness. When anaesthetising the area for a patient who is awake, it is recommended to begin by using a fine needle away from any inflammation or sensitive tissue, raising a 'bleb' under the skin, and allowing time for it to take effect before injecting it intracutaneously along the proposed line of incision which will cause a raised area similar in appearance to orange peel, then changing to a larger longer needle which will enable deeper infiltration (AORN 2007, Kirk 2010, Phillips 2013, Fencl 2015).

Local anaesthetic should be administered slowly as it is painful and can gauge the resistance of tissue; the practitioner should aspirate prior to each injection. The risk of infection can be introduced by administering local anaesthetic; this can be minimised by the use of proper equipment and sterile technique. Local anaesthetics are capable of blocking nerve impulses only if they are injected in close vicinity to the nerve and with a sufficient dose of the drug; a failure to achieve an effective block is mainly due to an inadequate dose of the drug or the practitioner's technical failure (Parry 2011, Phillips 2013, BNF 2016).

Guidelines and documentation

Healthcare providers should have guidelines in place for the selection of patients who are appropriate for local anaesthesia procedures and what the appropriate monitoring should be. The drug dosage, type, route, time of administration, patient monitoring used and its results should be documented. Documentation should include the preoperative assessment, consciousness level of the patient, vital signs, dosage, route, time and effect of anaesthetics, any untoward patient reactions, what practices were carried out to resolve them and a postoperative assessment based on the information from the preoperative assessment. It is necessary to develop policies and procedures for patients receiving local anaesthetic, which should be reviewed and revised by the multidisciplinary team and available for consultation in the practice setting (AORN 2007, Fencl 2015).

67 Injection of Local Anaesthetic for Wound Infiltration – Caution and Complications

The types and uses of local anaesthetics were discussed in Chapter 66. However, it is important for the practitioner to also have a knowledge of the potential complications of local anaesthetic and the cautions to be aware of.

Toxicity

Normal doses of local anaesthetic are very safe; however, there are factors which affect the potential for toxicity (the dose injected, how fast it is absorbed and the site and method of administration), as some sites have a more rapid absorption rate and toxicity can occur if large amounts of local anaesthetics are used in these areas. To help overcome this problem, use a local anaesthetic that contains adrenaline and slows absorption. Toxicity may be seen rapidly if local anaesthetic is injected intravascularly which leads to high levels of local anaesthetic in the blood; therefore, it is recommended that prior to injection, the practitioner should aspirate to ensure the needle tip isn't in a vessel. Toxicity is rare if the maximum dose is not exceeded; any practitioner who is infiltrating local anaesthetic should be aware of the appropriate dosage (Bourne *et al.* 2010, Mercado and Weinberg 2011, Fencl 2015).

Allergies to local anaesthetics

Allergy to the local anaesthetic is rare. The symptoms of an allergic reaction include dizziness, anxiety, nausea, rash, urticarial, bronchospasm, erythema and oedema (Caron 2007, Fuzier *et al.* 2009, Bhole *et al.* 2012, Batinac *et al.* 2013). Management is the same treatment as with any allergy.

Signs and symptoms of toxicity and allergic reactions of local anaesthetic

The practitioner administering local anaesthetic should be aware of the signs and symptoms of toxicity.

Rapid Perioperative Care, First Edition. Paul Wicker and Sara Dalby.

If the heart and brain have significant levels of a local anaesthetic drug, the drug will have the same membrane-stabilising effect as on the peripheral nerve which will cause progressive depression of function:

- Initial signs are numbness or tingling for the tongue or around-the-mouth area. This is because these areas have a good blood supply; subsequently, there is enough drug distributed to these areas to affect the nerve endings. Other possible signs include one or a combination of the following: anxiety, light-headedness, drowsiness or tinnitus. Increasing doses may cause the patient to lose consciousness and/or have convulsions.
- Cardiovascular effects consist of hypotension, bradycardia, heart block, cardiac arrest and ventrical tachycardia and fibrillation. Central nervous system effects incorporate agitation, euphoria, respiratory depression, twitching, convulsions and sensory disturbances (AORN 2007, AAGBI 2010, Parry 2011, Fencl 2015).

If a patient has symptoms of toxicity, the administration of the drug should be stopped immediately, oxygen administered and the monitoring continued. The ABC of basic life support should be started, treatment of any convulsions or cardiac problems should be treated, and correct any subsequent electrolyte abnormalities. In the event of local anaesthetic-induced cardiac arrest, standard cardiopulmonary resuscitation should be initiated immediately. Lidocaine must not be used as anti-arrhythmic therapy.

As outlined in the BNF (2016): If the patient does not respond rapidly to standard procedures, 20% lipid emulsion such as Intralipid (unlicensed indication) should be given intravenously at an initial bolus dose of 1.5 mL/kg over 1 min, followed by an infusion of 15 mL/kg/h. After 5 min, if cardiovascular stability has not been restored or circulation deteriorates, give a maximum of two further bolus doses of 1.5 mL/kg over 1 min, 5 min apart, and increase the infusion rate to 30 mL/kg/h. Continue infusion until cardiovascular stability and adequate circulation are restored or a maximum cumulative dose of 12 mL/kg is given.

Standard cardiopulmonary resuscitation must be maintained throughout lipid emulsion treatment. Systemic toxicity is rare in instances where local anaesthetics are used for regional anaesthesia; however, systemic toxicity due to local anaesthetic needs to be treated quickly. It is particularly complicated to treat patients who have suffered cardiovascular collapse from ropivacaine, bupivacaine or levobupivacaine. The Association of Anaesthetists have provided guidelines for the management of severe local anaesthetic toxicity which provide a step-by-step management programme which practitioners administrating local anaesthetics need to be familiar with (AAGBI 2010, Parry 2011).

Patient factors to consider

Some medical conditions need to be taken into account:

- Patients with coagulation problems or patients on anticoagulants are a contraindication for some techniques, such as subarachnoid or epidural blocks, due to local bleeding.
- *Hypotension*: Because of the risk of a drop in blood pressure, an epidural block should be avoided on patients with hypotension or hypovolemia.
- Any signs of local infection near the puncture wound of the needle should be avoided as it may spread the infection and reduces the effectiveness of the local anaesthetic.
- The age of the patient affects toxicity; practitioners should be especially cautious when administering local anaesthetic to either the very young or the elderly as they are more susceptible to toxicity than their body weight may indicate. Patients who are chronically incapacitated or acutely ill are more at risk of toxicity.
- Finally, most amide local anaesthesia are metabolised by the liver; therefore, practitioners need to be cautious with doses with patients who have liver failure or are on medications which affect liver metabolism (Parry 2011).

Local factors to take into account with toxicity

Local factors which influence toxicity are the site of injection, as sites which have an increased blood flow such as the head, pelvic floor and neck result in quicker absorption and high blood levels. When topical application is used, the upper respiratory tract and an inflamed urethra have a swift absorption rate. The use of vasoconstrictor agents slows the absorption rate, reducing the blood level achieved; subsequently, the maximum safe dose of the local anaesthetic may be increased. This lengthens its action, and the use of hyaluronidase with the local anaesthetic will increase the spread of injected fluid through tissues, thereby increasing the area the drug reaches and therefore the rate of absorption of the drug, but it makes toxicity more likely (Bourne *et al.* 2010, Mercado *et al.* 2011).

Caution when using local anaesthesia

The practitioner needs to be aware of the complications of local anaesthesia in order to try to minimise the chance of these occurring. Complications can be local or systemic, and causes include mechanical effects of needles and pharmacological effects of the administered drug. The prevention of complications can be achieved through patient assessment and preparation, an understanding of anatomy and physiology, appropriate selection of the drug and equipment and perpetual patient monitoring (Phillips 2012).

It is important to note that local anaesthetics do not rely on the circulatory system to transport them to the appropriate site, but their uptake into the circulatory system is relevant to ending their action and toxicity. After the use of local anaesthetic regionally, maximum arterial plasma concentrations of anaesthetic will develop within 10–25 min; therefore, the patient should be carefully monitored for the effects of toxicity within an hour of having the local anaesthetic administered (BNF 2016).

Contraindications of local anaesthesia

The contraindications for local anaesthetics are:

- Allergy to local anaesthetics (as discussed in this chapter).
- Patient choice should take into consideration; confused patients or children may be frightened and unable to comprehend or stay still during the procedure. The benefit of local anaesthesia may be in addition to a general anaesthetic for postoperative pain relief.
- The length of time that the proposed procedure will take, as many procedures will take too long for the duration of the drug or may require a patient to stay in an awkward position which is uncomfortable. In some instances, this may be helped by sedation.
- Action of local anaesthetics is affected by the pH levels of extracellular fluid. The pH of infected tissue is lower than normal, so this reduces the action of local anaesthetic; and as local infection causes vasodilatation the drug is removed faster from the area, leading to a shorter duration of action. Therefore, local anaesthetics shouldn't be injected into infected or inflamed tissues as the absorption of the drug into the bloodstream may increase the incidence of systematic side effects, and the effects of the drug may be reduced due to the change of pH.
- Local anaesthetics should not be used in the middle ear as they can be ototoxic; and if used in the oral cavity, the patient needs to be monitored due to the increased chance of aspiration.
- Not to be used on patients with complete heart block.

- Although it is rare that they cause any clinical problems, interactions between local anaesthetics and other drugs can occur. The toxicity of ester drugs is increased if the patient is taking anti-cholinesterase for myasthenia or concomitant administration of other drugs hydrolysed by plasma cholinesterase.
- Damage to nerves may occur due to intra-neural injection, needle breakage, damage to blood vessels incurring haematoma, direct needle puncture, inadvertent thermal injury to anaesthetised area, nerve compression due to poor patient positioning and ischaemia and necrosis following incorrect use of a vasoconstrictor around an end artery or because of the pressure effect of injected local anaesthetic (AORN 2007, BNF 2016).

68 Camera Holding

Introduction

Healthcare professionals with advanced surgical skills are able to hold cameras during laparoscopic surgery. It is important that the healthcare professional understands the need to hold the camera in the correct way, with patient safety being paramount. This will enable the surgeon to be able to undertake the surgery in a safe and effective way. Performance in laparoscopic surgery is affected by the help of a well-trained assistant, with good visualisation of the operating field being essential and only achieved through adequate camera holding (Shetty *et al.* 2012).

Laparoscopic surgery

Laparoscopic surgery has now become commonplace in most surgical specialities as it has many advantages over open surgery; however, it is more stressful than open surgery, partly due to the lack of stereoscopic vision. An effective camera holder can help to make the procedure less stressful. It requires expertise in psychomotor skills which are very different from those for open procedures. This is due to a change from a three-dimensional operating field to a two-dimensional monitor, altered depth perception and spatial awareness, distortion of hand–eye coordination, loss of binocular vision, and diminished tactile feedback whilst manoeuvring long instruments in a restricted space with an amplified tremor (Schreuder *et al.* 2011).

There are numerous benefits to laparoscopic surgery:

- Reduced morbidity
- Shorter hospital stays
- Better cosmetic results
- Earlier return to normal activities
- Decreased postoperative pain
- Reduction of excessive handling and retraction of internal organs.

The disadvantages of laparoscopic surgery:

- Longer learning curves
- Reduction in tactile feedback
- Limited working area
- Potential damage to internal organs outside of optical vision.

Laparoscopic equipment

It is important that both the surgeon and the assistant are familiar with the working properties of the laparoscopic set-up and the potential hazards, which ensures patient safety.

- Screen
- Insufflator

Rapid Perioperative Care, First Edition. Paul Wicker and Sara Dalby.

- Camera
- Light source.

Telescopes

Telescopes are available in two sizes, 10 mm and 5 mm, with varying degrees of camera angles; larger telescopes provide enhanced vision and carry more light for illumination, and therefore they are more frequently used. Zero-degree telescopes are forward viewing and are commonly used, whereas 30° and 45° telescopes are oblique and allow vision from different angles of an operating field. Angled scopes require more complex visuospatial skills due to the addition of off-axis viewing. Each camera has an orientation mark at the 12 o'clock position which allows correct orientation of the image. For angled laparoscopes, it is important to keep the camera in a 'true' upright position, altering the field of view by rotating the laparoscope with the light post whilst maintaining the camera. To look down the light, the post is positioned up, and to look up it is positioned down. Looking down is considered the best for generalised explorations as it delivers the surgeon's viewpoint of an open laparotomy.

Camera set-up

Five steps are suggested for setting up the 10 mm telescope before inserting into the port:

- The light cable is connected and turned on confirmation of attachment prior to turning on the light source is important for patient safety as the end can become heated and potentially burn through the drapes causing a fire hazard.
- Ensure attachment of the camera to the endoscope, making sure they are clean and free of moisture.
- Focus the camera.
- 'White balance' to correct colour sensitivity.
- Pre-warm the scope with saline, applying antifogging solution to the tip.

All the equipment needed should be checked prior to use, including the stack system, telescope and light cable.

Light intensity

Light intensity improves depth perception and image detail, with too much illumination washing out the image. Light is transported from the light source to the laparoscope via a fibre-optic cable. All connections should be checked; a loose connection leads to a significant loss of light reaching the surgical field. Light leads need to be handled with care as they may endure some damage to the optical fibres which decreases light transmission.

Skills necessary for camera holding

The camera holder should achieve the following:

- Maintain a correct horizon.
- Centre the operating field.
- Ensure appropriate focus.
- Maintain a steady image.
- Track instruments in motion (Shetty *et al.* 2012).

Poor camera holding

Poor camera holding can result in:

- Poor visualisation
- Frustration for the surgeon

- Longer operating time
- Increased errors.

Challenges for the camera holder

Neuromuscular and arthritic symptoms are experienced by practitioners undertaking laparoscopic surgery due to the working position; the incomplete ergonomic design of instruments and the lack of three-dimensional full perceptions can cause muscular fatigue and injuries due to the use and tension of muscles. Therefore, camera holding can be mentally draining for the assistant but also can be a physical strain (Kong *et al.* 2010).

Training and learning curve of camera holding

For development of endoscopic skills, including camera skills, simulators are safe and effective for training; this ensures that patients are not harmed. Box trainers allow practitioners to master camera holding through practicing their camera skills, particularly of the 30° camera. As mentioned in this chapter, camera holding is a technically challenging skill requiring dexterity and concentration. Practitioners need to learn psychomotor skills to overcome the challenges of the two-dimensional environment, restricted movement and a fixed access point. The camera holder needs to maintain a steady view of vision whilst maintaining a correct horizon. An understanding of the surgical procedure to be undertaken is also imperative for a camera holder. However, to achieve competence, there can be a prolonged learning curve enhanced by repetition (Larsen *et al.* 2009, 2012, Schreuder *et al.* 2011, Janse *et al.* 2013).

Camera holding is a technically challenging skill which is often underestimated. It requires a lot of mental concentration and can be physically straining. It is imperative for patient safety and the success of the surgical procedure that the camera holder can manipulate the camera effectively to allow visualisation of the operating field.

References and Further Reading

55. Legal, Professional and Ethical Issues

References

Carey B (2009) Consent and Refusal for Adolescents: The Law. *British Journal of Nursing* **18** (22) 1366–1368.

Department of Health (DH) (2009) *Reference Guide to Consent for Examination or Treatment*, 2nd ed. London, Department of Health.

Dimond B (2011) *Legal Aspects of Nursing*, 6th ed. Essex: Pearson Education Ltd.

Health and Safety Executive (HSE) (2014) Risk Assessment: A Brief Guide to Controlling Risks in the Workplace. Available at http://www.hse.gov.uk/pubns/indg163.pdf (accessed 25 January 2016)

Nursing and Midwifery Council (NMC) (2012) *Record Keeping Guidance for Nurses and Midwives*. London, Nursing and Midwifery Council.

Nursing and Midwifery Council (NMC) (2015) *The Code: Professional Standards of Practices and Behaviour for Nurses and Midwives*. London, Nursing and Midwifery Council.

Perioperative Care Collaborative (PCC) (2012) First Surgical Assistant Formerly Advanced Scrub Practitioner. PCC Position Statement. Available at www.afpp.org.uk (accessed 15 December 2015)

Further Reading

Beauchamp TL and Childress JF (2009) *Principles of Biomedical Ethics*, 6th ed. Oxford, Oxford University Press.

Pirie S (2011) Legal and Professional Issues for the Perioperative Practitioner. *Journal of Perioperative Practice* **22** (2): 57–62.

Websites

Health and Care Professionals Council: www.hcpc-uk.co.uk

Nursing and Midwifery Council: www.nmc.org.uk

56. Surgical First Assistant

References

Brame K (2011) The Advanced Scrub Practitioner Role: A Student's Reflection. *The Journal of Perioperative Practice* **21** (4): 118–122.

Deighton C (2007) A Reflection on the Development of the Advanced Scrub Practitioner. *The Journal of Perioperative Practice* **17** (10): 485–492.

Department of Health (2007) *European Working Time Directive*. London, Department of Health.

Halliwell GL (2012) Becoming an Advanced Scrub Practitioner: My Personal Journey. *The Journal of Perioperative Practice* **22** (12): 393–397.

Mardell A (2004) Why Are We Having This Discussion? *British Journal of Perioperative Nursing* **14** (1): 4–5.

Perioperative Care Collaborative (PCC) (2012) First Surgical Assistant formerly Advanced Scrub Practitioner. PCC Position Statement. Available at www.afpp.org.uk (accessed 14 October 2015)

Sutton J (2003) On Course: The Ethics of Theatre Nurse Practice under the Microscope. *British Journal of Perioperative Nursing* **13** (10): 405–413.

Timpany M and McAleavy J (2010) Perioperative Role Development Evaluating a Fast Track Approach to Advanced Scrub and/or Dual Role Practitioner Training. *The Journal of Perioperative Practice* **20** (1): 13–17.

Rapid Perioperative Care, First Edition. Paul Wicker and Sara Dalby.

Further Reading

Al-Hashemi J (2007) The Role of the Advanced Scrub Practitioner. *The Journal of Perioperative Practice* **17** (2): 76–80.

57. Surgical Care Practitioner

References

Christiansen A, Vernon V and Jinks A (2012) Perceptions of the Benefits and Challenges of the Role of Advanced Practice Nurses in Nurse-Led Out-of-Hours Care in Hong Kong: A Questionnaire Study. *Journal of Clinical Nursing* **22**: 1173–1181.

Department of Health (2007) *European Working Time Directive*. London, Department of Health.

Lowe G, Plummer V, O'Brien AP and Boyd L (2011) Time to Clarify – the Value of Advanced Practice Nursing Roles in Health Care. *Journal of Advanced Nursing* **68** (3): 677–685.

Quick J (2013) The Role of the Surgical Care Practitioner within the Surgical Team. *British Journal of Nursing* **22** (13): 759–765.

Royal College of Surgeons (RCS) (2014) Surgical Care Practitioner National Curriculum. Available at https://www.rcseng.ac.uk/surgeons/training/docs/surgical---care---practitioner---curriculum (accessed 15 June 2015)

Further Reading

Kumar R, DeBono L, Sharma P and Basu S (2013) The General Surgical Care Practitioner Improves Surgical Outpatient Streamlining and the Delivery of Elective Surgical Care. *The Journal of Perioperative Practice* **23** (6): 138–141.

Nicholas M (2010) The Surgical Care Practitioner: A Critical Analysis. *The Journal of Perioperative Practice* **20** (3): 94–99.

58. Pre and Postoperative Visiting

References

Arnold A and Underman Boggs K (2011) *Interpersonal Relationships: Professional Communication Skills for Nurses*, 6th ed. St. Louis, Elsevier Saunders.

Berry D (2006) *Health Communication: Theory and Practice*. London, Open University Press.

Ellis RB, Gates B and Kenworthy N (2003) *Interpersonal Communication in Nursing: Theory and Practice*, 2nd ed. London, Churchill Livingstone.

Holmes J (2005) Preoperative Visiting: Landmarks of the Journey. *Journal of Perioperative Practice* **15** (10): 434–443.

Hurley C and McAleavy J (2006) Preoperative Assessment and Intraoperative Care Planning. *Journal of Perioperative Practice* **16** (4): 187–194.

Further Reading

Alanazi AA (2014) Reducing Anxiety in Preoperative Patients: A Systematic Review. *British Journal of Nursing* **23** (7): 287–303.

Daykin S (2003) Implementation of Pre-Operative Visiting for Critical Care Patients. *Nursing Times* **99** (41): 26–28.

59. Retraction

References

Kotcher Fuller J (2010) *Surgical Technology: Principles and Practice*, 5th ed. St. Louis, Saunders Elsevier.

Paige JT (2009) Tissue Handling. In Rothrock JC and Seifert PC (eds) *Assisting in Surgery: Patient Centered Care*. Denver, Competency & Credentialing Institute, pp. 74–106.

Perioperative Care Collaborative (PCC) (2012) First Surgical Assistant Formerly Advanced Scrub Practitioner. PCC Position Statement. Available at www.afpp.org.uk (accessed 15 December 2015)

Spera P, Lloyd JD, Hernandez E, Hughes N, Petersen C, Nelson A and Spratt DG (2011) AORN Ergonomic Tool 5: Tissue Retraction in the Perioperative Setting. *AORN Journal* **94** (1): 54–58.

Steele PRC, Curran JF and Mountain RE (2013) Current and Future Practices in Surgical Retraction. *The Surgeon* **11** (6): 330–337.

Further Reading

Tamhankar A, Kelty C and Jacob G (2011) Retraction-Related Liver Lobe Necrosis after Laparoscopic Gastric Surgery. *JSLS* **15** (1): 117–121.

60. Cutting of Sutures

References

Guglielmi C and Hunter S (2011) Sutures, Needles and Instruments. In Rothrock JC (ed) *Alexander's Care of the Patient in Surgery*, 14th ed. St. Louis, Elsevier Mosby, pp. 174–203.

Kirk RM (2010) *Basic Surgical Techniques*, 6th ed. Edinburgh, Churchill Livingstone.

Kotcher Fuller J (2010) *Surgical Technology: Principles and Practice*, 5th ed. St. Louis, Saunders Elsevier.

Muffly TM, Cook C, Distasio J, Bonham AJ and Blandon RE (2009) Suture End Length as a Function of Knot Security. *Journal of Surgical Education* **66** (5): 276–280.

Perioperative Care Collaborative (PCC) (2012) First Surgical Assistant Formerly Advanced Scrub Practitioner. PCC Position Statement. Available at www.afpp.org.uk (accessed 14 October 2015)

Phillips N (2012) *Berry and Kohn's Operating Room Technique*, 12th ed. St. Louis, Elsevier.

Whalan C (2006) *Assisting in Surgical Operations: A Practical Guide*. Cambridge, Cambridge University Press.

Wicker P and O'Neill J (2010) *Caring for the Perioperative Patient*, 2nd ed. London, Wiley-Blackwell.

Further Reading

Davis NB (2015) Suturing Materials and Techniques. In Rothrock JC and Seifert PC (eds) *Assisting in Surgery: Patient Centered Care*. Denver, Competency & Credentialing Institute, pp. 195–243.

McCarthy J (2015) Sutures, Needles and Instruments. In Rothrock JC (ed) *Alexander's Care of the Patient in Surgery*, 14th ed. St. Louis, Elsevier Mosby, pp. 186–210.

61. Suture Materials

References

Andrews S and Cascarini L (2008) *Principles of Surgery*. Shrewsbury: tfm Publishing Ltd.

Davis NB (2009) Suturing Materials and Techniques. In Rothrock JC and Seifert PC (eds) *Assisting in Surgery: Patient Centered Care*. Denver, Competency & Credentialing Institute, pp. 195–242.

Goodman T and Spry C (2014) *Essentials of Perioperative Nursing*, 5th ed. Burlington MA, Jones & Bartlett Learning.

Hamlin L, Richardson-Trench M and Davies M (2010) *Perioperative Nursing: An Introductory Text*. Sydney, Elsevier Australia.

Hussey M and Bagg M (2011) Principles of Wound Closure. *Operative Techniques in Sports Medicine* **19**: 206–211.

Kirk RM (2010) *Basic Surgical Techniques*, 6th ed. Edinburgh, Churchill Livingstone.

Phillips N (2012) *Berry and Kohn's Operating Room Technique*, 12th ed. St. Louis, Elsevier.

Price CJ and Sinclair R (2008) *Fast Facts: Minor Surgery*, 2nd ed. Oxford, Health Press Limited.

Further Reading

Guglielmi C and Hunter S (2011) Sutures, Needles and Instruments. In Rothrock JC (ed) *Alexander's Care of the Patient in Surgery*, 14th ed. St. Louis, Elsevier Mosby, pp. 174–203.

62. Surgical Needles

References

Andrews S and Cascarini L (2008) *Principles of Surgery*. Shrewsbury: tfm Publishing Ltd.
Davis NB (2015) Suturing Materials and Techniques. In Rothrock JC and Seifert PC (eds) *Assisting in Surgery: Patient Centered Care*. Denver, Competency & Credentialing Institute, pp. 195–243.
Goodman T and Spry C (2014) *Essentials of Perioperative Nursing*, 5th ed. Burlington MA, Jones & Bartlett Learning.
Hamlin L, Richardson-Trench M and Davies M (2010) *Perioperative Nursing: An Introductory Text*. Sydney, Elsevier Australia.
Kirk RM (2010) *Basic Surgical Techniques*, 6th ed. Edinburgh, Churchill Livingstone.
Phillips N (2012) *Berry and Kohn's Operating Room Technique*, 12th ed. St. Louis, Elsevier.

Further Reading

Guglielmi C and Hunter S (2011) Sutures, Needles and Instruments. In Rothrock JC (ed) *Alexander's Care of the Patient in Surgery*, 14th ed. St. Louis, Elsevier Mosby, pp. 174–203.

63. Wound Closure

References

Davis NB (2015) Suturing Materials and Techniques. In Rothrock JC and Seifert PC (eds) *Assisting in Surgery: Patient Centered Care*. Denver, Competency & Credentialing Institute, pp. 195–243.
Kirk RM (2010) *Basic Surgical Techniques*, 6th ed. Edinburgh, Churchill Livingstone.
Phillips N (2012) *Berry and Kohn's Operating Room Technique*, 12th ed. St. Louis, Elsevier.

Further Reading

Barnes TG and Sheikh AA (2013) Suture Material, Knot Tying and Wound Closure in Surgery. *Journal of Operating Department Practitioners* **1** (1): 15–20.
Hochberg J, Meher KM and Marion MD (2009) Suture Choice and Other Methods of Skin Closure. *Surgical Clinics of North America* **89**: 627–641.

64. Suturing Methods

References

Davis NB (2015) Suturing Materials and Techniques. In Rothrock JC and Seifert PC (eds) *Assisting in Surgery: Patient Centered Care*. Denver, Competency & Credentialing Institute, pp. 195–243.
Guglielmi C and Hunter S (2011) Sutures, Needles and Instruments. In Rothrock JC (ed) *Alexander's Care of the Patient in Surgery*, 14th ed. St. Louis, Elsevier Mosby, pp. 174–203.
Kirk RM (2010) *Basic Surgical Techniques*, 6th ed. London, Churchill Livingstone.
Phillips N (2012) *Berry and Kohn's Operating Room Technique*, 12th ed. St. Louis, Elsevier.
Price CJ and Sinclair R (2008) *Fast Facts: Minor Surgery*, 2nd ed. Oxford, Health Press Ltd.
Thomas WEG (2013) Basic Surgical Skills and Anastomoses. In Williams NS, Bulstrode CJK and O'Connell PR (eds) *Bailey & Love's Short Practice of Surgery*, 26th ed. Kent, CRC Press, pp. 33–49.

Further Reading

McCarthy J (2015) Sutures, Needles and Instruments. In Rothrock JC (ed) *Alexander's Care of the Patient in Surgery*, 15th ed. St. Louis, Mosby, pp. 186–210.
Tajirian AL and Goldberg DJ (2010) A Review of Sutures and Other Skin Closure Materials. *Journal of Cosmetic and Laser Therapy* **12**: 296–302.

65. Alternative Methods of Wound Closure

References

Davis NB (2015) Suturing Materials and Techniques. In Rothrock JC and Seifert PC (eds) *Assisting in Surgery: Patient Centered Care*. Denver, Competency & Credentialing Institute, pp. 195–243.

DeBoard RH, Rondeau DF, Kang CS, Sabbaj A and McManus JG (2007) Principles of Basic Wound Evaluation and Management in the Emergency Department. *Emergency Medicine Clinical North America* **25**: 23–39.

Dignon A and Arnett N (2013) Which Is the Better Method of Wound Closure in Patients Undergoing Hip or Knee Replacement Surgery: Sutures or Skin Clips? *The Journal of Perioperative Practice* **23** (4): 72–76.

Dowson CC, Gilliam AD, Speake WJ, Lobo DN and Beckingham IJ (2006) A Prospective Randomised Controlled Trial Comparing n-butyl Cyanoacrylate Tissue Adhesive (Liquiband) with Sutures for Skin Closure after Laparoscopic General Surgical Procedures. *Surgical Laparoscopy, Endoscopy & Percutaneous Techniques* **16**: 146–150.

Goodman T and Spry C (2014) *Essentials of Perioperative Nursing*, 5th ed. Burlington MA, Jones & Bartlett Learning.

Hochberg J, Meyer KM and Marion MD (2009) Suture Choice and Other Methods of Skin Closure. *Surgical Clinics of North America* **89**: 627–641.

Hussey M and Bagg M (2011) Principles of Wound Closure. *Operative Techniques in Sports Medicine* **19**: 206–211.

Kirk RM (2010) *Basic Surgical Techniques*, 6th ed. London, Churchill Livingstone.

Lloyd JD, Marque MJ and Kacprowicz RF (2007) Closure Techniques. *Emergency Medicine Clinical North America* **25**: 73–81.

Sajid MS, Siddiqui MR, Khan MA and Baig MK (2009) Meta-Analysis of Skin Adhesives versus Sutures in Closure of Laparoscopic Port Site Wounds. *Surgical Endoscopy* **23**: 1191–1197.

Further Reading

Guglielmi C and Hunter S (2011) Sutures, Needles and Instruments. In Rothrock JC (ed) *Alexander's Care of the Patient in Surgery*, 14th ed. St. Louis, Elsevier Mosby, pp. 174–203.

66. Injection of Local Anaesthetic for Wound Infiltration

References

Anaesthesia UK (2016) Pharmacy of Regional Anaesthesia. Available at http://www.frca.co.uk/article.aspx?articleid=100816 (accessed 10 February 2016)

Association of Operating Room Nurses (AORN) (2007) Recommended Practices for Managing the Patient Receiving Local Anaesthetic. *AORN Journal* **85**(5): 965–971.

British National Formulary (BNF) (2016) Local Anaesthesia. Available at http://www.evidence.nhs.uk/formulary/bnf/current/15-anaesthesia/152-local-anaesthesia (accessed 10 February 2016)

Clark MK (2008) Lipid Emulsion as a Rescue for Local Anaesthetic-Related Cardiotoxicity. *Journal of Paranaesthesia Nursing* **23** (2): 111–121.

Cox F and Bhudia N (2009) Anaesthetic Medicines: Back to Basics. *The Journal of Perioperative Practice* **19** (11): 387–394.

Culp WC Jr, and Culp WC (2011) Practical Application of Local Anaesthetics. *Journal of Vascular Interventional Radiology* **22** (2): 111–118.

Fencl JL (2015) Guideline Implementation: Local Anaesthesia. *AORN Journal* **101**: 683–689.

Kirk RM (2010) *Basic Surgical Techniques*, 6th ed. Edinburgh, Churchill Livingstone.

Parry A (2011) Management and Treatment of Local Anaesthetic Toxicity. *Journal of Perioperative Practice* **21** (12): 404–409.

Phillips N (2012) *Berry and Kohn's Operating Room Technique*, 12th ed. St. Louis, Elsevier.

Further Reading

Cox F (2012) Pain Management. In In Woodhead K and Fudge L (eds) *Manual of Perioperative Care: An Essential Guide*. Chichester, Wiley-Blackwell, pp. 239–252.

Mehta V, Langford R and Haldar J (2013) Anaesthesia and Pain Relief. In Williams NS, Bulstrode CJK and O'Connell PR (eds) *Bailey & Love's Short Practice of Surgery*, 26th ed. Kent, CRC Press, 238–246.

67. Injection of Local Anaesthetic for Wound Infiltration – Caution and Complications

References

Association of Anaesthetists of Great Britain & Ireland (AAGBI) (2010) *AAGBI Safety Guideline: Management of Severe Local Anaesthetic Toxicity*. London, AAGBI.

Association of Operating Room Nurses (AORN) (2007) Recommended Practices for Managing the Patient Receiving Local Anaesthetic. *AORN Journal* **85** (5): 965–971.

Batinac T, Sotosek Tokmadzic V, Peharda V and Brajac I (2013) Adverse Reactions and Alleged Allergy to Local Anaesthetics: Analysis of 331 Patients. *Journal of Dermatology* **40** (7): 522–527.

Bhole MV, Manson AL, Seneviratne SL and Misbah SA (2012) IgE-Mediated Allergy to Local Anaesthetics: Separating Fact from Perception: A UK Perspective. *British Journal of Anaesthesia* **108** (6): 903–911.

Bourne E, Wright C and Royse C (2010) A Review of Local Anaesthetic Cardiotoxicity and Treatment with Lipid Emulsion. *Local Regional Anaesthesia* **3** (11): 11–19.

British National Formulary (BNF 2016) Local Anaesthesia. Available at http://www.evidence.nhs.uk/formulary/bnf/current/15-anaesthesia/152-local-anaesthesia (accessed 10 February 2016)

Caron AB (2007) Allergy to Multiple Local Anaesthetics. *Allergy and Asthma Proceedings* **28** (5): 600–601.

Fencl JL (2015) Guideline Implementation: Local Anaesthesia. *AORN Journal* **101**: 683–689.

Fuzier R, Lapeyre-Mestre M, Mertes PM, Nicolas JF, Benoit Y, Didier A *et al.* (2009) Immediate- and Delayed-Type Allergic Reactions to Amide Local Anaesthetics: Clinical Features and Skin Testing. *Pharmacoepidemiology and Drug Safety* **18** (7): 595–601.

Mercado P and Weinberg GL (2011) Local Anaesthetic Systemic Toxicity: Prevention and Treatment. *Journal of Anaesthesiology, Clinical Pharmacology* **29** (2): 233–242.

Parry A (2011) Management and Treatment of Local Anaesthetic Toxicity. *Journal of Perioperative Practice* **21** (12): 404–409.

Phillips N (2012) *Berry and Kohn's Operating Room Technique*, 12th ed. St. Louis, Elsevier.

Further Reading

Di Gregorio G, Neal JM, Rosenquist RW and Weinberg GL (2010) Clinical Presentation of Local Anaesthetic Systemic Toxicity: A Review of Published Cases, 1979 to 2009. *Regional Anaesthesia and Pain Medicine* **35** (2): 181–187.

Lui KC and Chow YF (2010) Safe Use of Local Anaesthetics: Prevention and Management of Systematic Toxicity. *Hong Kong Medical Journal* **16** (6): 470–475.

68. Camera Holding

References

Janse JA, Hitzerd E, Veersema S, Brockmans FJ and Schreuder HWR (2013) Correlation of Laparoscopic and Hysteroscopic 30 Degree Camera Navigation Skills on Box Trainers. *Gynecological Surgery* **11**: 75–81.

Larsen CR, Oestergaard J, Ottesen BS and Soerensen JL (2012) The Efficacy of Virtual Reality Simulation Training in Laparoscopy: A Systematic Review of Randomised Trials. *Acta Obstetricia et Gynecologica Scandinavica* **91**: 1015–1028.

Larsen CR, Soerensen JL, Grantcharov TP, Dalsgaard T, Schouenborg L, Ottosen C *et al.* (2009) Effect of Virtual Reality Training on Laparoscopic Surgery: Randomised Controlled Trial. *BMJ* **388**: 1802–1808.

Kong S-H, Oh B-M, Yoon H, Ahn HS, Lee H-J, Chung SG, *et al.* (2010) Comparison of the Two- and Three-Dimensional Camera Systems in Laparoscopic Performance: A Novel 3D System with One Camera. *Surgical Endoscopy* **24**: 1132–1143.

Schreuder HWR, Van der Berg CB, Hazebroek EJ, Verheijen RHM and Schijven MP (2011) Laparoscopic Skills Training Using Inexpensive Box Trainers: Which Exercises to Choose When Constructing a Validated Training Course. *BJOG* **118** (13): 1576–1584.

Shetty S, Panait L, Baranoski J, Dudrick SJ, Bell RL, Roberts KE and Duffy AJ (2012) Construct and Face Validity of a Virtual Reality-Based Camera Navigation Curriculum. *Journal of Surgical Research* **177**: 191–195.

Further Reading

Franzeck FM, Rosenthal R, Muller MK, Nocito A, Wittich F, Maurus C, *et al.* (2012) Prospective Randomised Control Trial of Simulator-Based versus Traditional In-Surgery Laparoscopic Camera Navigation Training. *Surgical Endoscopy* **26**: 235–241.

Zevin B, Levy JS and Satava RM (2012) A Consensus-Based Framework for Design, Validation and Implementation of Simulation-Based Training Curricula in Surgery. *Journal of the American College of Surgeons* **215** (4): 580–586.

SECTION 6

Recovery

Paul Wicker

69 Recovery Room Design

When patients spend time in the recovery room (also called the Post Anaesthetic Care Unit (PACU)), it can sometimes be a grim and dreary place because of the lack of pictures or paintings, windows and bright lights; reduced numbers of staff; noisy equipment and so on. However, in modern days the recovery room has changed a lot to help patients relax more (Wicker and Cox 2010, Haruguchi 2011). There are several new devices or changes, including:

- *Alcohol-based hand sanitiser pumps*: These are used to clean hands and reduce the chance of infection in patients.
- *Private rooms*: This reduces the risk of airborne infections, and it helps to ensure comfortable resting (because of lack of talking or shouting by other patients) and better chances of sleeping.
- *Introduction of carpeting*: This is to reduce injuries from trips and falls and increase the chance of visitors staying longer (HFT 2014).
- *A room with a view*: A window which shows a garden, trees or countryside helps the patients to relax better because of natural lighting and helps to reduce pain, nausea and other minor problems.
- *Equipment beside the bed*: This includes IV pumps, ventilators, monitors, suction machines and so on. This reduces the need for the patients to move around the hospital and reduces errors or miscommunication among recovery staff (Wicker and Cox 2010).
- *Music*: High-density fiberglass tiles on the ceiling reduce noise levels, and music helps to provide the patient with distraction from pain, stress, anxiety and so on, allowing them to rest better and sometimes helping them to sleep.

The improvement in recovery rooms over the past years has allowed patients to recover faster and spend less time in recovery (Hatfield and Tronson 2014). The rest of this chapter describes some of the more important features of the recovery room.

Recovery bays

Each recovery bay needs utilities to support the patient; normally, these will be located at the head of the bed or attached to the wall (Haruguchi 2011). These may include:

- Oxygen outlets – complete with flow meters
- Suction machines – including tubing and suction catheters
- Electrical sockets – for the use of equipment
- Mobile lamp – to provide light while examining the patient
- Shelves – to store equipment or accessories
- Storage cupboards – for the patient's use and for any other items required
- IV drip stands.

Rapid Perioperative Care, First Edition. Paul Wicker and Sara Dalby.

It is also essential that equipment is close to the patient, especially if the patient has had major surgery or is suffering from after-effects postoperatively (Wicker and Cox 2010, Hatfield and Tronson 2014). These may include:

- Sphygmomanometer – for recording of blood pressure, attached to the wall close to the bed. This will also require a stethoscope.
- Sterile disposable gloves – for use by practitioners when caring for patients
- Pressure infusion bag – used to increase the rate of IV fluids
- A moveable bed–table – to allow the patient to sit up in bed, and help them to eat or drink
- Oxygen equipment – including tubes, clear masks and humidifiers
- Suction equipment – with various suction catheters and tubing
- Guedel airways – including oral and nasal airways
- Airway devices – for example, a self-inflating bag, T-pieces (for intubated patients), oral airways, intubating equipment and so on
- Pulse oximeter – to measure the patient's level of oxygenation
- Bowls or kidney dishes – in case the patient vomits
- Other items – for example, hand towels, scissors, syringes, tissues and so on.

Recovery room facilities

Recovery room facilities are slowly improving over time to provide better comfort and safety for patients (HFT 2014). Air conditioning is normally present in recovery rooms, and temperatures should remain around 21 to 24 °C to ensure the patient does not become hypothermic. Air conditioning is essential to ensure that anaesthetic gases exhaled by patients leave the room because of the air flows (Haruguchi 2011). Other facilities that are needed in recovery rooms include (Hatfield and Tronson 2014):

- *Power supplies*: This will include sockets in every bay and also sockets in rooms where devices need batteries powered up. Battery-powered lights should also be available in case of power cuts.
- *Emergency station*: This is an emergency trolley which covers equipment such as intubation equipment, defibrillators and other pieces of equipment. This should be easily accessible in case of patient emergencies.
- *Non-slip flooring*: This is essential in case of practitioners or patients slipping and hurting themselves. The floor colour should be clear with no patterns or shapes to identify when objects have been dropped or lost (HFT 2014).
- *Hand washing*: Ideally, a hand basin would be part of the patient's bay so practitioners can wash their hands to prevent infecting the patient (Dzubow 2011). This will include hot water, soap, paper towels and a waste bin.
- *Drug cupboards*: Drugs need to be easily identified once the cupboard is unlocked, so that patients can receive drugs quickly. A drug list may also be useful to identify which drugs are available. Normally, a wide range of drugs are required in the recovery room for postoperative patients (Wicker and Cox 2010).
- *Linen cupboards*: To provide sheets, blankets, pillows and so on for patients. Also, laundry bins for soiled sheets or clothing would be needed.
- *Lighting*: Lights should not be too bright as they affect the patient or the practitioners when checking patients. Walls should be painted with a neutral colour, with or without pictures, and ideally windows would be available to encourage normal daylight. The overall idea is to reduce the patient's anxiety caused by intense lighting or intense colours.

Other items found in a recovery room can include toilets, disposable rooms, telephones, electric cables, notice boards and so on (Dzubow 2011). It is important that essential facilities are clean, effective and easily available, so practitioners may support patients during their recovery.

Recovery room equipment

Recovery practitioners provide care for postoperative patients by using the correct equipment and ensuring it is working well. Examples of essential equipment include oxygen supplies, suction, electrocardiograph (ECG) monitors, SPO_2 monitors, intubation equipment, cardiac arrest trolley and patient heating devices. There are many other pieces of equipment used in recovery rooms because of the needs of the patient who is recovering from both anaesthesia and surgery (Hatfield and Tronson 2014).

Other examples of equipment needed include:

- *Blood warmers*: Postoperative patients often suffer from hypothermia because of blood loss, anaesthetic drugs and exposure of the body or organs during surgery. Blood warmers help prevent hypothermia and also reduce pain on transfusion. Blood warmers can also reduce the viscosity of blood and help to reduce blood clots.
- *Emergency alarm*: This is often attached to the bed or within reach of the patient. The purpose of this is to call for help immediately if the patient needs urgent help because of serious problems arising.
- *Emergency trolleys*: These are also called *crash carts*, which are located within the recovery area. Emergency trolleys contain equipment, machines and drugs to help solve issues such as vomiting, emergency airway problems, insertion of drains, vascular access and anaphylaxis.
- *Monitors*: At least one monitor is needed in every bay and normally provides details on heart rhythm, pulse, blood pressure, oxygen saturation, expired carbon dioxide, breathing rates and so on. The patient will need to be connected to the monitor using devices such as blood pressure cuffs, ECG electrodes and wires, pulse oximeter and so on (Gordon 2007).
- *Refrigerator*: This will be needed to store drugs that need to stay cold, and other items such as ice if needed for local anaesthetic blocks. Blood may also be stored in a fridge, but it is important that it is thermostatically controlled and alarms are activated in case the temperature rises or falls beyond normal limits (Dzubow 2011).
- *Warming cabinet*: This is often used to warm blankets to keep the patient warm, and also for IV fluids, especially if the patient is hypothermic. Again, temperatures must be monitored and regulated within normal limits.
- *Airway equipment*: This may include respirators, ventilators and equipment such as laryngoscopes, endotracheal tubes, laryngeal mask airways (LMAs), syringes and so on. The purpose of this is to ensure the patient is breathing well; if not, then intubation may be required (Wicker and Cox 2010).
- *Sharps disposal*: Safely disposing of sharps is important to prevent harm to the patient and possible infection to the practitioner. Sharps include needles, glass ampules, blades and so on. The sharps should be placed in the 'sharps bucket' and sealed when full. They are then incinerated by the hospital.

Conclusion

When patients enter recovery, they are usually still under the effects of anaesthesia, and may be anxious, delirious, or confused. If the recovery room is calm and relaxing, with a minimum amount of noise, then this may help the patient to recover quicker from the anaesthetic and surgery (Hatfield and Tronson 2014). For example, painting walls and ceilings in soft and pleasing colours, such as light blue or yellow, helps to encourage relaxation (Gordon 2007).

Indirect lighting is also good to use because harsh lighting can affect the health of patients as they recover. Most modern equipment is now quiet to prevent disturbing the patients and staff (Wicker and Cox 2010). When the patient recovers and calms down, recovery practitioners tell them where they are and what is being done to help them recover, for example wound checking or delivery of IV fluids. Once the patient has fully recovered, the ward staff will receive information before the patient leaves the recovery room.

70 Patient Handover

Careful transfer of the patient from the operating room to recovery room is essential in order to ensure discussion between the anaesthetist, surgeon, scrub practitioner and recovery practitioner. Transferring of patients to the recovery room occurs immediately following surgery and, normally, once the drugs have been reversed and the patient is semiconscious. The anaesthetist will formally hand over information about the patient to a qualified member of the recovery room staff, and the scrub practitioner will usually give information about the surgical procedure (Hatfield 2014).

Following recovery of the patient in the operating room, the patient will be transferred to the recovery room, supported by suitable equipment such as providing oxygen via an oxygen mask and cylinder, and monitoring of oxygen levels, pulse, blood pressure and so on (Hatfield 2014). The care taken for the patient will depend on how close the recovery room is to the operating room, the patient's level of consciousness and his or her respiratory and cardiovascular status. If the recovery room is not immediately alongside the operating theatre, then the patient will need complete monitoring and safe care until they enter the recovery room. The anaesthetist has the responsibility to ensure the transfer is safe and the patient is kept comfortable and pain free.

The patient's handover

The patient handover involves giving information about the patient to the recovery practitioner to support the patient's health and safety. This process also hands over responsibility for the care of the patient to the recovery practitioner. Handovers involve discussions with the recovery staff and also showing the patient's records during anaesthesia and surgery.

However, the handovers can often take place in a comprehensive environment where staff are under pressure and there are distractions because of other patients or staff members. This may lead to communication failures, omission of content, lack of critical information and the like. Lack of effective face-to-face communication and misunderstanding of notes written during anaesthesia or surgery can lead to poor handovers which can result in harm to the patient (Catchpole *et al.* 2007). At times these handovers can also be unstructured, informal and error prone, leading to poor practice and problems for the patient. Improvements to patient handovers may include the use of checklists which will improve the discussion, leading to a focus on important details.

Effective handovers

Nagpal *et al.* (2010) stated that information is best passed on by using checklists or information technology, in order to improve communication between the anaesthetist and the recovery staff. Also the handover processes within hospitals are often being scrutinised following reports from organisations such as the Care Quality Commission (CQC). There are many ways to improve communication during handover, for example:

- *Standardise handover information*: Hospitals should develop a policy that provides a standardised approach to patient handover. This would offer the opportunity for questions

Rapid Perioperative Care, First Edition. Paul Wicker and Sara Dalby.

to be asked, for communication to be listened to carefully and for both parties to gain up-to-date information about the patient.

- *Effective communication*: This would include providing clear information regarding the care of the patient, the treatment needed, any changes that may occur due to the patient's health, feedback on patient results, and any services that may be required (e.g. x-ray).
- *Minimise interruptions during talking*: This is to prevent staff from informing the anaesthetist, and vice versa, about issues regarding the patient. Interruptions can result in information not being passed on or possibly being forgotten about later (Hatfield 2014).
- *Improve communication*: This would involve listening to the anaesthetist and also informing the anaesthetist of any issues. Both parties need to listen to their colleagues in these cases.
- *Ask and respond to questions*: This applies to both the anaesthetist and the recovery staff. Questions may be important, especially if the recovery practitioner has no understanding of the issues being discussed.
- *Historical data*: Including previous care, treatment and services that the patient received in the past.

Effective handover process

Catchpole *et al.* (2007) developed a protocol to provide an efficient handover for patients following anaesthesia and surgery. This was modelled on aviation modules and consists of four phases which can help to provide the best care possible for the postoperative patient. The four areas are discussed in this section.

Pre-handover

This includes informing recovery staff about the patient transfer at least 30 min before the patient is transferred to the recovery room. This would prepare the recovery staff for receiving the patient and setting up the recovery bay in preparation for his or her arrival.

Equipment and technology handover

This includes a check of the equipment being used and removal if necessary. The anaesthetist will check the patient is being ventilated and monitored and is stable. Any issues with equipment may be solved by exchanging devices so they can be used effectively.

Information handover

Under normal circumstances, the anaesthetist and the surgeon will speak together to provide relevant information about anaesthesia and surgery (Hatfield 2014). They should not be interrupted by recovery staff at this point, so the staff can listen and collect information as needed. After the discussion has finished, the recovery practitioner can check the information and ask questions about the patient. Examples of the anaesthetic handover may include (Catchpole *et al.* 2007):

- Checking the name, age and number of the patient
- Explaining medical conditions – for example, anxiety, pain and vomiting
- Details of vital signs – including cardiovascular status, temperature, circulatory status, use of IV fluids, medications given and so on
- Urine output
- Wound care – dressing used, drains and so on
- Monitoring required in recovery
- Recommended analgesics and anti-emetics.

The recovery practitioner may also need to maintain the patient's airway during handover and also discuss with the anaesthetist or surgeon any actions that recovery practitioners need to take during the recovery period. The anaesthetist and surgeon should also let the recovery practitioner know how to get in touch with either of them in case of serious problems arising (Smith and Mishra 2010).

Discussion and plan

The surgeon, anaesthetist and recovery team will then discuss the patient's status and needs during recovery. The recovery staff will then acknowledge their responsibility for the patient's care.

Catchpole *et al.* (2007) found that the organised method of handover reduced the duration of the handover and also reduced the number of errors by 40%. This will significantly reduce the risks of harm to the patient and may result in the patient recovering well and leaving the recovery room within a shorter time.

Smith and Mishra (2008) carried out a research study of patient handovers between anaesthetists and recovery staff and analysed the results. One of the issues they discovered was that many different members of staff were involved with patients which caused distraction and interferences during the handover, leading to poor quality of information exchange. Problems associated with the patient during anaesthesia and surgery are also often not discussed, even though there may be implications postoperatively. However, it is important that anaesthetists or practitioners highlight these points to a specific recovery practitioner, for example hypoxia due to blockage of airways, in case the same things happen during the patient's recovery (Smith and Mishra 2008).

Conclusion

Lack of communication and lack of transfer of patient data to recovery staff can lead to major adverse events happening to the patient. It is therefore important that staff engage fully during communication, listening to each other as well as speaking with each other, and ensuring that handovers are not interrupted by other practitioners. Well-structured handovers, using paperwork, forms, medication allergies, imaging, results from surgery and so on, can help to save serious problems with patients by decreasing the number of 'never events' and serious incidents, and increasing the value of communication between the theatre staff and the recovery staff.

71 Postoperative Patient Care

Recovery staff are responsible for providing care to the patient as soon as they enter the recovery room and the patient handover has been completed. Patients often have major concerns because of the anaesthesia and surgical procedures; these may include airway problems, postoperative pain, poor mental status because of anaesthetic drugs, and problems with wounds. Patients may also develop other problems because of past history of illness or disease, or because of issues following on from their recovery, including diabetes, retention of urine, deep venous thrombosis (DVT), circulation problems, allergies, and hypothermia or hyperthermia. The rest of this chapter highlights some of the actions needed regarding postoperative patient care.

Airway care

Following completion of the surgical procedure, patients are usually extubated and allowed to recover a little from their anaesthetic before arriving in the recovery room. On arrival in the recovery room, patients should be placed on their sides until they are fully recovered to prevent inhalation of phlegm or sputum, and also to prevent inhalation of vomit (Scott 2012). Intubation during anaesthesia may cause patients to cough for up to 24 h after extubation. However, patients who have smoked or have airway problems such as asthma or bronchitis may be subject to coughing for much longer periods until the airway becomes clear (Hatfield 2014). If patients have constant coughing, due to smoking or airway problems, then an inspirometer may be used to measure the volume, force and frequency of a patient's inspirations (AAGBI 2013).

Patients who suffer from hypoxic dyspnoea or non-hypoxic dyspnoea will be identified by using pulse oximetry arterial blood gas tests (AAGBI 2013). Undertaking a chest x-ray will also help to identify lung fluid overload caused by atelectasis. Atelectasis is the result of collapse or closure of the lung, resulting in reduced or absent gas exchange which may affect part or all of one lung, resulting in deflation of the alveoli. Dyspnoea is defined as an uncomfortable awareness of breathing by the patient. If dyspnoea occurs postoperatively, it results in low levels of breathing, anxiety or distress for the patient, and it is usually associated with disease of the heart or lungs or surgery on the chest or abdomen (Scott 2012). This can result in non-hypoxic dyspnoea, where the patient still has adequate oxygen levels, or hypoxic dyspnoea which results in hypoxemia which is a result of low oxygen levels in the blood, usually caused by pulmonary dysfunction (Jevon and Ewans 2007).

Sedation using drugs may cause hypoxaemia which often results in dyspnoea (difficult breathing) or tachypnoea (rapid breathing). Therefore, it is normal for patients under sedation to be monitored using pulse oximetry or capnometry to measure their oxygen and carbon dioxide levels. Patients who have cardiac problems, kidney disease or fluid overload may result in hypoxic dyspnoea which can result in serious problems in terms of the oxygen levels in their bloodstream (Hatfield 2014). This can be treated by increasing oxygen levels and ensuring the oxygen mask remains in place. Non-hypoxic dyspnoea can be treated using anxiolytics (to relieve anxiety) or analgesics (to relieve pain) (Hatfield 2014).

Rapid Perioperative Care, First Edition. Paul Wicker and Sara Dalby.

Pain relief

Once patients are conscious, they may start experiencing pain caused by their surgical procedure. To prevent pain, opioids are usually the first choice, although other drugs can also be given either orally, intramuscularly or intravenously.

Opioids are the best painkillers to give to patients, although they do have serious side effects, such as respiratory depression, bradycardia, pruritus, sedation, nausea and vomiting, hypotension and reduction in bowel function (Wicker and Cox 2010). Treating nausea and pruritus with antihistamines may also lead to effects on sedation and respiratory depression. Respiratory depression is one of the most serious complications of opioids which may lead to morbidity or mortality in postoperative patients.

Examples of drugs used include:

- *Systemic opioids*: Morphine, meperidine and fentanyl; may be administered via several different routes, such as oral, rectal, sublingual, transdermal, subcutaneous, intramuscular, intrathecal, epidural, inhalational or intravenous routes.
- *Nonsteroidal anti-inflammatory drugs (NSAIDS)*: Diclofenac, ibuprofen, naproxen and aspirin. NSAIDS are commonly used to treat inflammation and pain. NSAIDS inhibit the COX-2 enzyme which reduces the production of prostaglandins (Ramsay 2000) which helps to reduce pain, fever and vasodilatation.
- *Regional techniques*: Epidural and spinal opioids can provide good levels of analgesia, although side effects can still occur. Local anaesthetics do reduce or eliminate pain but may cause hypotension or muscle weakness in the patient.
- *Non-pharmacologic techniques*: These may include electrical stimulation of peripheral nerves which may affect pain inhibitory pathways, acupuncture or massage which can help to reduce pain (Jevon and Ewans 2007, Wicker and Cox 2010, Leigh *et al.* 2011).

As time progresses, there are different drugs being produced and advances in postoperative pain control that may result in reduced postoperative pain in patients.

Mental health

Anaesthetic drugs sedate patients and make them unconscious, and when they wake up they are often confused for a short while until the effects of the drugs wear off. Elderly patients are especially susceptible, although the use of magnesium tablets has been shown to alleviate the effect of anaesthetic drugs and reduce the chances of dementia following anaesthesia (Vizcaychipi 2013). Anticholinergics are particularly dangerous for elderly patients, even though they may be used before anaesthesia to decrease secretions in the upper airway; however, they should not be given to elderly patients unless they are essential for their safety. Opioids and H2 blockers can also lead to delirium in the elderly (Hatfield 2014). Recovery practitioners should assess the mental state of patients postoperatively, and if there are problems, then inform the anaesthetist, discuss the stopping of drugs and increase the level of oxygenation to ensure that oxygenation is at a good level. Patients who are demented or in delirium need careful observation and assessment of their physiological state, and they may need to be restricted in case of harm to themselves, other patients or staff members (Wicker and Cox 2010).

Wound care

Under normal circumstances, the wound is dressed in the operating room and remains in place for 24 h. However, if there is leakage or the dressing moves, then it may by changed during the recovery period. Antibiotics may be given to the patient postoperatively to reduce the risk of infection, and drain tubes may be used to help exudate flow out of the wound. The drain tubes will be observed to prevent excess fluid loss, excess blood loss or the like.

It is also possible that wounds may split open, and the patient may need re-suturing or insertion of skin clips; this is normally carried out by the surgeon.

Deep venous thrombosis

There may always be a risk of DVT after surgery because of the long time spent lying supine or because of the effects of surgery. Patients who undergo major surgery should therefore receive thromboprophylaxis using either medications or mechanical means (NICE 2011). Low-molecular-weight heparin, warfarin or aspirin is often given to patients who are assessed as being at risk of DVT or pulmonary embolism prior to surgery. Chemoprophylaxis requires the use of anticoagulant treatment to reduce the likelihood of coagulation (Narani 2010). Some of the drugs used, such as aspirin, may cause side effects such as an increased risk of bleeding, which could be a problem for the patient during surgery (Augistinos and Ouriel 2004). Intermittent pneumatic compression (IPC) devices, such as compression stockings or intermittent compression devices, are often used alongside various medications. Anaesthetists or surgeons may recommend heparin to be started soon after surgery has completed to prevent DVT or to help remove blood clots. Postoperatively, it is best practice for patients to begin moving their limbs as soon as they have recovered from anaesthesia and have returned to the ward.

Fever

High doses of anaesthesia or complex surgery can result in the patient undergoing stress which raises their metabolic rate, leading to hyperthermia (Jevon and Ewans 2007). Hyperthermia can also be caused by wound infections, anaesthetic drugs, pneumonia or urinary tract infections. Hyperthermia is a rare inherited disease and may lead to morbidity or death in some patients. The drug dantrolene sodium can be given to reduce temperatures, and other actions such as removing bed coverings, giving cold fluids and applying fans may be used (Wicker and Cox 2010).

Other problems

Patients in recovery can be susceptible to many problems which need to be assessed and actioned by the recovery staff. If the issues are important or dangerous, then the recovery staff needs to contact the anaesthetist or surgeon to help the patient to recover. Other issues include:

- *Orthopaedic surgery*: May require patients to be placed in appropriate positions so they don't cause pain or dislocate joints.
- *Major surgery*: Doctors and staff must be careful about moving the patient depending on the type of surgery that has been carried out. For example, if cardiac surgery has been carried out, the patient should not be placed on their left or right side, only in the supine or sitting position on the bed.
- *Urinary retention*: Patients must be monitored and may need catheterisation if they are unable to urinate. This may be caused by the use of anticholinergics or opioids, immobility and decreased oral intake (AAGBI 2013).
- *Reduction in strength*: This can be caused by loss of muscle mass, especially in patients who have undertaken prolonged bed rest. Patients should be encouraged to sit up in bed, transfer to a chair, stand and exercise as much as possible; this may occur during recovery if they have been in the recovery for several hours, or it can be encouraged once they return to the ward. It is also important that once the patient has recovered, they take fluids and food to maintain their nutritional and fluid levels. Tube feeding or parenteral feeding may be necessary if the patient has had surgery on the oesophagus, stomach, intestines or the like (Hatfield 2014).

Conclusion

Once the patient has recovered, they will be discharged from the recovery room and sent to the ward or other unit, depending on their health status. The actions discussed in this chapter show a selection of issues that can be faced in recovery; however, patients may be susceptible to many problems, all of which need actions in order to maintain their health. This Recovery section of the book will also describe other problems which occur in recovery and the actions that need to be taken.

72 Postoperative Patient Monitoring and Equipment

The purpose of the recovery room is to help the patient recover from anaesthesia and surgery, and to do this the staff need the suitable equipment for monitoring the patient to help prevent postoperative complications. Ideally, the recovery room is fully staffed and equipped with modern and up-to-date equipment and facilities, which provides the best environment for postoperative patients. The most common problems in recovery arise from the patient's airway, breathing and circulation. Identifying these early can be rectified quickly before the patient suffers serious harm. In 2013, the Association of Anaesthetists of Great Britain and Ireland (AAGBI 2013) published recommendations on 'Immediate Post-anaesthesia Recovery', including completion of patient records (Table 72.1), patient observation and provision of equipment (Table 72.2) and discharge criteria (Table 72.3).

Monitoring equipment

The need for efficient and effective monitoring equipment is essential for postoperative patients to optimise their safety and improve their recovery. The recovery practitioner will observe and assess the patient and decide which monitors are needed for the patient. Depending on the patient's clinical status, the recovery practitioner may need to monitor and regularly assess respiratory and cardiovascular function, neuromuscular function, mental status, temperature, pain, nausea and vomiting, drainage and bleeding, and urine output (AAGBI 2013) (Photo 8).

Respiratory monitoring

- *Pulse oximeter*: This device assists in the early detection of hypoxaemia by monitoring the patient's O_2 saturation (Hatfield 2014). The pulse oximeter is placed on the patient's fingertip, toe or earlobe. It then passes two wavelengths of light through the tissue to a photodetector on the opposite side of the device. The pulse oximeter then measures the oxygen in the haemoglobin in the artery or arteriole. The pulse oximeter then assesses the oxygen in the bloodstream and displays it on the screen. Normal oxygen levels should be 93% or higher.
- *Clinical observation*: The practitioner also checks breathing, chest movement and signs of cyanosis in the patient (Hatfield 2014).

Monitoring levels of oxygenation (SPO_2) and ventilation is important until the patient recovers from their anaesthetic drugs, or if the patient remains intubated until they wake up. Recovery practitioners may be trained to extubate patients during recovery, but they need confirmation from the hospital to be able to do this.

Rapid Perioperative Care, First Edition. Paul Wicker and Sara Dalby.

Table 72.1 Adapted from: AAGBI (2013) *Immediate Post-anaesthesia Recovery 2013*. London, Association of Anaesthetists of Great Britain and Ireland

Patient records

- Level of consciousness
- Patency of the airway
- Respiratory rate and adequacy
- Oxygen saturation
- Oxygen administration
- Blood pressure
- Heart rate and rhythm
- Pain intensity on an agreed scale
- Nausea and vomiting
- Intravenous infusions
- Drugs administered
- Core temperature
- Other parameters depending on circumstances (e.g. urinary output, central venous pressure, expired CO_2 and surgical drainage volume)

Table 72.2 Adapted from: AAGBI (2013) *Immediate Post-anaesthesia Recovery 2013*. London, Association of Anaesthetists of Great Britain and Ireland

Essential postoperative observations

- Oxygen administration
- Oxygen saturation
- Respiratory frequency
- Blood pressure and heart rate
- Conscious level
- Pain score
- Operation site review
- Temperature
- Urine output where necessary
- Drugs or fluids administered

Table 72.3 Adapted from: AAGBI (2013) *Immediate Post-anaesthesia Recovery 2013*. London, Association of Anaesthetists of Great Britain and Ireland

Discharge criteria (examples)
Ensure the patient:

- Is conscious and maintaining a clear airway
- Has protective airway reflexes
- Has satisfactory breathing and oxygenation (above 93%)
- Has a stable pulse and blood pressure
- Is pain free, with pain controlled through the use of analgesics
- Has body temperature within acceptable limits
- Does not have postoperative nausea and vomiting, and any PONV is controlled with an anti-emetic
- Has surgical drains and catheters checked
- Has good peripheral perfusion using intravenous infusions
- Has all records complete
- Has medical notes present.

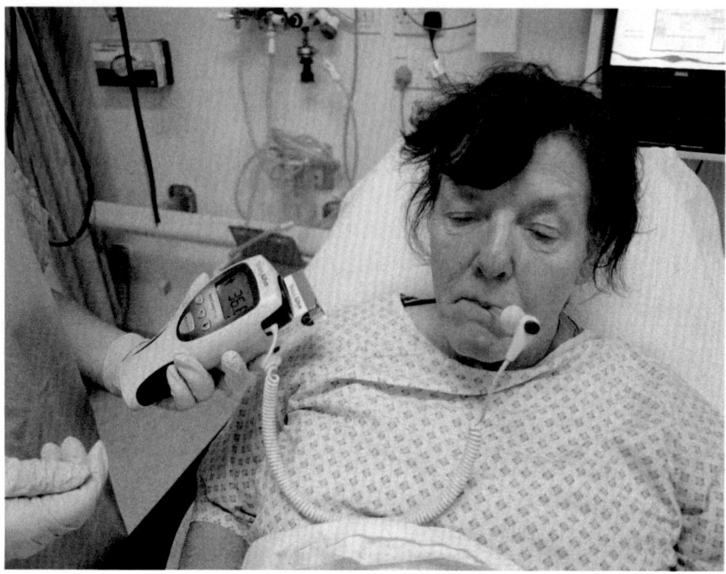

Photo 8 Monitoring the patient's temperature. Courtesy of Liverpool Women's Hospital

Cardiovascular monitoring

- *Electrocardiograph (ECG) machine*: The heart produces electrical impulses which spread through the heart muscle to make the heart contract. An ECG records the electrical activity of the heart, and the impulses are detected by the ECG monitor. The electrical activity is picked up by electrodes connected to the upper and lower parts of the chest. The heart disorders that can be detected include:
  - Abnormal heart rhythms – showing characteristic ECG patterns
  - Myocardial infarction – detected by abnormal ECG patterns
  - An enlarged heart – produces larger impulses than normal.

The ECG machine also records and monitors pulse rate, blood pressure (connected to a blood pressure cuff) and oxygen saturation (connected to a pulse oximeter). ECG monitoring detects cardiovascular complications, such as abnormal rhythm, and so it should always be used during the patient's recovery phase.

Neuromuscular monitoring

- *Nerve stimulator*: Neuromuscular blocking agents paralyse muscles, allowing anaesthesia and surgery to progress effectively. Once the patient is awake, and if he or she appears to have muscle weakness, the anaesthetist may apply the nerve stimulator which provides electrical stimulation to nerves and records the muscle responses. Assessment of neuromuscular function helps to identify problems such as difficulty in breathing or moving limbs (AAGBI 2013).

Patients who received long-acting non-depolarising neuromuscular blocking agents, or who have medical conditions associated with neuromuscular dysfunction, may need these tests to assess their health status.

Psychological monitoring

The patient's mental and psychological condition may be affected by anaesthetic drugs, such as propofol or ketamine, leading to anxiety, distress, anger and disruption (RCPRCP 2003). Ongoing assessment of the patient's mental status and behaviour may reduce postoperative complications, such as agitation, wound damage, or removal of catheters by the patient. The Joanna Briggs Institute (JBI 2011) describes several types of scoring systems to assess the patient's psychological status to reduce the possibility of harm to the patient.

Temperature monitoring

- Skin core temperature-corrected liquid crystal thermography
- Axillary electronic thermometer
- Oral electronic thermistor readings
- Infrared tympanic membrane thermometry

Regular measurement of the patient's body temperature in recovery is essential to prevent either low or high temperatures, leading to prolonged stay in the recovery room (Hatfield 2014). The oral method is more accurate and has greater precision than either the liquid crystal or axillary methods. The patient's temperature can change because of the effects of anaesthetic drugs and the surgical procedure. In recovery, the patient temperature may also reduce rapidly because of issues such as the administration of cold IV fluids, the lack of warming blankets or the effects of surgery (AAGBI 2013). Delivering regular assessment of the patient's temperature may help reduce serious postoperative complications such as shivering, hypothermia or hyperthermia (Bernard 2014). Assessment of patient temperature, therefore, detects complications and may reduce adverse outcomes during recovery.

Pain monitoring

Patients often undergo pain postoperatively because of the effects of the surgical procedure, and sometimes because of stress and anxiety. Anaesthetists may give analgesics during surgery, but their effects may reduce during recovery, leading to postoperative pain. Pain in the patient is assessed by asking the patient about their pain, or by asking them to complete a numerical assessment form (Rawlinson *et al.* 2012). The pain score of 10 is high and indicates the patient needs analgesia quickly. A pain score of 1 or 2 does not usually cause problems but may need small doses of analgesics. Regular monitoring of the patient and assessment of pain by the recovery practitioner will help to keep the patient pain free and comfortable during their recovery phase.

Nausea and vomiting

Thirty percent of postoperative patients suffer from postoperative nausea and vomiting (PONV) (Smith *et al.* 2012). When vomiting occurs, the patient may suffer from anxiety, aspiration into the lungs, poor analgesia (due to vomiting of the tablets), dehydration and damage to surgical wounds. Detecting complications and improving patient outcomes are essential by regularly assessing and monitoring any nausea and vomiting, and also assessing the patient's condition. Risk assessment of PONV can also be carried out before surgery (Rawlinson *et al.* 2012). Ondansetron is a strong anti-emetic drug given to patients to prevent vomiting. Unconscious patients should always be turned on their side to reduce the chance of inhaling vomit into their trachea, bronchus or lungs.

Fluid monitoring

Fluid balance refers to the input and output of fluids in the body to assist metabolic processes. The key features of assessment and monitoring of fluid balance include capillary refill, blood pressure, dry mouth, oedema, urine output and fluid balance charts.

Central venous pressure is one of the first signs of reduction in intravascular volume, leading to changes in skin pallor (possibly blue skin caused by low circulation), pulse rate, sweating and a fall in blood pressure, resulting in major patient issues. However, if the peripheries are pink and warm caused by rapid capillary refill, then this suggests that there is adequate circulation. Monitoring and assessment of pulse, blood pressure and urine output help to identify the level of fluids and electrolytes. However, if the patient is seriously ill, then invasive techniques may be required to assess cardiovascular function (Shepherd 2011).

Regular postoperative assessment of the patient's hydration status and fluid management reduces problems and improves the patient's comfort and satisfaction. Surgical procedures which involve significant loss of blood or fluids may need extra fluid management.

Urine output

Patients undergoing urological surgery, or who have low fluid imbalances, will be assessed for their levels of urine output during recovery (Hatfield 2014). Assessment of urine output may be more important in some patients. Oliguria is the low output of urine; it can lead to dehydration, renal failure, hypovolaemic shock, urinary tract infection and several other problems (Chenitz and Lane-Fall 2012). When low levels of urine output are detected, it is important to inform the anaesthetist and/or surgeon so that actions can be taken. Oliguria may be caused by several problems, such as low perfusion of the kidney, bleeding problems, dehydration, renal damage or obstruction of urine flow (e.g. due to an enlarged prostate gland) (AAGBI 2013). Often, patients who have had major surgery will have experienced fluid and blood loss which will also decrease urine output. In such cases, it is likely that fluids will be administered to restore intravascular volume. Scanning of the kidney may also be carried out if urine output does not increase once fluid levels have been restored (Chenitz and Lane-Fall 2012).

Drainage and bleeding

Patients undergoing major surgery may have drains inserted into their wounds to help drain blood and fluids. Recovery practitioners must assess and monitor any drainage and bleeding which will help to reduce adverse outcomes. Drainage can originate from chest or wound drains; any excessive blood loss in either case needs referring to the surgeon or anaesthetist so action can be taken if needed. Fluid or blood loss must be recorded in the patient's notes and be regularly monitored when issues arise.

Discharge

Every patient is continuously monitored and observed until they are considered fit for return to their ward. Discharge criteria vary between individuals, depending on their level of anaesthesia or surgery. Criteria assessed before patients leave the recovery area would include:

Being fully conscious
Capable of protective reflexes (e.g. vomiting safely and not inhaling vomit into the lungs)
Maintaining a clear airway

Breathing appropriately
Maintaining oxygen levels (93% or more)
Ensuring a stable pulse rate
Normal blood pressure and normal temperature
Being pain free (Hatfield 2014).

If the patient had major surgery and is still potentially likely to have problems on the way to the ward, they may still be connected to monitors and have an oxygen mask over their face as well as support offered from the anaesthetist, recovery practitioner and ward nurse.

73 Maintaining the Airway

Anaesthetic drugs used during anaesthesia and surgery can affect the patient postoperatively as they interfere with their ventilation by affecting their airway muscles and restricting breathing, leading to respiratory complications. It is also possible for patients to have airway obstruction, for example because of their tongue falling backwards into their trachea or epiglottis. Examples of partial airway obstruction include chest or sternum problems (following surgery on the chest), snoring, stridor, hypoxaemia (low levels of oxygen) and hypercarbia (high carbon dioxide levels) (Dalal and Taylor 2004). Complete airway obstruction may be caused by the inability to breathe, damage to the sternum and ribs, blockage of airways caused by phlegm or sputum, or inhalation of vomit (Scott 2012).

Patient assessment

Before anaesthesia begins, it is important that patients are assessed for any problems related to their airways. This is usually carried out by the anaesthetist, but certain problems can also be discussed with the patient by the anaesthetic practitioner. Any problems regarding airways should be mentioned and discussed with the anaesthetist to ensure the patient doesn't have the risk of increased airway management problems. Some of the risk factors which could affect the airway include a past history of problems during anaesthesia, such as stridor, arthritis, stiff neck, tumours in the head or neck, being obese, being elderly and so on (Scott 2012).

Assessing the patient's airway includes checking the patient's mouth and airways, and any physiological problems leading to respiratory complications (Hatfield 2014). Any issues discovered should be documented in the patient's record. Examples of the areas to examine include:

- *Mouth cavity*
    - Small mouth opening (less than 3 cm in an adult)
    - Missing, loose or capped teeth
    - Dental appliances, including crowns, bridges or dentures
    - Enlarged tonsils
    - Non-visible uvula
    - Presence of a tumour or growth that may block the air flow (Scott 2012).
- *Temporomandibular joint*: Most adults normally have a mouth opening of 4 to 6 cm. Pain, limited range of motion or temporomandibular joint disease can result in the patient having an opening smaller than 4 cm (Dalal and Taylor 2004). This can result in the patient being unable to use oral airways during respiratory distress.
- *Neck stiffness*: The anaesthetist may assess the movement of the neck via the atlanto-occipital joint by flexing it, extending it and moving it from side to side. This would assess the level of movement in the neck and any problems that might arise. Endotracheal tube (ETT) intubation requires the anaesthetist to align the oral, pharyngeal and laryngeal anatomical parts of the airway, to ensure the ETT is placed correctly.
- *Physical appearance*: Preoperatively, patients should be assessed for any physical problems leading to airway difficulties. For example:

Rapid Perioperative Care, First Edition. Paul Wicker and Sara Dalby.

- Obesity in the neck and face
- High, arched palate in the mouth
- Large tongue that can block the airway
- Short, immobile or stiff neck
- Mouth that cannot open wide
- Protruding teeth, broken teeth, loose teeth, sore teeth and so on
- A jaw that is either recessed or protruding (Scott 2012, Hatfield 2014).

- *Mallampati Airway Score*: In anaesthesia, the Mallampati score is used to predict the ease of intubation. A high Mallampati score, which is based on Class 3 or 4, is associated with more difficult intubation (Figure 73.1). The Mallampati score assesses the height of the mouth; the distance from the tongue base to the roof of the mouth, and therefore the amount of space in which there is to work when carrying out intubation. The anatomy of the oral cavity is assessed to see whether the base of the uvula, facial pillars (the arches in front of and behind the tonsils) and soft palate are visible (Hatfield 2014). The Mallampati scoring system is as follows:
  - Class 1: Soft palate, uvula, facial pillars visible
  - Class 2: Soft palate, uvula, facial pillars less visible
  - Class 3: Soft palate, base of uvula visible
  - Class 4: Only hard palate visible (Scott 2012).

Basic airway management

Observation of respiratory function in recovery patients is essential, and actions are taken when problems arise leading to hypoxaemia. Initially, suction may be used if the patient is coughing or choking due to inhalation of sputum, phlegm or vomit. However, other actions may need to be taken following initial actions. The anaesthetist needs to be informed in these situations, so he or she can help the patient as soon as possible.

Manual techniques

If the patient is drowsy or sedated and lying supine in recovery, the tongue relaxes and tends to fall backwards towards the oropharynx. The epiglottis may also fall backwards and obstruct the pharynx (Dalal and Taylor 2004). When the patient is seen to be not breathing, a jaw thrust or chin lift may be used to open the airway and improve breathing:

- *Jaw thrust*: The jaw is moved forward which also brings the tongue forward and stops obstruction of the airway. The recovery practitioner should stand at the head of the bed,

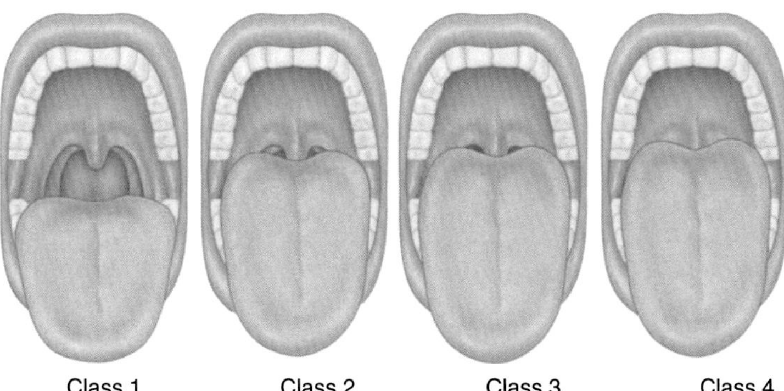

Figure 73.1 Mallampati score.

place the middle finger of each hand at the angle of the patient's jaw and the head is then tilted backwards to elevate the mandible.
- *Chin lift*: The fingers of both hands are placed under the mandible to gently lift it upwards, and the thumbs are used to open the mouth.

Reversing sedatives

Antagonist drugs may be used to reverse the effects of opioids and benzodiazepines to revitalise the patient and improve their airway and breathing problems. Naloxone may be used to reverse opioids, and flumazenil can be used to reverse benzodiazepine which is a sedative used during general anaesthesia. Once the patient wakes up or is stimulated by these medicines, then the airway passages should be improved.

Airway equipment

Patients who still find breathing a difficulty, or are still under the effects of anaesthetic drugs, may be given oropharyngeal or nasopharyngeal airways to improve their breathing and oxygenation. They may also be intubated using an endotracheal tube (ETT) or laryngeal mask airway (LMA). The oral and nasal airways prevent the tongue from falling backwards against the posterior pharyngeal wall, thereby keeping the airways open.

While the oral airways are useful for most patients, they can lead to problems such as airway obstruction if they slip too far backwards, incorrect sizes, trauma to soft tissues and inducing vomiting. Nasal airways can also cause damage to nasal tissues leading to bleeding, and if the nasal airway is too long it may enter the oesophagus rather than staying in the posterior pharynx (Hatfield 2014).

- *Oropharyngeal airway*: The most common oral airway used is the Guedel airway which is a curved, firm and hollow tube made from plastic, with a rectangular opening that prevents the tube from being squashed by the teeth. The airway is inserted upside down, pushed backwards into the mouth and then reversed when it touches the back of the throat. Oral airways come in various sizes (from 50 mm to 100 mm) depending the age and size of the patient. The oral airways have a flange on the proximal end to prevent over-insertion of the airway and to prevent the airway from slipping further down the trachea. Oral airways should only be used for unconscious or unresponsive patients so that the patient does not start coughing or generating a gag reflex. When the patient wakes up and becomes agitated, it is possible for the oral airway to cause vomiting and aspiration.
- *Nasopharyngeal airway*: The nasal airway is normally a soft rubber tube which is passed through the nose and into the posterior pharynx just above the epiglottis; these are better tolerated by patients as they cause minimum disruption to their airways. The nasal airway may be used when the patient is awake or their jaw is clenched because of issues the patient is having due to airway problems.
- *Endotracheal tube (ETT)*: An ETT would be used for a postoperative comatose patient to enable ventilation. The ETT is the best method used to provide a patent airway and to prevent aspiration for the patient.
- *Laryngeal mask airway (LMA)*: An LMA can be inserted into the lower oropharynx if the recovery patient is comatose and suffering from airway problems. There are also newer models which have a channel that can guide an ETT into the trachea. The LMA does not require laryngoscopy for insertion.

Bag–Valve–Mask (BVM) ventilation

Knowing how to provide BVM ventilation for patients who have difficult airways is essential for doctors and recovery practitioners. BVM enables doctors and practitioners to support patients with airway problems and enable them to inhale oxygen to prevent hypoxaemia from occurring (Hatfield 2014). The next step, once the anaesthetist arrives, may be to

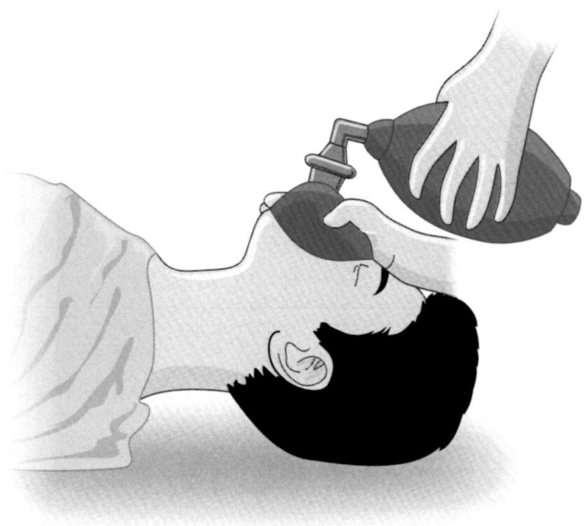

Figure 73.2 The face mask is placed over the patient's open mouth and the balloon is attached to oxygen. The bag must be squeezed slowly by the recovery practitioner every 5 seconds to enable the patient to inhale oxygen and to remain alive.

insert an ETT or LMA. Both doctors and practitioners should practice the BVM technique regularly, either on patients or in a simulated environment, in order to ensure they carry out the procedure correctly and to the best of their abilities.

The three main actions to take when performing BVM ventilation are (Scott 2012):

- *Ensure the airway is open*: Use oral or nasal airways, and the jaw thrust or chin lift if necessary.
- *Suitable mask size*: Ensure the mask is the correct size for the patient and that it is placed in the correct position and held correctly to prevent leakage of oxygen from the mask (Figure 73.2).
- *Appropriate ventilation*: Ensure that mask ventilation is carried out with lack of errors:
  - Do not provide the patient with excessive tidal volumes – this may damage the airway, chest, ribs or lungs.
  - Do not force air too quickly – squeeze the bag slowly and carefully over a period of 1–3 sec.
  - Ventilate at normal levels – normal ventilation will be around 10 to 12 breaths per minute (Scott 2012).

Conclusion

Recovery rooms set criteria for discharge of patients, which would include that patients are conscious, are able to breathe and maintain their own airway, have reduced pain, are normothermic and are free of cardiovascular problems. A handover will also be given to the ward nurse explaining anaesthesia and surgery, any perioperative complications and the anaesthetist's and also the surgeon's postoperative care instructions.

74 Diagnosis and Management of Postoperative Infection

Patients need clear and consistent advice about the risk of surgical site infection and how to manage it. Patients will also need advice on how to care for their wounds after discharge, especially if infection develops. This may include telling them how to recognise when wound infection develops, and to contact their GP or surgeon if they have concerns. Patients also need to be informed later that they have been given antibiotics during surgery, especially if there have been problems during the procedure.

Preoperative infection prevention

Various actions should be taken preoperatively to help ensure the patient doesn't become infected. This involves ensuring the patient is clean, free from infection and less likely to acquire infection during surgery (NICE 2008). Preoperative actions to take include:

- *Preoperative showering*: The day before or the morning before surgery.
- *Hair removal (within area of surgery)*: Use electric clippers with a single-use head on the day of surgery. Razors should not be used as they may 'scrape' or scratch the skin, increasing the risk of surgical site infection.
- *Patient theatre wear*: Including patient gown, socks, slippers, dressing gown and so on. Consider the patient's comfort and dignity, and ensure they are kept warm.
- *Staff theatre wear*: All circulating staff will wear theatre suits and must remain outside of the sterile area. Theatre staff should also change their suits if they move in or out of the operating department.
- *Nasal decontamination*: Should not be used to eliminate *Staphylococcus aureus* unless essential for nasal surgery (NICE 2012).
- *Mechanical bowel preparation*: Should not be used because of the risk of damage to the bowels and increased risk of surgical site infection (NICE 2012).
- *Hand jewellery, artificial nails and nail polish*: Patients and theatre staff should remove these items before entry into the operating department (Goodman and Spry 2014).
- *Antibiotic prophylaxis*: At the jurisdiction of the anaesthetist. May be given before anaesthesia for trauma patients, contaminated surgery, contaminated wounds, sick patients and so on (WHO 2006).

Intraoperative infection prevention

Caring for the patient intraoperatively is important to ensure they don't become contaminated, and this is a requirement of the surgeons, anaesthetists and theatre staff. Patients with an operative site infection need treatment with antibiotics, such as cephalosporins (e.g. cefoxitin or cefotaxime) and penicillins (e.g. ampicillin or piperacillin) (NICE 2012). Actions needed during surgery to reduce the chances of infection may include:

Rapid Perioperative Care, First Edition. Paul Wicker and Sara Dalby.

- *Hand decontamination*: The theatre team should clean their hands using alcohol hand rub before entering the operating room. Scrub staff will scrub hands and arms using an aqueous antiseptic surgical solution, following the hospital scrub guidelines. This is normal practice before every surgical operation.
- *Incise drapes*: Non-iodophor-impregnated incise drapes may increase the risk of surgical site infection during surgery, so they should not be used. Iodophor-impregnated drapes do reduce the risk of surgical site infection (Dewan *et al.* 1987, Makki *et al.* 2015). However, removal of incise drapes during wound closure may also increase the risk of contamination (Makki *et al.* 2015).
- *Sterile gowns*: The surgical team wears sterile gowns during surgery.
- *Gloves*: Normally, surgical staff wear two pairs of sterile gloves to reduce the risk of contamination caused by perforation of the outer glove.
- *Antiseptic skin preparation*: Povidone–iodine and chlorhexidine are used to reduce the risk of infection around the surgical site (Goodman and Spry 2014). It is important that alcohol-based solutions are dried before using electrosurgery; otherwise, the solution may ignite, leading to major problems for the patient and staff.
- *Patient temperature*: This should be maintained around 37 °C, plus or minus 1 °C. Any changes to the patient's temperature will need actions such as warming or cooling the patient.
- *Patient oxygenation*: This needs to be monitored regularly to ensure oxygenations stays around 95% or more during surgery and recovery.
- *Perfusion during surgery*: Ensure the patient is given appropriate levels of fluids and electrolytes during surgery to ensure their circulation and oxygenation are maintained correctly.
- *Wound irrigation*: This should only be used if essential due to the surgical procedure. Wound irrigation and cavity lavage can lead to more chance of wound infection because of the mix of fluids: blood, pus and so on.

Management of postoperative infection

Postoperative patients who suffer from infection following surgery need to be monitored and treated urgently to prevent further issues with their health and well-being. Patients who have infections before surgery need to be treated to prevent further problems. The surgeon should also avoid the risk of infection during surgery to reduce postoperative infection. For example, opening the bowel can lead to infection in the abdomen. Also, obese patients require closure of the lower half of the subcutaneous layer of their abdomen to reduce the likelihood of dehiscence, wound infection, haematoma and seroma (a pocket of clear serous fluid that may develop after surgery). Patients undergoing pelvic surgery, for example caesarean section or hysterectomy, should receive prophylactic antibiotics which decrease the number of the bacteria, make the body less hospitable for the growth of bacteria and enhance the phagocytosis (destruction) of pathogenic bacteria.

One of the best drugs to use for prophylaxis (prevention of disease) is cefazolin (given as 1 g intravenous or intramuscular). If the patient is allergic to this drug or has a sensitive reaction to it, then an alternate drug is doxycycline, which is given as 100 mg intravenously. Usually, the patient needs only a single dose of antibiotics for treatment. For patients undergoing obstetric or gynaecologic procedures, it is best to administer antibiotics before surgery rather than following the surgery (Goodman and Spry 2014). Prophylaxis, luckily, does not normally increase the chance of urinary tract infection.

Postoperative care

Infection prevention and control (IPC) is very important in the perioperative environment due to infections such as hepatitis B, tuberculosis, multi-resistant staphylococcus aureus (MRSA) and human immunodeficiency virus (HIV). Infection control policies designed by hospitals therefore aim to reduce the risk of cross-infection in the operating department. Recovery practitioners can use 'Standard Precautions' (WHO 2006) to assess the safety of activities they are undertaking, regardless of whether the patient is infected or not (CDC 1998, Goodman and Spry 2014). The recovery room may contain bacteria and viruses in the airstreams and also contains the risk of infection because of blood and body fluids; therefore, it is a high-risk environment for patients and staff. Recovery practitioners therefore need to be aware of standard precautions, national guidelines (e.g. NICE 2012) and local policies on infection control. Examples of actions to take in postoperative care include:

- *Changing dressings*: Use an aseptic non-touch technique, including wearing gloves and an apron, for checking or removing wound dressings.
- *Postoperative cleansing*: Sterile saline is the best solution to use for wound cleansing immediately after surgery if the wound is still not healed. Once the wound has healed, tap water may be used.
- *Showers*: Patients can shower safely after 48 h following surgery.
- *Antibiotics*: Topical antimicrobial agents should not normally be used for open wounds or they may lead to wound infection.
- *Wound dressings*: Eusol and gauze, or moist cotton gauze or mercuric antiseptic solutions, should also not be used for primary or secondary wound healing. An appropriate dressing should be used to manage secondary surgical wounds.
- *Antibiotic treatment of wound site*: The patient may require an antibiotic if the wound site appears to be infected. Microbiological tests can help in choosing the correct antibiotic.

Conclusion

The provision of wound care is important for patients with large wounds, or wounds that are susceptible to infection. A structured approach to care, which includes preoperative assessments and postoperative assessments, is needed to improve the management of surgical wounds (Goodman and Spry 2014). Postoperative infections must be treated urgently by using antibiotics to cover the range of possible pathogens. To support the patient, practitioners needs training and understanding of the methods used to care for wounds.

75 Postoperative Pain Management

Postoperative patients often suffer from pain because of their surgery. Ensuring that pain is controlled and managed is therefore essential to provide excellent care for the patient. If pain is not managed, then patients may suffer from morbidity or mortality. The use of local anaesthetics is often considered to be the most effective analgesic technique; however, other drugs such as opioids and nonsteroidal anti-inflammatory agents are also used effectively for patients in pain (Malcolm 2015).

Managing postoperative pain will improve patient comfort and satisfaction with their own care, and it will provide earlier mobilisation, fewer complications and a faster recovery. If recovery practitioners fail to provide pain relief, this may be because of lack of understanding, poor pain assessment and inadequate staffing, leading to intense work for every practitioner.

Pain assessment

Assessment tools can be used to assess pain and also to understand the pain from which the patient is suffering (Carr *et al.* 2010). Normally, a 10-point pain assessment scale is used, the lowest levels (1–3) indicate there is no pain, whereas higher levels of 8–10 indicate high levels of pain (Hatfield 2014). The rating is usually agreed between the practitioner or doctor and the patient. The patient's pain rate and also any other complications associated with pain should be recorded in their notes, so further action can be taken if necessary.

When the practitioner understands the patient's pain, then pain therapy may be changed to support the patient better. Actions that can be taken include (Wicker and O'Neill 2010):

- Note the source of the pain and its severity.
- Understand the reason for the anatomical source of the pain.
- Understand the patient's anxiety, stress or fear, and attempt to treat if possible.
- Reassess the patient's score on a regular basis so side effects of the treatment may be helped, for example sedation, nausea, or pruritus.
- Check if the patient is satisfied with the outcome.

Analgesia can be administered during anaesthesia and before surgery starts, which helps to prevent or reduce postoperative pain. Pain assessment and treatment will therefore help the patient to understand that pain is treated and also helps the patient to relax more and be comfortable following surgery (Malcolm 2015).

Side effects of pain

It is essential that postoperative pain management relieves pain, but also reduces side effects to a minimum. Opioids are analgesics that relieve pain effectively; however, they also have side effects such as sedation, respiratory depression, nausea and vomiting and hypotension, amongst others (Hatfield 2014).

Rapid Perioperative Care, First Edition. Paul Wicker and Sara Dalby.

Using opioids can result in respiratory depression which can be a major life-threatening problem for the patient. Severe respiratory depression can occur when patients use patient-controlled analgesia pumps. If the patient is in severe pain, they may press the button several times, leading to high doses of opioids. It is therefore essential that the patient is monitored and observed in case of issues arising. The pulse oximeter is often used to monitor respiratory depression when opioids are being given. However, the pulse oximeter only measures levels of oxygen in the blood and does not measure poor breathing, even if the patient has an oxygen mask in place. The pulse oximeter therefore would detect low respiration much later. The oxygen mask will provide oxygen, but due to low breathing levels the patient may develop high levels of CO_2 in the blood vessels. Problems with ventilation can result in poor breathing and little air movement, leading to hypoxia. It is therefore essential for the recovery practitioner to clinically monitor the ventilation and breathing rate of the patient and also record the respiratory rate and level of sedation in the patient's charts. If the patient has ventilation or breathing problems, then the anaesthetist must be called to support the patient and prevent hypoxaemia.

Systemic opioids

Opioids are useful to relieve patients from pain; they act as agonists on opioid receptors. Opioids are given via oral, rectal, sublingual, transdermal, subcutaneous, intramuscular and intravenous pathways (Carr *et al.* 2010). Under normal circumstances, opioids are given either intravascularly or intramuscularly. The drugs commonly used include morphine, meperidine, fentanyl and hydromorphone. All the opioids can result in side effects despite the relief of pain (Malcolm 2015). For example, meperidine may cause seizures, and in elderly patients meperidine may cause psychosis or delirium because of its effects on the central nervous system (Hatfield 2014).

Patients undergoing pain often use a patient-controlled analgesia machine (PCA) which allows them to press a button to inject small amounts of analgesics into their bloodstream (Mitchell 2010). Patients can therefore obtain pain relief without having to wait for a recovery practitioner, and painful injections are also not required. To ensure that this device is safe, the pump needs to work effectively and the pump is also controlled by the patient themselves, not by family members. The patient therefore has to be conscious and not suffering from sedation or delirium in order to activate the system. Patients should also be assessed after using the PCA to see if they are still in pain or whether the PCA pump can be removed.

Oral opioids are also effective for patients, and they relieve the use of painful injections, allowing earlier discharge from the hospital. Oxycodone is an example of a controlled-release tablet which provides good pain control for up to 12 h.

Nonsteroidal Anti-inflammatory Drugs (NSAIDS)

NSAIDS treat pain and inflammation; they are less potent than the narcotics but do not have the same effects (Malcolm 2015). Over time, more potent NSAIDS have been produced, for example ketorolac, which is useful in managing the pain following minimally invasive surgery. There are, however, some side effects, including peptic ulcer disease, gastrointestinal haemorrhage or renal dysfunction. Depending on the health and physiology of the patients, these drugs may not always be used postoperatively. NSAIDS inhibit the enzyme cyclooxygenase (COX), which synthesises prostaglandins, which are responsible for pain, fever and vasodilatation in patients suffering from trauma (Hatfield 2014). A major problem with using these drugs is that they can reduce the effects of the prostaglandins and decrease tissue inflammation.

There are two forms of COX called COX-1 and COX-2 (Carr *et al.* 2010). COX-1 is found in most tissues, uses prostaglandin to protect the gastric mucosa, improves renal perfusion and preserves platelet function. COX-2, however, is induced by pain and inflammation, and COX-2 inhibitors therefore reduce pain and inflammation. COX-2 inhibitors are available for oral use and can also be used parenterally. The new NSAIDS may be safer and will help the management of postoperative pain (Hatfield 2014).

Regional techniques

Epidural and spinal analgesia may improve surgical outcomes in postoperative patients, especially elderly patients, by reducing the chances of intraoperative blood loss and deep vein thrombosis, and also improving blood flow and pulmonary function (Wicker and O'Neill 2010, Malcolm 2015). Epidural and spinal opioids provide good pain relief but also provide side effects such as respiratory depression or pruritus; therefore, regular observation and monitoring are definitely required.

Local anaesthetics may also cause hypotension and muscle weakness in patients; therefore, low concentrations of local anaesthetics should be used to avoid problems for the patient.

When epidural catheters are placed, they may result in developing a spinal haematoma, especially in patients receiving anticoagulant therapy. Neurological monitoring may be required once patients have had an epidural catheter inserted in order to detect the formation of an epidural haematoma. The epidural clot is normally removed quickly to prevent further problems once it has been detected.

Two effective drugs

Two drugs that may provide better therapeutic benefits are dexmedetomidine and remifentanil (Ramsay *et al.* 1998, Hall *et al.* 2000, Carr *et al.* 2010, Hatfield 2014).

Dexmedetomidine

Dexmedetomidine is an alpha-2-adrenergic agonist that provides the patient with sedation and analgesia, but does not cause ventilatory depression. Infusion of the drug at 0.2 to 0.7 μg/kg/h maintains pain relief, some sedation and no respiratory depression (Hall *et al.* 2000). This drug can be used intravenously in the recovery room and provides a good level of safety compared to opioids.

Remifentanil

Remifentanil acts as an m-opioid receptor agonist, which can provide good analgesia depending on the rate of infusion. Remifentanil, however, is a potent narcotic and may lead to respiratory depression (Ramsay *et al.* 1998). In recovery, it needs to be closely monitored and carefully titrated to provide appropriate pain relief for postoperative patients, without ongoing sedation.

Conclusion

Pain management drugs are improving and changing over time, including advances in pharmacology, leading to even better management of postoperative pain. Recovery practitioners therefore need to address education issues and postoperative patient care to improve pain management and provide the best possible care to postoperative patients.

76 Fluid Balance in Postoperative Patients

Managing fluid balance in postoperative patients involves providing fluid via intravenous infusion and replacing intraoperative fluid losses caused by blood loss, fluid redistribution and evaporation. Using 0.9% sodium chloride or 5% dextrose is normal, although infusing Hartmann's solution (compound sodium lactate) to the patient is common if he or she has high fluid losses (Gau and Bartel 2015).

The main goal of perioperative fluid management is to create a balance between providing too little fluid or a fluid overload. When fluids in the patient's body are low, it is likely that hypotension, increased postoperative nausea, inadequate organ perfusion and reduced tissue oxygenation may occur (Clancy *et al.* 2002). Infusing the patient with too much fluid can cause oedema, poor wound healing, delayed gastric emptying, prolonged resumption of bowel function and heart failure (Bamboat and Bordeianou 2009). The main objectives of fluid management are therefore to preserve good tissue perfusion, ensure adequate oxygen delivery, preserve normal electrolyte concentration and maintain normoglycaemia and pH of the blood (Clancy *et al.* 2002).

Possible actions to preserve fluid balance in postoperative patients include:

- Correcting any pre-existing deficit of fluids and electrolytes
- Supplying basic needs for intravenous fluids
- Replacing unusual fluid losses (e.g. because of surgical drains or pyrexia).

The oral route should be used when possible, if the patient is fully conscious, although this is unlikely immediately following surgery. Some patients may benefit from aggressive preoperative fluid loading guided by invasive monitoring. In some cases, due to stress-related changes in endocrine function, many patients do better when water and sodium intake is restricted. However, it is important to avoid hypovolaemia in the patient during their early postoperative phase. Postoperative management of fluid balance by recovery practitioners, especially in emergency cases, poses a complex problem in finding the right fluid balance. This is because sometimes not all the volumes that have been lost and replaced will be understood by the recovery practitioners or the anaesthetists (Gau and Bartel 2015).

To preserve suitable fluid levels, the recovery practitioner must consider the following points:

- Replacement of the preoperative shortfall caused by preoperative fasting
- Assess the likelihood of the patient being dehydrated for several days before surgery due to illness or disease.
- Give large amounts of fluid postoperatively if the patient had a long period of illness before the surgery.
- Assess the fluid balance and health of the patient after delivering fluid intravenously.
- Assess fluid loss from wound drains, bleeding, urination and so on.
- If the patient is hypothermic, deliver warm intravenous fluids.

Rapid Perioperative Care, First Edition. Paul Wicker and Sara Dalby.

- As the patient warms up, more fluid volume is needed because the circulation improves (Gau and Bartel 2015).

There are different ways to deliver different types of fluids, slow or fast, depending on the state of the patient (SIGN 2004). Actions to consider include:

- If the patient is hypovolaemic because of fasting and surgery, provide the fluid at a high rate as a fluid bolus, but keep the patient under direct observation in case of problems arising.
- Create a maintenance schedule to plan for the appropriate levels and types of fluids.
- Observe the patient's responses; these may include (SIGN 2004):
    - Depressed eyes returning to normal
    - Increased blood pressure
    - Urine output
    - Slowing of tachycardia
    - Skin pallor returning to normal.

Maintenance fluids

Maintaining fluids is used for most patients following trauma or major surgery. The intravenous route is most often used rather than enteral (food or drug administration) maintenance or rehydration treatment, because of the high workloads and actions that recovery staff need to take, utilising their valuable time during recovery. Modern infusion pumps (e.g. MCM 500 by Fresenius) are often used for the delivery of fluids in postoperative patients, and they are considered safe because they also monitor the fluid being delivered and control the quantity of fluids being given to the patient (Wikipedia 2014). It is possible that there may be miscalculations of the infusion rates and possible mistakes regarding dosage errors for additives, for example too much water, or too much salt or electrolytes in the circulation. Under normal circumstances, patients may need:

- 3 L a day for an adult, equivalent to 125 ml/h
- Change 1 L litre bags every 8 h.
- To provide normal body electrolytes – infuse normal saline first, then 5% dextrose (glucose) and finally Ringer's lactate, every 24 h.
- Patients with high electrolytes – may be given 5% glucose which is a replacement for water (Wikipedia 2014).

Other fluid losses can be replaced using solutions containing sodium (normal saline or Hartmann's solution), and potassium at 20 mmol/L can also be added if required (Clancy *et al.* 2002). The fluid regime is normally provided by the anaesthetist, who also gives instructions about the rate and volume to give to the patient. If the patient's condition changes, then the recovery practitioner would need to contact the anaesthetist, so he or she can assess the patient's condition and reorder the necessary fluid needed. Blood transfusions are only given if necessary because of blood loss, and also the potential risk of reactions or infections caused by infusing the blood.

Samples of the patient's blood can be sent to laboratories to estimate the levels of sodium and potassium in the few days following surgery (Gau and Bartel 2015). Normal levels of sodium and potassium are (Bamboat and Bordeianou 2009):

- Sodium: 125–145 mmol/L
- Potassium: 3.5–5.5 mmol/L (potassium supplements may be needed if the quantity is less than 3.5 mmol/L).

Fluid balance chart

The fluid balance chart is used to measure the patient's hourly fluid intake and output while the patient recovers from anaesthesia and surgery. On return to the ward following 24 h, the anaesthetist or ward staff will measure the output (e.g. urine and wound drains) and subtract it from the amount of fluids given to the patient, such as intravenous infusion or oral intake of fluids (Gau and Bartel 2015). The result of the calculation is called the fluid balance.

If the records indicate a positive fluid balance, in other words the fluids and electrolytes in the patient's body are at a high level, then there is more intake than output and the patient may suffer from over-hydration by accumulating water. Outputs such as faeces, sweat, evaporation and conduction cannot be measured, and so they are called insensible losses. A normal healthy adult has a fluid balance of about 1–1.5 L a day to maintain normal fluid levels (Clancy *et al.* 2002).

However, in postoperative patients in recovery, who have been fasting and undergoing anaesthesia and surgery, the fluid balance chart may show high levels of fluids, up to 10 L in the normal adult. During the patient's recovery on the ward, fluid balance needs to revert to the normal 1–1.5 L per day over the following few days (SIGN 2004). However, a severely ill patient may maintain a high level of fluid balance each day, which indicates that an ongoing condition, such as renal failure, is not resolving.

Care of the infusion site

Care of the infusion site is essential to ensure that postoperative infusions continue, to preserve the patient's health (Wikipedia 2014). Issues, such as infusions stopping because the fluid bag is empty, can result in the patient developing hypotension and cardiovascular problems, possibly leading to morbidity on the first night after major surgery. Secure and effective placement of the intravenous cannula, bag and giving set is important. The correct actions to take include:

- Use a vein in a safe position that is secure for the recovery area and the ward.
- Secure the cannula and giving set, carefully using tape or Opsite dressing.
- Use tape that sticks to the skin, and use the wings or other large part of the IV cannula for attachment.

Conclusion

Patients who have undergone major surgery over a long period of time, and have been subject to anaesthetic drugs, can have fluid and electrolyte disorders resulting in morbidity within the hospital. Therefore, maintenance and observation of a patient's fluid levels are essential to support and care for the patient. The use of medicines postoperatively in the recovery can also affect the patient's fluid balance and electrolytes. Recovery practitioners should identify prompt recognition and treatment of severe fluid deficits in postoperative patients, and manage the situation accordingly with the help of the anaesthetist and the surgeon.

77 Postoperative Medications

Medications are given to patients before, during and after surgery, and the types of drugs given to patients vary widely. For example, the anaesthetic drugs received by patients depend on medical conditions they may have. The patient must tell the surgeon and anaesthetist about drugs they have been taking before surgery, because some medications can change the effectiveness of anaesthesia, or may stimulate bleeding during the procedure (Lubin *et al.* 2003).

The drugs that patients receive postoperatively therefore depend on the anaesthesia and surgery that they were undergoing. Various drugs may be given postoperatively, including antibiotics, antifungal agents, analgesics, anticoagulants, anti-emetics and diuretics. The variety of drugs given postoperatively can be very detailed and complex (Hatfield 2014).

Antibiotics

Antibiotics destroy bacteria that cause infection in patients because of surgery or wound infections (Lubin *et al.* 2003). Patients receive antibiotics orally, in pill form or intravenously. During postoperative care. antibiotics would normally be given intravenously; however, antibiotics could also be given to the patient as pills. The antibiotic used depends on the type of surgery, the infection of the wound by particular bacteria, and the physiology of the patient (Hudsmith *et al.* 2004). There are many types of antibiotics which may be given to the patient, including:

- Amoxicillin
- Ampicillin
- Cephalexin
- Piperacillin
- Rifampin
- Vancomycin.

Antifungals

Antifungal medicines are used to treat fungal infections which are most commonly found on the skin, hair and nails (Hatfield 2014). Antifungal drugs treat fungal infections in the body, such as aspergillosis (fungal infection of the lining of the lungs), candidiasis (yeast) or cryptococcal meningitis. Antifungal agents may be given intravenously or in a pill form. Antifungal medicines work by destroying the fungal cells by affecting a substance in the cell walls, causing the contents of the fungal cells to leak out and the cells to die (Hatfield 2014). The antifungal agents can also prevent the fungal cells from growing and reproducing. Some of the most common antifungal agents include:

- Amphotericin (Amphotericin B)
- Flagyl (Metronidazole)
- Nystatin
- Clotrimazole

Rapid Perioperative Care, First Edition. Paul Wicker and Sara Dalby.

- Terbinafine
- Fluconazole
- Ketoconazole.

Analgesics

Recovery practitioners often monitor and watch patients who are in pain and take actions to lower their pain levels. Analgesics control pain before surgery starts, during surgery and after surgery if the pain persists (Radford *et al.* 2004). Analgesic drugs are available to give to the patient in several different ways, for example intravenously, in pill form, as a lozenge, as a suppository, as a liquid taken by mouth or as a skin ointment which is absorbed through the skin.

Analgesics vary in their ability to prevent pain from happening. For example, opioids are strong analgesics which can stop patients from feeling pain; but on the other hand aspirin, which is a nonsteroidal anti-inflammatory drug (NSAID), may only reduce pain a little (Hatfield 2014). Sometimes, this also depends on the dosage which is prescribed to the patient, as these can be different between different patients. Therefore, the medication prescribed depends on the condition of the patient. Many postoperative analgesics are given to patients who are in severe pain in which case opioids are often used, either with or without other analgesics such as paracetamol or NSAIDs. Examples of analgesics used for postoperative patients who are in pain include:

- Codeine
- Meperidine
- Hydromorphone
- Fentanyl
- Hydrocodone
- Morphine
- Oxycodone
- Tramadol.

IV Fluids and electrolytes

Postoperative patients receive intravenous fluids for two main reasons:

- To replace fluids they have lost by fasting before surgery, or because of blood or fluid loss during surgery
- IV fluids are provided because patients cannot drink fluids immediately postoperatively.

Patients in recovery are often prescribed different solutions, depending on their anaesthesia, the length of surgery or the state of their health (Yentis *et al.* 2009). The solution may also change periodically during their stay in recovery, depending on their fluid and electrolyte balance. Patients who are able to take water orally will not need IV fluids as much, and they may be stopped if fluid levels become too high. Examples of fluids delivered to patients include:

- Half-normal saline (0.45% NaCL)
- Normal saline (0.9% NaCl)
- Lactated Ringer's
- 5% Dextrose (Yentis *et al.* 2009).

Electrolytes are minerals that are integrated into fluids and include calcium, chloride, magnesium, phosphate, potassium and sodium (Yentis *et al.* 2009). They are found in blood, body fluids and urine. Postoperative patients absorb electrolytes via IV infusions, medicines and drug supplements. Electrolytes are found in the blood and can support an electrical charge for nerves and especially for helping the heart to maintain its normal rhythm. However, if electrolytes increase or decrease, this can cause disruptions in the heart's function. Electrolytes also help to control fluid balance in the body and are important elements in providing muscle contraction, energy generation and practically every major biochemical reaction in the body (Barone *et al.* 2003, Lubin *et al.* 2003).

Anticoagulants

Anticoagulants are agents that are used to prevent the formation of blood clots or emboli in patients, especially postoperatively if they have been lying supine on the operating table for several hours. Examples of anticoagulant drugs include intravenous heparin which inactivates thrombin and other clotting factors, and oral anticoagulants such as warfarin and dicumarol, which act by inhibiting the liver's production of vitamin K to prevent the formation of blood clots (Yentis *et al.* 2009).

Monitoring and observation of patients to identify blood clots or deep venous thrombosis (DVT) in the legs are important after surgery, because the effects of the surgical procedure may result in blood clots forming in the bloodstream (Hatfield 2014). Anticoagulants may be given during or after surgery, normally using intravenous injections, to prevent blood clots from forming and causing complications such as a stroke or pulmonary embolus. Examples of IV anticoagulants include:

- Argatroban (an anticoagulant used in the prophylaxis and treatment of heparin-induced thrombocytopenia)
- Warfarin
- Heparin
- Enoxaparin (low-molecular-weight heparin).

Diuretics

Diuretics promote the formation of urine by the kidney and therefore increase urination. The use of diuretics causes the patient to reduce in fluids and sodium, but there is relatively little loss of potassium (Barone *et al.* 2003). Diuretics work in different ways and can have different effects on fluid and electrolyte balance, and in some cases they can relieve hypertension (Barone *et al.* 2003). Diuretics also stimulate kidney function and increase the flow of urine. Examples of diuretics include:

- Frusemide (inhibits sodium and potassium)
- Hydrochlorothiazide (HCTZ) (a thiazide diuretic that helps prevent the body from absorbing too much salt)
- Dopamine (promotes sodium excretion)
- Acetazolamide (inhibits H^+ secretion)
- Mannitol (promotes osmotic diuresis).

There are potential effects of diuretics in postoperative patients, which may include hypovolemia, hypokalaemia, hyperkalaemia, hyponatremia, metabolic alkalosis, metabolic acidosis and hyperuricemia (an abnormally high level of uric acid in the blood) (Hudsmith *et al.* 2004).

Antacids

Antacids control acid levels in the patient's stomach. Antacids neutralise the acid in the patient's stomach and help reduce the symptoms of heartburn and provide relief from stomach pain (Hatfield 2014). Antacids can also coat the surface of the oesophagus to protect it against stomach acid. Antacids may be given to patients to help recovery from surgery, because stomachs often continue to produce stomach acids which can lead to nausea, vomiting and gastric pain (Lubin *et al.* 2003). To prevent this from happening, antacids are given. Antacids are available for postoperative patients in liquid form or as chewable tablets. The common ingredients of antacids include aluminium hydroxide, magnesium carbonate and magnesium trisilicate (Hatfield 2014). Examples of antacids include:

- Pepcid
- Cimetidine
- Dulkolax
- Isopan
- Sodium citrate
- Milk of magnesia
- Magnesium oxide.

Mouth care

Mouth care is an important element to consider after surgery, especially for patients who are on a ventilator or who are still unconscious (Hatfield 2014). The recovery practitioner will ensure good mouth care, for example rinsing the mouth with a solution that helps kill bacteria. This can help to prevent pneumonia which may happen if the patient has been intubated and placed on a ventilator. Examples of drugs used for mouth care include:

- Chlorhexidine (an antibacterial agent used as a disinfectant)
- Lidocaine hydrochloride (rapid onset, local anaesthetic)
- Clindamycin (used only for serious bacterial infections)
- Morphine sulphate (only for adults who have moderate to severe mouth pain).

Conclusion

Recovery staff need to understand drugs before offering them to the patient; they need to know how they work, and why they may interact with anaesthetic agents or drugs given during surgery. If the staff do not know about the pharmacological principles of drugs, then they may cause the patient harm. After drugs are given to the patient, they may react quickly and lead to either the patient getting better or negative effects that may lead to morbidity or mortality. However, given the problems associated with the health of the patient following anaesthesia and surgery, it is important to have available a wide range of drugs in the recovery room to support the patient in the best possible way.

78 Managing Bleeding Problems

Recovery practitioners who identify bleeding in patients need to contact the anaesthetist and surgeon urgently to address the issues. The recovery practitioner, however, can manage haemorrhage by using several methods. When identifying bleeding, it is seen as being either local (e.g. a superficial wound haemorrhage) or general (e.g. internal in the abdomen). Haemorrhage is classified at three levels (Daqi 2005):

- Primary haemorrhage (when bleeding occurs during the surgery)
- Reactionary haemorrhage (occurs within the first 24 h of the operation)
- Secondary haemorrhage (occurs up to 10 days following the operation).

Local bleeding is often seen close to the operative site or the wound itself. Bleeding from the wound site may be caused because of excessive movement or stress on the wound site, or infection in the wound. If the wound is internal, it may be caused by gastrointestinal haemorrhage which was caused by rupture of the intestines or leakage from internal surgery. Bleeding that occurs in several different sites, for example the oozing of fresh and unclotted blood from wound edges or bleeding from intravenous cannulae, may be caused by a coagulation problem which may need medication for the patient (Baljinder *et al.* 2010).

Patients who have primary or reactionary bleeding might occur from a blood vessel that was not properly ligated, or was not ligated at all, indicating wrong ligation techniques. During surgery, there may be no bleeding of the blood vessel because of hypotension; although once the patient is in recovery, IV fluids are given and blood pressure rises again, bleeding may well start from an unligated blood vessel. Secondary haemorrhage may be caused by infection which erodes the blood vessel leading to bleeding, caused by rupture of the artery or vein. This may occur when a contaminated wound is closed immediately after surgery, leading to infection and damage of blood vessels. However, it is possible to prevent bleeding by delaying wound closure for a day or more so the wound can be treated by antibiotics (Koh and Hunt 2003).

Postoperative haemorrhage

Postoperative haemorrhage can occur in various ways, including wound bleeding, internal abdominal bleeding, gastrointestinal haemorrhage and various other sites caused by problems with haemostasis. Management of the bleeding will depend on the health of the patient and assessment of the areas that are bleeding. Examples of bleeding problems include:

- A patient with a blood-soaked dressing covering the wound site
- A hypotensive patient with high levels of blood oozing from the wound or collecting in the chest drain or wound drain (Koh and Hunt 2003)
- A patient with a low platelet count resulting in generalised bleeding in several different areas (Hatfield 2014).

Rapid Perioperative Care, First Edition. Paul Wicker and Sara Dalby.

Recovery practitioners may remove the bloody or wet dressing and apply a different dressing to prevent the bleeding by applying pressure. If the surgeon is present, it is likely that he or she will remove the dressing and inspect the wound to try to establish a way of preventing further bleeding. Patients who have a major internal bleed may be taken back to the operating room for internal exploration of the bleeding to prevent it from leading to major complications. Patients with problems because of anticoagulation defects may need medical treatment urgently to prevent constant haemorrhage in all parts of the body (Baljinder *et al.* 2010).

Assessment of postoperative haemorrhage in a patient would be based on clinical observation of bleeding points. Also, practitioners need understanding of the surgical procedure that was carried out, the patient's postoperative progress or lack of progress, and assessment of the patient's vital signs such as blood pressure, circulation, pulse and so on (Parker and Wagner 2015). Any treatment undertaken would depend on the blood loss being identified and any underlying causes. If the patient is hypovolaemic and has circulatory failure, then replacement of fluids will be essential to maintain oxygenation and circulation (Daqi 2005, Kumar and Yeung 2010). Further surgery may be needed if bleeding cannot be stopped or the patient continues to suffer from hypovolaemia or circulatory problems.

Actions to prevent haemorrhage

Recovery practitioners must constantly monitor and observe patients during the recovery phase to assess any problems that may arise. Various actions may need to be taken if haemorrhage occurs or if the patient appears to have low blood pressure and poor circulation. Actions that can be taken by the doctors or the recovery practitioners may include (Koh and Hunt 2003, Daqi 2005, Hatfield 2014):

- Monitor a patient every 15 min as a minimum on entry to the recovery room in case of reactionary haemorrhage, especially monitoring the patient's pulse and blood pressure regularly (Kumar and Yeung 2010). Bleeding may occur because of rupture of a blood vessel, slipped ligature, infected wound or eroded blood vessel.
- When a patient's wound starts to bleed, apply local pressure and packing to reduce blood flow. Minor bleeding is likely to stop after time. If bleeding does not stop, the surgeon should be contacted, and the patient may return to the operating room for further surgery. If the wound is infected, then the patient will need antibiotics.
- The patient's blood pressure may fall postoperatively (Hatfield 2014) because of hypovolaemia as a result of:
  - Bleeding during surgery which has not been replaced
  - Fluid lost during surgery because of removal of tissues or organs
  - Deep anaesthesia leading to depressed respiration, causing hypoxaemia and hypotension
  - Opioids, such as morphine or pethidine, may have been given in large doses because of possible postoperative pain.
  - The patient may have developed septicaemia because of bowel problems or rough handling while moving from the operating table to the trolley.
- The patient needs blood volume restored, fluids and electrolytes replaced and legs raised to improve blood flow in the abdomen and chest (Koh and Hunt 2003).
- The patient may suffer from shock, which may be caused by a fast pulse, pallor, abdominal distension or increased blood loss into a drain incision (Hatfield 2014). This may be the result of bleeding inside their abdomen. Blood transfusion of up to two units may be needed, and if this doesn't work then the patient may need further surgery to prevent and control the bleeding.
- Bleeding from a nasogastric tube may result after surgery on the stomach. If the patient has slightly reduced blood pressure, gastric lavage can be performed every 30 min with iced water containing 8 mg of noradrenalin which should assist in preventing bleeding

(Daqi 2005). If bleeding persists, then further surgery may be required to repair any bleeding problems.

- If the patient's bowels bleed a few days after the surgery, it may be caused by development of an ulcer, or a pre-existing ulcer, perhaps caused by stress or anxiety. This can lead to serious problems such as morbidity and mortality. The patient will need monitoring and observation of his or her pulse, blood pressure and urine output. IV infusions should also be used to maintain fluid and electrolyte balance, and the patient will require his or her haematocrit (the volume of red blood cells in the total volume of blood in his or her body) to be measured every 3 h. Blood bags need to be easily available and cross- matched so they are ready for use if necessary. Cold saline or water containing noradrenalin 8 mg may be irrigated in his or her stomach to reduce the chances of bleeding. (Daqi 2005, Baljinder *et al.* 2010)

Conclusion

Postoperative bleeding can occur immediately following surgery or several days later, both at the incision site or internally inside the body. Because of the loss of blood, postoperative bleeding may lead to morbidity or mortality in the patient. Surgical problems are often the cause of postoperative bleeding, because of vessels not being closed or sudden ruptures following surgery, or organ damage which was not discovered during surgery. Problems such as liver or kidney disease, or haemophilia, can also lead to bleeding disorders in recovery. Various medicines can also lead to bleeding disorders; for example, aspirin can make blood less cohesive and may prevent blood clots. Vitamins and herbs such as vitamin E, ginkgo biloba, ginseng or feverfew can also reduce clotting factors. Following postoperative bleeding, the patient may notice blood soaking through the bandage, develop anxiety and breathe faster, as well as not voiding urine. Postoperative bleeding may be treated by blood transfusion, and clotting factors may be given such as platelets and plasma. Anti-fibrinolytic (inhibitors of fibrinolysis) medicines (Baljinder *et al.* 2010) may also be given to reduce bleeding, and alternatively surgery may be recommenced to discover the cause of bleeding or to repair the blood vessel or organ.

79 Managing Postoperative Nausea and Vomiting

Postoperative nausea and vomiting (PONV) may occur soon after anaesthesia and surgery and can affect up to 30% of patients, although up to 80% of patients at high risk can also develop PONV (Kovac 2000). PONV can be caused by anaesthetic drugs as well as the effects of surgical procedures. This may result in patient discomfort and dissatisfaction as well as higher costs because of extended time spent in the hospital (Chung and Mezei 1999). Patients who vomit may also develop major complications such as aspiration of vomit into their lungs, leading to major airway complications.

PONV is therefore a significant problem for patients, and most patients are often more concerned about PONV than pain. It is therefore important that recovery practitioners monitor and observe patients who suffer from PONV and take actions to treat them to encourage them to be safe and comfortable (Chung and Mezei 1999).

The physiology of PONV

Nausea and vomiting happen because of the effect of anaesthetic drugs and surgery that may affect the stomach or vagus nerve. Vomiting is controlled by the vomiting centre which is located in the medulla. There are five different pathways which stimulate the vomiting centre (Pierre and Whelan 2013, Lewis *et al.* 2015):

- *The chemoreceptor triggering zone*: Found in the medulla oblongata which receives inputs from blood-borne drugs or hormones, and communicates with other structures in the vomiting centre to initiate vomiting
- *The vagal mucosal pathway in the gastrointestinal system*: Where the vagus nerve coordinate responses to intestinal stimuli via the dorsal vagal complex in the brain
- *Neuronal pathways from the vestibular system*: This system contributes to a sense of balance in the human body.
- *Reflex afferent pathways from the cerebral cortex C2,3*: Neuronal pathways leaving the brain and affecting the vomiting centre
- *Midbrain afferents*: Pathways leaving the midbrain and affecting the vomiting centre.

When one or more of these pathways is activated, the vomiting centre is stimulated by receptors such as cholinergic (muscarinic), dopaminergic, histaminergic or serotonergic receptors (Kovac 2000).

The management of PONV

The use of medicines to treat PONV can lead to high costs and sometimes provides risks due to adverse effects of the drugs, especially if they interact with anaesthetic drugs given during surgery. Patients who have minimum effects of PONV don't require medicines, but patients

Rapid Perioperative Care, First Edition. Paul Wicker and Sara Dalby.

who are at high risk due to the effects of anaesthesia and surgery, and potential illness, should be given suitable drugs to oppose the effects of PONV. The estimated probability of PONV can vary from 10% to 78% because of the risks associated with patients (Smith *et al.* 2012). The greatest risk is the use of opioids. There are four main risk factors associated with PONV (Pierre and Whelan 2013):

- *Female*: Women tend to be a bit sicker than men because of possible anxiety levels.
- *Prior history of motion sickness or PONV*: Caused by travelling in cars or previous cases of PONV
- *Non-smoker*: Patients who smoke are less likely to develop PONV due to the drugs within the tobacco, especially nicotine.
- *The use of postoperative opioids*: These can lead to PONV (Chatterjee *et al.* 2011).

Risk factors associated with PONV

There are several risk factors associated with PONV; these are based on patients, anaesthetics and surgery. Examples of possible risks include:

- *Patients*: Female gender (Apfel *et al.* 1999), non-smokers, previous history of PONV or motion sickness
- *Anaesthesia*: Use of volatile anaesthetics for more than 2 h, use of nitrous oxide, use of intraoperative and postoperative opioids, high doses of neostigmine
- *Surgery*: Long duration of surgery, surgery on the stomach or intestines, and surgery on the vagus nerve (Apfel *et al.* 1999).

Surgeons, anaesthetists and recovery practitioners need to be aware of the risk factors associated with PONV, which should then be reduced as much as possible to prevent the onset of PONV.

Reducing PONV in the perioperative period

Some perioperative factors undertaken during anaesthesia and surgery may reduce the risk of PONV (Kovac 2000). This includes several factors:

- Administering regional anaesthetic reduces the chance of PONV compared to general anaesthesia.
- Patients undergoing general anaesthesia should be given propofol which is effective in reducing the risk of PONV compared to other induction agents.
- Avoiding intraoperative and postoperative opioids reduces PONV. The use of NSAIDs decreases the risk of PONV (Miniche *et al.* 2003).
- The appropriate use of oxygen during surgery reduces PONV by reducing the chance of hypoxia or stomach tissues and organ damage.
- Intravenous fluid administration during surgery reduces PONV (Magner *et al.* 2004). Lack of fluids and electrolytes may cause the release of serotonin because of low perfusion in the intestines and a fall in blood pressure caused by induction agents.
- Neostigmine, which reverses non-depolarising muscle relaxants, can result in the increased possibility of PONV, and so should be avoided if possible.

Anti-emetics

The two main groups of anti-emetics are antagonists and agonists. Antagonists include dopaminergic, cholinergic, histaminergic, 5-HT3 and NK-1 drugs (Smith *et al.* 2012, Lewis *et al.* 2015). Antagonists are chemicals that reduce the physiological activity of chemical substances (such as opiates) which act by blocking receptors within the nervous system. Agonists are medications which combine with a receptor on a cell and initiate a reaction or activity that prevents neurotransmitter release to the chemoreceptor trigger zone or vomiting centre in the brain. Agonists include dexamethasone and cannabinoids (Hill *et al.* 2000).

Examples of anti-emetics

1. Ondansetron is used to prevent nausea and vomiting, and can also support headaches, reduce liver enzymes and stop constipation (Lewis *et al.* 2015).
2. Dexamethasone is a corticosteroid which is administered at a dose of 8–10 mg IV and prevents PONV. Smaller doses of 2.5–5 mg may be used, depending on the status of the patient. Dexamethasone helps to release endorphins which elevate the patient's mood and also help to stimulate appetite (Chandrakantan and Glass 2011). There are few adverse effects related to the use of dexamethasone in the management of PONV.
3. Droperidol can be used to block dopamine receptors in the chemoreceptor trigger zone (CTZ). Droperidol is similar to ondansetron for the treatment of PONV. However, droperidol can cause problems in some patients, including heart problems when the QT interval (which represents electrical depolarisation and repolarisation of the ventricles) is elongated and can cause ventricular tachycardia (Lewis *et al.* 2015).
4. Metoclopramide is a drug which is used to block dopamine receptors in the CTZ and vomiting centre. Doses of 50 mg are used to reduce PONV; however, it does produce side effects which can be harmful to the patient, so it tends not to be used as much as ondansetron to prevent PONV.
5. Dimenhydrinate is a commonly used antihistaminic which works efficiently by affecting the high concentration of histamine and muscarinic cholinergic receptors within the vestibular system (Wilhelm *et al.* 2007).
6. Promethazine and prochlorperazine are phenothiazines which act on the central anti-dopaminergic mechanism in the CTZ. However, these drugs are rarely used now because they can cause side effects such as sedation, dizziness and extrapyramidal symptoms (Wilhelm *et al.* 2007).
7. Scopolamine is an anticholinergic that blocks emetic muscarinic receptors in the cerebral cortex and is useful in preventing PONV. However, its use is limited because it can take up to 4 h before it becomes effective and it can also cause side effects (Chandrakantan and Glass 2011).

In high-risk patients, the available agents displayed above are not necessarily effective in the prevention of PONV for the patients. A combination of agents works better since there are four major receptor systems (see above) involved in the development of PONV. Combining 5-HT3 receptor antagonists with ondansetron, droperidol and dexamethasone makes the curing of PONV more effective. It is advisable therefore that a combination of anti-emetics is given to patients to reduce the risk of PONV (Chatterjee *et al.* 2011, Lewis *et al.* 2015).

Other methods for reducing the risk of PONV include the use of acupuncture, ginger root and cannabinoids. Acupoint electrical stimulation may also be used as an alternative therapy for the prevention of PONV.

Rescue treatment for PONV

When the patient has persistent nausea and vomiting, certain drugs should be withheld, such as patient-controlled morphine analgesia; and the presence of blood in the pharynx, or an abdominal obstruction, should be managed before 'rescue therapy' is initiated. If treatment for a particular drug fails, such as dexamethasone or scopolamine, then it should not be repeated, and other anti-emetics should be used instead (Hill *et al.* 2000). If a patient does not recover from the drugs given, then treatment using a 5-HT3 receptor antagonist (e.g. 1 mg ondansetron) may be considered (Hill *et al.* 2000, Lewis *et al.* 2015).

Conclusion

Postoperative nausea and vomiting is a common complication following surgery and anaesthesia, leading to other problems which can cause the patient discomfort and pain, and prolong their stay in Recovery. It is essential therefore that recovery practitioners are aware of PONV issues and take steps to support the patient and reduce the possibility of major complications. In most situations, it is highly effective to use a combination of drugs that have different mechanisms of action to reduce the possibility of PONV by increasing their anti-emetic properties. Practitioners can improve patient satisfaction and reduce direct costs of PONV by monitoring and taking actions for patients who are at risk of nausea and vomiting.

80 Critical Issues in Postoperative Care

Seriously ill patients often undergo high-risk general surgery in every major acute hospital. High-risk patients undergoing major surgery, such as gastrointestinal and vascular procedures, may have up to a 50% risk of complications (ASGBI 2012). Patients who need emergency surgery may develop complications that have to be managed by theatre staff, using many critical care resources and leading to high financial costs (Hatfield 2014).

It is essential that patients who have undergone emergency surgery need efficient and effective management that is patient centred and aimed at reducing their problems. Patient outcomes can vary between patients, especially if problems are not known or understood by recovery practitioners. Hospitals need to identify the clinical pathway for critical patients to ensure that patients at high risk undergo diagnostic tests, have access to anaesthetist and surgeons, have appropriate surgery and are prepared for immediate postoperative care on completion of their surgery (NICE 2007, Peden 2009).

The numbers of practitioners in the NHS are now falling, creating the possibility that surgical patients will receive poor-quality care which has severe implications for patients and the NHS. According to Jhanji *et al.* (2008), over 170,000 patients in the United Kingdom are susceptible to high-risk surgery every year. Almost half of these patients develop significant problems which result in over 25,000 deaths (Jhanji *et al.* 2008). In reality, patients undergoing general surgery because of sudden illness or trauma provide a large percentage of all surgical deaths (ASGBI 2012).

Complications may occur in 50% of patients who undergo normal procedures, resulting in huge increases in their length of stay in the hospital and cost. Because of the rise in the number of elderly people in the United Kingdom, many patients have comorbidities, and those who are over 80 years old normally have emergency surgery rather than elective, leading to higher risks (Hatfield 2014). Postoperative care is therefore essential for all patients to increase the likelihood of quick recovery and safe and comfortable experiences.

Managing sepsis

Surgical patients can become critically ill because of emergency surgery following a major accident, or complications that follow from the surgical procedure. The patient may need urgent help from doctors and practitioners, or help from the cardiac arrest team. However, a patient developing sepsis, which is the development of harmful bacteria and toxins sometimes because of infection in their wound, results in serious complications which are not always treated in the best way, leading to adverse outcomes (ASGBI 2012).

It is therefore a fundamental principle for recovery practitioners to identify critically ill patients at an early stage to provide effective treatment of sepsis and other complications. Guidelines have been written by NICE (2007) and the Department of Health (2009) which offers guidelines for practitioners looking after critically ill patients. Surgical patients can develop serious problems compared to non-surgical patients, including urgent treatment and possibly more complex surgical interventions following assessment of their condition.

Rapid Perioperative Care, First Edition. Paul Wicker and Sara Dalby.

Immediate postoperative care

The care given by the recovery practitioner for the postoperative patient is assessed according to the patient's critical situation. The postoperative pathway would identify the risk of death and serious complications that the patient has succumbed to, and the recovery practitioner must have the appropriate knowledge and skills to deal with critically ill surgical patients (ASGBI 2012).

Following surgery, doctors and recovery staff must assess the level of critical care needed by the patient, and failing to understand the critical physiological state or the level of organ dysfunction may lead to the patient's death. Critical care is therefore essential for seriously ill patients and should be carried out immediately on entry to the recovery room. However, staff may be relatively inexperienced with treating patients needing critical care, or they may be tired or dealing with issues they are not familiar with. Therefore, it would be logical to assess the patient near to the end of surgery in order to set up a plan for the patient's care. Examples of assessment of the patient include the Apgar score (Gawande 2007) or the surgical assessment developed by Peden (2009) which identifies, by a preoperative assessment, the risk of morbidity or mortality and the chances of deteriorating during the surgical procedure. Actions to take postoperatively in a high-risk patient may include:

- Risk assessment for likelihood of mortality above 5% (high risk)
- Assess arterial blood gases and oxygen, lactate in blood and acid–base status.
- Assess fluid and electrolyte levels, and identify continuing fluid needs.
- Reverse muscle relaxant drugs by using neostigmine and a nerve stimulator to assess muscle reactions.
- Assess the patient's temperature, and treat the patient as needed (Peden 2009).

Following assessment of the patient's high risk in the recovery room, the surgeon and anaesthetist may decide on the patient being admitted to an intensive care unit (ICU) to support as much as possible the patient's condition (DoH 2009). The above criteria will act as an addition to existing assessment within the ICU.

Postoperative care

Skills in delivering critical care are essential to provide suitable postoperative care for high-risk patients, so complications can be identified early and patients do not undergo major problems. High-risk patients are often managed after surgery in an intensive care bay in the recovery room. Hospitals need to prepare critical care resources and bays to fully support high-risk patients. Examples of the levels of care needed for high-risk or critical care patients may include frequent observations, basic resuscitation, high dependency needs or transport to an ICU for multiple organ support (TICS 2009).

High-risk postoperative patients need to have an updated clinical management plan which would involve haemodynamic and blood gas parameters, continuing antibiotics, nutrition and thromboembolic prophylaxis (TICS 2009). Also, practitioners must be aware of any deterioration in organ function so that timely intervention will help to optimise the patient's health. Monitoring high-risk patients may be difficult in a recovery room if the staffing ratio is not adequate, given the potential number of patients and the reduction in staffing levels across the NHS. The hospital therefore has to address issues regarding staff shortages in order to deliver a reliable care pathway for the patient.

Postoperative care of the high-risk patient would include a clinical pathway. A basic example of actions to take may include:

Principles of Care

Develop a postoperative plan that includes the diagnosis, the surgical procedure and the patient's clinical condition.

Constantly monitor the patient for early detection of acute organ dysfunction.
Provide mobilisation at the earliest opportunity.

Interventions

Carry out a minimum of once-hourly observations following surgery.
Provide antibiotic therapy, dependent on surgical diagnosis.
Provide chest physiotherapy and mobilisation when suitable.
Provide a nutritional regime when suitable.
Provide DVT prophylaxis following assessment of poor circulation.
Monitor fluid balance regularly.
Provide postoperative pain relief when needed, regularly.
Consider admission to a critical care unit or ICU following assessment of the patient's condition (Nice 2007, Peden 2009, Hatfield 2014).

Conclusion

Postoperative care of high-risk patients requires overall recognition and a strategy for the care of all patients at high risk of death and complications. Identifying high-risk patients must be a formal part of preoperative and postoperative patient assessment and be included in the preoperative checklist. Forming a clinical pathway for such patients can help to identify major problems and ways to solve them. This clinical pathway should identify:

- Risk of death
- The needs of the patient
- Diagnostic tests
- Timing of surgery and postoperative location of care (Recovery, Intensive Care Unit or Critical Care Ward) (TICS 2009).

The surgeon and anaesthetist would assess the patient's risks and health status and provide guidance for recovery staff on the treatment and care of the patient. One of the major risks for patients is the development of sepsis, which can be severe enough to cause mortality or severe morbidity.

As healthcare increases in complexity and the ageing population grows, patients need a high level of care to ensure they recover safely from their surgery and anaesthesia. Recovery staff therefore need knowledge and skills to assess, recognise and manage the patient's deterioration quickly; otherwise, it may result in unnecessary deaths. Junior members of staff may not recognise the patient's deteriorating physiology and signs of clinical deterioration, and they may misunderstand the need for oxygen therapy, management of fluid balance and so on. It is therefore essential that recovery staff are fully trained and knowledgeable about the health of patients to ensure their health and well-being following anaesthesia and surgery.

81 Enhanced Recovery

Introduction

Enhanced recovery provides better care for patients and is used in many hospitals throughout the NHS to help patients recover faster and to be safer. However, some patients are not suitable for enhanced recovery, and also some hospitals do not provide enhanced recovery.

After enhanced recovery was developed, it was offered to healthy patients to increase their recovery rates. This made an impact on recovery practitioners, who understood the advantages of faster recovery compared to normal recovery rates. The enhanced recovery programme (ERP) is now used in many hospitals for patients having major operations, to provide better care to patients and to reduce the time spent in the hospital (RCA 2012).

There are two important elements related to enhanced recovery, in order to provide the best care to the patients. These include clear communication with the patient, which provides the best information and explanation of the anaesthesia or surgery, and an organised sequence of postoperative care in the form of a care pathway (RCA 2012). The established care pathway enables all practitioners to work well together following the same pathway. Communication would allow patients to be involved in their treatment and to know what was happening at every stage of their recovery (Cottle 2013). This would result in less anxiety and fear and reduced stress following the operation (Hollins and Mavrommatis 2012). This pathway leads to the patient being more confident with the recovery and also feeling better physically. Information about ongoing treatment should therefore be provided to the patient at every stage of the pathway to ensure they fully understand the actions to be taken (Archer *et al.* 2014).

Communication

The enhanced recovery team communicates with patients in several different ways to provide them with the information they need about preoperative care. The steps required include:

- A specialist doctor or nurse will tell the patient of the benefits of surgery and also any risks they may meet. The patient will agree or disagree to the surgery depending on the outcomes (Hollins and Mavrommatis 2012, Cottle 2013).
- The patient will be advised to improve their recovery period; this may include not smoking, staying physically active, checking blood pressure and not taking alcohol (RCA 2012).
- The patient is informed at a pre-assessment clinic about the expected anaesthetic drugs to be given, and methods of pain relief.
- Enhanced recovery care pathways provide paper for the patient to write down their progress and concerns on a day-to-day basis (DoH 2010).
- Information about caring for the patient at home is provided, for example food, water, resting, not smoking, no alcohol and so on. This may help the patient's confidence and well-being at home, with the help of family members (Archer *et al.* 2014).

Rapid Perioperative Care, First Edition. Paul Wicker and Sara Dalby.

Enhanced recovery

There are six sections of enhanced recovery (RCA 2012) to guide theatre and recovery staff in preparing the patient for surgery and for postoperative recovery:

1. Referral from primary care: involvement of the GP
2. Preoperative care by the hospital team
3. Admission to hospital
4. Care during the operation by the surgeon and the anaesthetist
5. Postoperative care in the hospital
6. Follow-up – rehabilitation and going home (RCA 2012).

Step one: Referral from primary care: Involvement of the GP

Patients should be as healthy as possible before surgery to improve their recovery following surgery. Health checks could include diseases or illnesses the patient already has, such as heart disease, asthma or high blood pressure, which should be managed as well as possible by the GP (DoH 2010). Recovery is also faster and safer if certain activities are stopped before surgery, for example stopping smoking or drinking alcohol. Staying active is also beneficial for postoperative recovery; regular and moderate exercising helps to keep the patient healthy and fit before surgery (RCA 2012). Tests may also be needed before surgery, for example anaemia, regular blood loss, poor diet, low iron levels, or a range of chronic diseases such as diabetes or allergies (RCA 2012). Patients with diabetes need support from GPs, doctors or specialist diabetes nurses in order to control blood sugar levels as much as possible. They may suggest the patient loses weight and increases their physical activity, which can help reduce diabetic problems.

Step two: Preoperative care by the hospital team

Patients need to understand the processes for anaesthesia and surgery, how they will feel postoperatively and actions that can be taken if things go wrong. This will make the patient feel more confident, relaxed and comfortable during their recovery, enabling a faster recovery time (Archer *et al.* 2014).

Patients have the right to ask questions to doctors and staff in order for them to understand the processes and actions that will be taken during perioperative care (RCA 2012). Patients who attend a pre-assessment clinic may ask various questions, including:

- *What is the status of my general health?* Nurses will give the patient information leaflets and will answer their questions.
- *What type of anaesthetic will I have?* This will be discussed by the anaesthetist.
- *Will I be in pain following surgery?* The nurse will outline details of pain medication and any further options.
- *How is my operation going to progress?* The surgeon will outline the details of surgery, the reasons for it and the advantages of the surgical procedure (Hollins and Mavrommatis 2012).
- *What happens after surgery?* Healthcare professionals (e.g. nurses, doctors, physiotherapists and occupational therapists) will provide information about caring following the surgical procedure, for example using crutches, how to sit down, use of a urinary catheter, changes to home life and so on (Hollins and Mavrommatis 2012).

Enhanced recovery pathways also provide new and different elements of care, compared to normal recovery. This could include drinking water up to 2 h before surgery, to prevent hypovolaemia. Water can also be taken following recovery from anaesthesia and surgery, normally on return to the ward (Cottle 2013). Preparation of the bowel, before bowel surgery, used to be a traditional method to empty faeces. However, nowadays this is less likely to occur because flushing of the bowels can lead to loose motions, dehydration and imbalance of salts in the blood (RCA 2012). On discharge, the recovery team will assess the patient's condition and give advice on actions to take if problems occur after leaving the recovery room or the hospital.

Step three: Admission to hospital

The enhanced recovery team advise the patient to sleep well the night before surgery and to enter the hospital on the day of surgery, so they are kept relaxed and at ease before surgery (Cottle 2013). When the patient arrives in the hospital admissions area, the surgeon, anaesthetist and enhanced recovery staff visit the patient to ensure that the patient is prepared for the surgery and to answer any questions asked by the patient. Small amounts of food, water or carbohydrate drinks can be given to the patient at least 2 h before surgery (Archer *et al.* 2014). The staff will also instruct the patient to stop drinking, eating, smoking and anything else that is necessary within 2 h before surgery. Pre-medication tablets or injections may be given to the patient to help them relax, especially if they are feeling anxious. The patient will probably walk to the operating theatre if he or she is capable of doing so.

Step four: Care during the operation by the surgeon and the anaesthetist

The surgeon, anaesthetist and theatre staff will take care of the patient during surgery, such as minimally invasive surgery, laparoscopic surgery, orthopaedic surgery and so on (Hollins and Mavrommatis 2012). This can include various actions including careful positioning, using head rests, adding deep vein thrombosis (DVT) stockings, placing jelly pads under certain parts of the body and so on. Other actions to be taken during surgery may also include:

- Ensuring the patient is comfortable on the operating table and does not suffer pain, for example due to joint stiffness, pressure sores or neck pain.
- *Fluid balance therapy*: This is managed by the anaesthetist to ensure fluid levels remain stable (Cottle 2013).
- *Anaesthesia*: The anaesthetist will give anaesthetic drugs which act quickly and allow faster recovery, for example propofol. Anti-emetic drugs may also be given, as well as local anaesthetics to prevent pain in the surgical site on awakening (Cottle 2013).
- *Preventing hypothermia*: This is essential during surgery because the patient may on occasion succumb to loss of body heat, leading to major problems regarding the cardiothoracic system. This may involve using a warm mattress, a Bair Hugger, heated irrigation fluids and warm blankets (Bernard 2014). The patient's temperature will be monitored regularly to maintain normal temperatures (RCA 2012).
- *Nasogastric tubes*: These are used when patients have abdominal surgery to help prevent aspiration of stomach contents into the lungs. However, they are uncomfortable for patients, so they may be avoided whenever possible (DoH 2010).

Step five: Postoperative care in the hospital (Photo 9)

Several actions can be taken to enhance the recovery of the patient in hospital the day after surgery has completed (RCA 2012). This may include:

- *Being active*: Encourage the patient to move around once they have recovered from the anaesthetic drugs and surgery. Walking around helps to prevent deep vein thrombosis and chest infection, and it encourages the stomach and bowel to accept and absorb food (Archer *et al.* 2014). The enhanced recovery team will encourage the patient to be active and may write down notes of examples of what the patient can do following

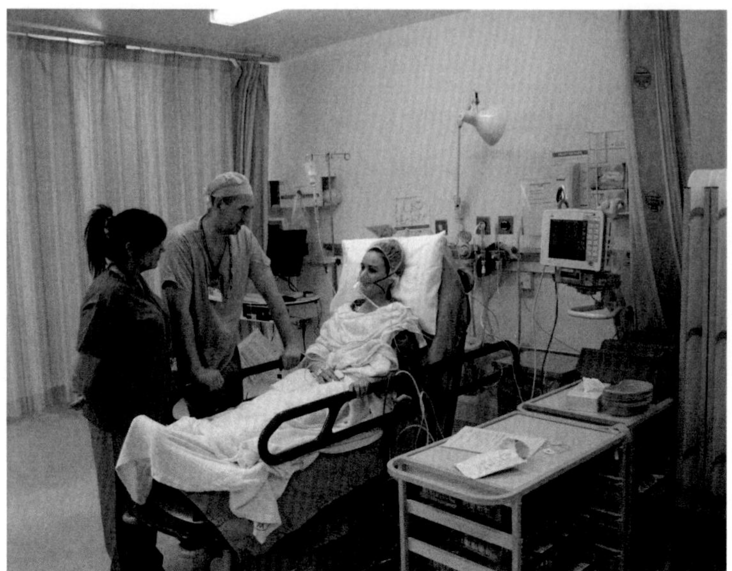

Photo 9 Moving to the ward. Courtesy of Aintree Hospital, Liverpool

recovery from surgery. The enhanced recovery team will also monitor levels of pain and treat them accordingly.

- *Eating and drinking*: This is encouraged as soon as the patient has fully recovered from anaesthesia and is capable of eating and drinking following surgery. The enhanced recovery team will specify the timing and type of food and drink which will provide nutrients for the patient to help them recover faster (Cottle 2013). Removing an IV line once the patient starts eating and drinking will enable them to move around more easily, use the toilet, take pain tablets and so on.

Step six: Follow-up – rehabilitation and going home

Even when patients leave the hospital, they need to be cared for by GPs, doctors or nurses at home to ensure they are kept safe and do not suffer any problems. This is normally planned out by the pre-assessment team and discussed further with the GP (RCA 2012). Two main examples of actions to take include:

- *Going home*: Discharge planning is undertaken by the pre-assessment team to ensure the patient is prepared for going home and has all the necessary medicines or equipment needed. The date of discharge will be given to the patient and his or her family, as well as any social services that are required.
- *24-hour telephone helpline* (DoH 2010): Patients need to know how to contact hospital staff urgently in case problems arise once they are home. This will enhance the patient's confidence and reduce anxiety. Sometimes, the enhanced recovery staff might contact the patient to ensure they are still safe and comfortable, and request any questions the patient may want to ask. The patient may also be encouraged to visit their GP or contact emergency services if there are problems arising.

Summary

The benefit of enhanced recovery is to improve the experience and health of patients undergoing major surgery. Enhanced recovery helps patients to recover from anaesthesia and surgery faster so that they can return home as quickly as possible to return to a normal life. The four main stages of enhanced recovery (pre-admission planning, reducing stress, perioperative management and early mobilisation) support patient care and enable them to recover quickly by acting on the enhanced recovery staff's suggestions, to bring them back to better health (DoH 2010).

References and Further Reading

69. Recovery Room Design

References

Dzubow L (2011) Room for Recovery: What the Hospital Room of the Future Looks Like. Available at http://www.oprah.com/health/Hospital-Room-Design-Better-Hospitals-Hospital-Room-Recovery_1 (accessed 18 February 2015)

Gordon D (2007) Preop, PACU, and Stage 2 Recovery. Healthcare Design. Available at http://www.healthcaredesignmagazine.com/article/pre-op-pacu-and-stage-2-recovery (accessed 18 February 2015)

Haruguchi K (2011) Improving Recovery Rooms with Design. Available at http://visualsyntax.net/wordpress/wp-content/uploads/2011/05/kousaku_haruguchi_mm_process_guide_2011.pdf (accessed 18 February 2015)

Hatfield A and Tronson M (2014) *The Complete Recovery Book*, 5th ed. Oxford, Oxford University Press.

Healthcare Facilities Today (2014) Hospital Room Design Boosts Patient Recovery Times. Available at http://www.healthcarefacilitiestoday.com/posts/Hospital-room-design-boosts-patient-recovery-times-Interior-Design–6721 (accessed 18 February 2015)

Wicker P and Cox F (2010) Patient Care during Recovery. In Wicker P and O'Neill J (eds) *Caring for the Perioperative Patient*. Chichester, Wiley-Blackwell, pp. 379–412.

Further Reading

Sullivan K (2014) Strategic Hospital Room Design Hastens Patient Recovery, Minimizes Staff Errors. Available at http://www.fiercehealthcare.com/story/strategic-hospital-room-design-hastens-patient-recovery-minimizes-staff-err/2014-08-25 (accessed 19 February 2015)

Wiklund PE (1965) Design of a Recovery Room and Intensive Care Unit. *Journal of the American Society of Anesthesiologists*. Available at http://anesthesiology.pubs.asahq.org/article.aspx?articleid=1965769 (accessed 19 February 2015)

Websites

Labor–Delivery–Recovery Room Design That Facilitates Non-pharmacological Reduction of Labor Pain: http://perkinswill.com/sites/default/files/ID%208_PWRJ_Vol0601_07_Labor-Delivery-Recovery%20Room%20Design.pdf (accessed 19 February 2015)

Recovery Room Care of the Surgical Patient: http://www.brooksidepress.org/Products/Nursing_Care_of_the_Surgical_Patient/lesson_3_Section_1.htm (accessed 18 February 2015)

Videos

A Look inside the New Oakville Hospital: https://www.youtube.com/watch?v=Zo8DUqeSslU (accessed 19 February 2015)

Post Anesthesia Care Unit: https://www.youtube.com/watch?v=ZrdaVEsz9MYandlist=PLojFpb1F-_7ZrlrUxjwdxX_AasR42tc6P (accessed 19 February 2015)

Post Anesthesia Care Unit 2013 – "I Want a Room with a View": https://www.youtube.com/watch?v=BsV0r9SWXbU (accessed 19 February 2015)

Postoperative Recovery: http://www.youtube.com/watch?v=BLKEUHYr9ls (accessed 19 February 2015)

Rapid Perioperative Care, First Edition. Paul Wicker and Sara Dalby.

70. Patient Handover

References

Catchpole KR, de Leval MR, McEwan A, Pigott N, Elliott MJ, McQuillan A *et al.* (2007) Patient Handover from Surgery to Intensive Care: Using Formula 1 Pit-Stop and Aviation Models to Improve Safety and Quality. *Paediatric Anaesthesia* **17** (5): 470–478.

Hatfield A (2014) *The Complete Recovery Book*, 5th ed. Oxford, Oxford University Press.

Nagpal K, Arora S, Abboudi M, Vats A, Wong HW, Manchanda C *et al.* (2010) Postoperative Handover: Problems, Pitfalls, and Prevention of Error. *Annals of Surgical Journal* **252**: 171–176.

Smith AF, Mishra K (2010) Interaction between Anaesthetists, Their Patients, and the Anaesthesia Team. *British Journal of Anaesthesia* **105** (1): 60–68.

Further Reading

Lipp A (2007) *Recovery for Day Surgery Units*. London, British Association of Day Surgery.

Smith AF, Pope C, Goodwin D, Mort M (2008) Interprofessional Handover and Patient Safety in Anaesthesia: Observational Study of Handovers in the Recovery Room. *British Journal of Anaesthesia* **101**: 332–337.

van Rensen EL, Groen ES, Numan SC, Smit MJ, Cremer OL, Tates K, Kalkman CJ (2012) Multitasking during Patient Handover in the Recovery Room. *Anesthesia and Analgesia Journal* **115** (5): 1183–1187.

Websites

A Framework for Clinical Handover: http://www.safetyandquality.gov.au/wp-content/uploads/2012/02/SHARED-communications.pdf (accessed 20 February 2015)

Handover in Recovery: http://www.medscape.com/viewarticle/725242_7 (accessed 20 February 2015)

Interprofessional Handover and Patient Safety in Anaesthesia: Observational Study of Handovers in the Recovery Room: http://bja.oxfordjournals.org/content/101/3/332.short (accessed 20 February 2015)

Videos

Handover in Recovery: https://www.youtube.com/watch?v=hHyLc_5DuFs (accessed 19 February 2015)

Know the Plan, Share the Plan, Review the Risk (Part 3 – Operating Theatre Recovery to Ward): https://www.youtube.com/watch?v=H6BSace51Zg (accessed 19 February 2015)

Nursing Communication: Handover from Theatres: https://www.youtube.com/watch?v=kXAeYe7i52o (accessed 19 February 2015)

POST OP Initial Assessment: https://www.youtube.com/watch?v=sdnM5ZuPfl0 (accessed 19 February 2015)

71. Postoperative Patient Care

References

The Association of Anaesthetists of Great Britain and Ireland (2013) *Immediate Post-anaesthesia Recovery 2013*. London, AAGBI. Available at http://www.aagbi.org/sites/default/files/immediate_post-anaesthesia_recovery_2013.pdf (accessed 21 February 2015)

Augistinos P, Ouriel K (2004) Treatment of Venous Thromboembolism. *Circulation* **110**: 1–27. Available at http://circ.ahajournals.org/content/110/9_suppl_1/I-27.full (accessed 22 February 2015)

Hatfield A (2014) *The Complete Recovery Book*, 5th ed. Oxford, Oxford University Press.

Jevon P and Ewans U (2007) *Monitoring the Critically Ill Patient*. Oxford, Blackwell Science Ltd.

Leigh KL, Jones C, Day A (2011) Optimising Perioperative Care: Enhanced Recovery following Colorectal Surgery. *Journal of Perioperative Practice* **21** (7): 239–243.

Narani KK (2010) Deep Vein Thrombosis and Pulmonary Embolism – Prevention, Management, and Anaesthetic Considerations. *Indian Journal of Anaesthesia* **54** (1): 8–17. Available at http://www.ncbi.nlm.nih.gov/pmc/articles/PMC2876903/ (accessed 22 February 2015)

National Institute for Health and Care Excellence (NICE) (2011) *Venous Thromboembolism: Reducing the Risk of Venous Thromboembolism (Deep Vein Thrombosis and Pulmonary Embolism) in Patients Undergoing Surgery*. London, NICE. Available at http://guidance.nice.org.uk/CG92 (accessed 22 February 2015)

Ramsay MAE (2000) Acute Postoperative Pain Management. *BUMC Proceedings Journal* **13** (3): 244–247. Available at http://www.ncbi.nlm.nih.gov/pmc/articles/PMC1317048/ (accessed 22 February 2015)

Scott B (2012) Airway Management in Post Anaesthetic Care. *Journal of Perioperative Practice* **22** (4): 135–138.

Vizcaychipi MP (2013) A Descriptive Review of Magnesium in Homeostasis. *Journal of Operating Department Practitioners* **1** (1): 2–7.

Wicker P and Cox F (2010) Patient Care during Recovery. In Wicker P and O'Neill J (eds) *Caring for the Perioperative Patient.* Chichester, Wiley-Blackwell, pp. 379–412.

Further Reading

Akhtar A, MacFarlane RJ, Waseem M (2013) Pre-Operative Assessment and Post-Operative Care in Elective Shoulder Surgery. *Open Orthopaedic Journal* **7**: 316–322. Available at http://www.ncbi.nlm.nih.gov/pmc/articles/PMC3788190/ (accessed 21 February 2015)

Liddle C (2013) Postoperative Care 1: Principles of Monitoring Postoperative Patients. *Nursing Times* **109** (22): 24–26.

Rhodes A and Cecconi M (2013) Can Surgical Outcomes Be Prevented by Postoperative Admission to Critical Care? *Critical Care Journal* **17**: 110.

Websites

Postoperative Care: http://www.who.int/surgery/publications/Postoperativecare.pdf (accessed 21 February 2015)

Postoperative Care: http://www.healthline.com/health/postoperative-care#Overview1 (accessed 21 February 2015)

Postoperative Care: http://www.surgeryencyclopedia.com/Pa-St/Postoperative-Care.html (accessed 21 February 2015)

Pre and Post Op Care: http://shswebspace.swan.ac.uk/HNHarveys/module%205/Pre%20and%20Post%20op%20Care.ppt (accessed 21 February 2015)

Videos

Caring for the Postoperative Patient: https://www.youtube.com/watch?v=0wSkUPiOQoA (accessed 21 February 2015)

General Postoperative Instructions: https://www.youtube.com/watch?v=m5uhJ1MDHfM (accessed 21 February 2015)

Postoperative Care Content Map: https://www.youtube.com/watch?v=ayYRWiyRlFUandlist=PLB8BC6E48B009AABB (accessed 21 February 2015)

Pre and Postoperative Care: https://www.youtube.com/watch?v=XZq1gExGh8k (accessed 21 February 2015)

72. Postoperative Patient Monitoring and Equipment

References

Association of Anaesthetists of Great Britain and Ireland (AAGBI) (2013) *Immediate Post-anaesthesia Recovery 2013*. London, AAGBI. Available at http://www.aagbi.org/sites/default/files/immediate_post-anaesthesia_recovery_2013.pdf (accessed 23 February 2015)

Bernard H (2014) The Importance of Patient Warming for Enhanced Recovery. *Journal of Operating Department Practitioners* **2** (4): 166–172.

Chenitz KB, Lane-Fall MB (2012) Decreased Urine Output and Acute Kidney Injury in the PACU. *Journal of Anesthesiology Clinics* **30** (3): 513–526.

Hatfield A (2014) *The Complete Recovery Book*, 5th ed. Oxford, Oxford University Press.

The Joanna Briggs Institute (JBI) (2011) Post-Anesthetic Discharge Scoring Criteria. *Best Practice Journal* **15** (17): 1–4.

Rawlinson A, Kitchingham N, Hart C, *et al.* (2012) Mechanisms of Reducing Postoperative Pain, Nausea and Vomiting: A Systematic Review of Current Techniques. *Journal of Evidence Based Medicine* **17**: 75–80.

Royal College of Physicians and the Royal College of Psychiatrists (2003) The Psychological Care of Medical Patients: A Practical Guide. Available at http://www.rcpsych.ac.uk/files/pdfversion/cr108.pdf (accessed 23 February 2015)

Shepherd A (2011) Measuring and Managing Fluid Balance. *Nursing Times* **107** (28): 12–16.

Smith HS, Smith EJ, Smith BR (2012) Postoperative Nausea and Vomiting. *Annals of Palliative Medicine* **1** (2): 94–102.

Further Reading

Reid J, Robb E, Stone D, Bowen P, Baker R, Irving S, *et al.* (2004) Improving the Monitoring and Assessment of Fluid Balance. *Nursing Times* **100** (20): 36–39.

Task Force on Postanesthetic Care (2002) Care Practice Guidelines for Postanesthetic Care. *Anesthesiology* **96**: 742–752.

Sign (2015) Principles of Postoperative Management. Available at http://www.sign.ac.uk/pdf/qrg77.pdf (accessed 23 February 2015)

Websites

Monitoring of Neuromuscular Block: http://ceaccp.oxfordjournals.org/content/6/1/7.full (accessed 23 February 2015)

Principles of Monitoring Postoperative Patients: http://www.nursingtimes.net/Journals/2013/05/31/g/l/a/050613-Principles-of-monitoring-postoperative-patients.pdf (accessed 23 February 2015)

Standards of Monitoring during Anaesthesia and Recovery: http://www.aagbi.org/sites/default/files/standardsofmonitoring07.pdf (accessed 23 February 2015)

Videos

Post-operative Invasive Cardiac Monitoring: https://www.youtube.com/watch?v=cFeH-a1ld3I (accessed 23 February 2015)

POST OP Initial Assessment: https://www.youtube.com/watch?v=sdnM5ZuPfl0 (accessed 23 February 2015)

Reducing the Incidence of Postoperative Cognitive Dysfunction: https://www.youtube.com/watch?v=XCmaq_D0IQ8 (accessed 23 February 2015)

The Role of Active Monitoring and Recognising Postoperative Complications: https://www.youtube.com/watch?v=ibDi0Xle9uU (accessed 23 February 2015)

73. Maintaining the Airway

References

American Heart Association (2005) Guidelines for Cardiopulmonary Resuscitation and Emergency Cardiovascular Care. Part 4: Adult Basic Life Support. *Circulation* **112**: IV-19–V-34.

American Heart Association (2005) Guidelines for Cardiopulmonary Resuscitation and Emergency Cardiovascular Care. Part 7.1: Adjuncts for Airway Control and Ventilation. *Circulation* **112**: IV-51–IV-57.

Dalal P and Taylor A (2004) *Essentials of Airway Management*. London, Greenwich Media Ltd.

Hatfield A (2014) *The Complete Recovery Book*, 5th ed. Oxford, Oxford University Press.

Scott B (2012) Airway Management in Post Anaesthetic Care. *Journal of Perioperative Practice* **22** (4): 13–38.

Further Reading

Euliano TY and Gravenstein JS (2004). *Essential Anesthesia: From Science to Practice*. Cambridge, Cambridge University Press, pp. 24–27.

Oakley M (2009) Airway Management in Recovery. *British Journal of Anaesthetic and Recovery Nursing* **5** (1): 5–8.

World Health Organization (2015) Postoperative Care. Available at http://www.who.int/surgery/publications/Postoperativecare.pdf (accessed 24 February 2015)

Websites

Airway Management Postoperatively: http://www.evidence.nhs.uk/search?q=airway%20management%20post%20op (accessed 24 February 2015)

Recovery Position: http://www.nhs.uk/Conditions/Accidents-and-first-aid/Pages/The-recovery-position.aspx (accessed 24 February 2015)

Sedation Airway Management: http://www.sgna.org/issues/sedationfactsorg/patientcare_safety/airway management.aspx (accessed 24 February 2015)

Videos

Airway Management with Simple Adjuncts – Respiratory Medicine: https://www.youtube.com/watch?v=U4FrtssdyEQ (accessed 24 February 2015)

Basic Airway Management 1: https://www.youtube.com/watch?v=etPa9oxVWyU (accessed 24 February 2015)

How to Open the Airways: https://www.youtube.com/watch?v=2fnS8mtqzms (accessed 24 February 2015)

Preoperative Airway Management Training: https://www.youtube.com/watch?v=HJddgaDaFNk (accessed 24 February 2015)

74. Diagnosis and Management of Postoperative Infection

References

Centre for Disease Control (CDC) (1998) Perspectives in Disease Prevention and Health Promotion Update: Universal Precautions for Prevention of Transmission of Human Immunodeficiency Virus, Hepatitis B Virus and Other Blood Borne Pathogens in Healthcare Settings. *Morbidity and Mortality Weekly Report* **37** (24): 377–388.

Dewan PA, Van Rij AM, Robinson RG, Skeggs GB, Fergus M (1987) The Use of an Iodophor-Impregnated Plastic Incise Drape in Abdominal Surgery – A Controlled Clinical Trial. *Australian and New Zealand Journal of Surgery* **57** (11): 859–863.

Goodman T and Spry C (2014) *Essentials of Perioperative Nursing*, 5th ed. Burlington MA, Jones and Bartlett Learning.

Makki D, Probert N, Gedela V, Kustos I, Thonse R, Banim R (2015) Lifting Incise Drapes off the Skin during Wound Closure Can Cause Contamination. *Journal of Perioperative Practice* **25** (5): 112–114.

National Institute for Health and Clinical Excellence (2008) Surgical Site Infection. Available at http://www.nice.org.uk/guidance/cg74/resources/guidance-surgical-site-infection-pdf (accessed 26 February 2015)

National Institute for Health and Clinical Excellence (2012) Infection: Prevention and Control of Healthcare-Associated Infections in Primary and Community Care. Available at http://www.nice.org.uk/nicemedia/live/13684/58656/58656.pdf (accessed 26 February 2015)

World Health Organization (2006) Key Elements of Standard Precautions. Available at http://www.who.int/csr/resources/publications/4EPR_AM2.pdf (accessed 26 February 2015)

Further Reading

Association of Peri-Operative Registered Nurses (AORN) (2012) *Perioperative Standards and Recommended Practices*. Denver, AORN.

Dinah F and Adhikari A (2006) Gauze Packing of Open Surgical Wounds: Empirical or Evidence-Based Practice? *Annals of the Royal College of Surgeons England* **88** (1): 33–36. Available at http://www.ncbi.nlm.nih.gov/pmc/articles/PMC1963638/ (accessed 26 February 2015)

Vermeulen H, Ubbink D, Goossens A, Vor R, Legemate D (2004) Dressings and Topical Agents for Surgical Wounds Healing by Secondary Intention. *Cochrane Database of Systematic Reviews* (2): CD003554.

World Health Organization (WHO) (2009) *WHO Guidelines on Hand Hygiene in Health Care*. Geneva, WHO.

Websites

Common Postoperative Complications: http://www.patient.co.uk/doctor/common-postoperative-complications (accessed 26 February 2015)

Fever in the Postoperative Patient: http://www.antimicrobe.org/e23.asp (accessed 26 February 2015)

Postoperative Infections: http://jama.jamanetwork.com/article.aspx?articleid=186132 (accessed 26 February 2015)
Standard Precautions and Infection Control: http://www.ashm.org.au/images/publications/monographs/HIV_viral_hepatitis_and_STIs_a_guide_for_primary_care/hiv_viral_hep_chapter_13.pdf (accessed 26 February 2015)

Videos

Ayliffe Hand Washing Technique: http://www.youtube.com/watch?v=EwjDShmfFHM (accessed 26 February 2015)
Infection Prevention in the Operating Room: http://www.youtube.com/watch?v=TuYEcS_bezU (accessed 26 February 2015)
Postoperative infection: https://www.youtube.com/watch?v=uk3_YX2mj28 (accessed 26 February 2015)
Surgical Site Infection: Where Are We Today?: https://www.youtube.com/watch?v=iMqrxfMHOEk (accessed 26 February 2015)

75. Postoperative Pain Management

References

Carr E, Layzell M, Christensen M (2010) *Advancing Nursing Practice in Pain Management*. Chichester, Wiley-Blackwell.
Hall JE, Uhrich TD, Barney JA, Arain SR, Ebert TJ (2000) Sedative, Amnestic, and Analgesic Properties of Small-Dose Dexmedetomidine Infusions. *Anesthesia and Analgesia Journal* **90**: 699–705.
Hatfield A (2014) *The Complete Recovery Book*, 5th ed. Oxford, Oxford University Press.
Malcolm C (2015) Acute Pain Management in the Older Person. *Journal of Perioperative Practice* **25** (7–8): 134–139.
Mitchell E (2010) Pain Control. In Smith FG and Yeung J (eds) *Core Topics in Critical Care Medicine*. Cambridge, Cambridge University Press.
Ramsay KJ, Ramsay MAE, Joshi G, Hein HAT, Bishara L, Cancemi E (1998) Remifentanil versus Thoracic Epidural Analgesia in Lung Transplantation. *Anesthesia and Analgesia Journal* **86**: S93.
Wicker P and O'Neill J (2010) *Caring for the Perioperative Patient*. Chichester, Wiley-Blackwell.

Further Reading

Hallingbye T, Martin J, Viscomi C (2011) Acute Postoperative Pain Management in the Older Patient. *Aging Health Journal* **7** (6): 813–828.
Lutz L (2015) Managing Pain in the Surgical Patient. Available at https://www.mnhospitals.org/Portals/0/Documents/ptsafety/ade/managing_surgical_pain.ppt (accessed 27 February 2015)
Pan PH (2006) Post Caesarean Delivery Pain Management: Multimodal Approach. *International Journal of Obstetric Anaesthesia* **15** (3): 185–188.

Websites

Management of Postoperative Pain: http://www.uptodate.com/contents/management-of-postoperative-pain (accessed 27 February 2015)
Neuropathic Pain – Pharmacological Management: http://www.nice.org.uk/guidance/cg173/resources/guidance-neuropathic-pain-pharmacological-management-pdf (accessed 27 February 2015)
Postoperative Pain Relief: http://www.who.int/surgery/publications/Postoppain.pdf (accessed 27 February 2015)

Videos

How to Best Manage Post-op Pain: https://www.youtube.com/watch?v=A7-87XULNSY (accessed 27 February 2015)
Management of Postoperative Pain with Acupuncture: https://www.youtube.com/watch?v=mKTOlk8BNtg (accessed 27 February 2015)
Nerve Blocks for Postoperative Pain Management: https://www.youtube.com/watch?v=mGR1esyQm9A (accessed 27 February 2015)
Postoperative Pain Management: https://www.youtube.com/watch?v=ElyXAaw2Ers (accessed 27 February 2015)

76. Fluid Balance in Postoperative Patients

References

Bamboat ZM and Bordeianou L (2009) Perioperative Fluid Management. *Clinics in Colon and Rectal Surgery Journal* **22** (1): 28–33.

Clancy J, McVicar AJ, Baird N (2002) *Perioperative Practice: Fundamentals of Homeostasis*. London, Routledge.

Gau E and Bartel B (2015) Fluid and Electrolyte Management. Available at http://samples.jbpub.com/9781449604783/04783_CH07_PASS01.pdf (accessed 28 February 2015)

Scottish Intercollegiate Guidelines Network (2004) Postoperative Management in Adults. Available at http://www.sign.ac.uk/pdf/sign77.pdf (accessed 1 March 2015)

Wikipedia (2014) Infusion Pump. Available at http://en.wikipedia.org/wiki/Infusion_pump (accessed 1 March 2015)

Further Reading

Chappell D, Jacob M, Hofmann-Kiefer K, Conzen P, Rehm M (2008) A Rational Approach to Perioperative Fluid Management. *Anesthesiology* **109** (4): 723–740.

Jeremy Powell-Tuck J, Gosling P, Lobo DL, Allison SP, Carlson GL, Gore M *et al.* (2011) British Consensus Guidelines on Intravenous Fluid Therapy for Adult Surgical Patients. Available at http://www.bapen.org.uk/pdfs/bapen_pubs/giftasup.pdf (accessed 1 March 2015)

Rassam SS and Counsell DJ (2015) Perioperative Electrolyte and Fluid Balance. *Continuing Education in Anaesthesia, Critical Care and Pain Journal* **5** (5): 157–160.

Websites

Approaches to Fluid Management: http://www.openanesthesia.org/w/index.php?title=Fluid_Management (accessed 28 February 2015)

Intraoperative Fluid Management and Blood Transfusion: http://www.ucdenver.edu/academics/colleges/medicalschool/education/degree_programs/MDProgram/clinicalcore/peri-operativecare/Documents/FluidMgmt.pdf (accessed 28 February 2015)

Videos

Fluid Electrolyte Balance: http://www.youtube.com/watch?v=pQe7Tb7NVYE (accessed 28 February 2015)

Homeostasis 2, Fluid Balance: https://www.youtube.com/watch?v=IoU3lKrOYMY (accessed 1 March 2015)

Perioperative Fluid Therapy: http://www.youtube.com/watch?v=LFz43_fKkIM (accessed 28 February 2015)

77. Postoperative Medications

References

Barone CP, Lightfoot ML and Barone GW (2003) The Postanesthesia Care of an Adult Renal Transplant Recipient. *Journal of Perianesthesia Nursing* **18** (1): 32–41.

Hatfield A (2014) *The Complete Recovery Book*, 5th ed. Oxford, Oxford University Press.

Hudsmith J, Wheeler D, Gupta A (2004) *Core Topics in Perioperative Medicine*. London, Greenwich Medical Media Ltd.

Lubin MF, Walker HK, Smith RB (2003) *Medical Management of the Surgical Patient*, 4th ed. Cambridge, Cambridge University Press.

Radford M, County B, Oakley M (2004) *Advancing Perioperative Practice*. Cheltenham, Nelson Thornes Ltd.

Yentis SM, Hirsch NP, Smith GB (2009) *Anaesthesia and Intensive Care A–Z*. Edinburgh, Elsevier Ltd.

Further Reading

Klein M, Gogenur I, Rosenburg J (2012) Postoperative Use of Non-steroidal Anti-inflammatory Drugs in Patients with Anastomotic Leakage Requiring Reoperation after Colorectal Resection: Cohort Study

Based on Prospective Data. *British Medical Journal* **345**: e6166. Available at http://www.bmj.com/content/345/bmj.e6166 (accessed 2 March 2015)

Kranke P, Eberhart LH, Roewer N, Tramer MR (2002) Pharmacological Treatment of Postoperative Shivering: A Quantitative Systematic Review of Randomized Controlled Trials. *Anaesthesia and Analgesia Journal* **94**: 453–460. Available at http://anaesthesie.uk-wuerzburg.de/fileadmin/uk/anaesthesie/_Dokumente/Kranke2002_Shivering_Treatment.pdf (accessed 2 March 2015)

McCracken G, Houston P, Lefebrve G (2008) Guideline for the Management of Postoperative Nausea and Vomiting. SOGC Clinical Practice Guideline. Available at http://sogc.org/wp-content/uploads/2013/07/gui209CPG0807E.pdf (accessed 2 March 2015)

Websites

Postoperative Acute Pain: http://www.webmd.com/drugs/condition-3081-Postoperative+Acute+Pain.aspx?diseaseid=3081anddiseasename=Postoperative+Acute+Painandsource=0 (accessed 2 March 2015)

Postoperative Care (Drugs): http://www.merckmanuals.com/professional/special_subjects/care_of_the_surgical_patient/postoperative_care.html (accessed 2 March 2015)

What Are the Treatment Options for Post-operative Shivering?: http://dig.pharm.uic.edu/faq/Dec10/shivering.aspx (accessed 2 March 2015)

Videos

How to Best Manage Post-op Pain: https://www.youtube.com/watch?v=A7-87XULNSY (accessed 2 March 2015)

Risk Factors for PONV: https://www.youtube.com/watch?v=ft58EsCi1bg (accessed 2 March 2015)

Shared Decision-Making Approaches for Medication Management in the Recovery Process:
https://www.youtube.com/watch?v=ac9cFz62tts (accessed 2 March 2015)

Vomiting and Antiemetic Drugs: https://www.youtube.com/watch?v=JsBafhi3W6k (accessed 2 March 2015)

78. Managing Bleeding Problems

References

Baljinder D, Wasim SK, Tailor H (2010) Management of Anticoagulation Therapy in the Perioperative Patient. *Journal of Perioperative Practice* **21** (8): 279–283.

Daqi TF (2005) The Management of Postoperative Bleeding. *Surgical Clinics of North America Journal* **85** (6): 1191–1213.

Hatfield A (2014) *The Complete Recovery Book*, 5th ed. Oxford, Oxford University Press.

Koh MB and Hunt BJ (2003) The Management of Perioperative Bleeding. *Blood Reviews Journal* **17** (3): 179–185. Available at http://www.ncbi.nlm.nih.gov/pubmed/12818228 (accessed 3 March 2015)

Kumar A and Yeung J (2010) Haemodynamic Monitoring. In Smith FG and Yeung J (eds) *Core Topics in Critical Care Medicine*. Cambridge, Cambridge University Press.

Parker WH and Wagner WH (2015) Management of Haemorrhage in Gynaecological Surgery. Available at http://www.uptodate.com/contents/management-of-hemorrhage-in-gynecologic-surgery (accessed 3 March 2015)

Further Reading

Asani S (2008) Cardiac Care: Managing Postoperative Bleeding.
Available at http://www.modernmedicine.com/modern-medicine/content/cardiac-care-managing-post operative-bleeding?page=full (accessed 3 March 2015)

Mannucci PM and Levi M. (2007) Prevention and Treatment of Major Blood Loss. *New England Journal of Medicine* **356** (22): 2301.

Gobble RM and Hoang MD (2012) A Meta-Analysis of Postoperative Bleeding with the Use of Toradol. *Plastic and Reconstructive Surgery Journal* **130** (5S-1): 66.

Websites

How Do I Manage Postoperative Bleeding following Periodontal Surgery?: http://www.oasisdiscussions.ca/2012/10/30/postop-bleed-perio-surg/ (accessed 3 March 2015)

Management of Intraoperative and Postoperative Bleeding. Available at http://www.expertconsultbook.com/expertconsult/ob/book.do?method=displayandtype=bookPageanddecorator=noneandeid=4-u1.0-B978-1-4377-0823-3..10230-9--s0030andisbn=978-1-4377-0823-3 (accessed 3 March 2015)

Postoperative Haemorrhage: http://www.ahrq.gov/professionals/systems/hospital/qitoolkit/d4g-postophemorrhage-bestpractices.pdf (accessed 3 March 2015)

Videos

Autologous Blood Transfusion: https://www.youtube.com/watch?v=MFXkgoqgYTI (accessed 3 March 2015)

The Incidence and Management of Postoperative Haemorrhage after Laparoscopic Gastric Bypass: https://www.youtube.com/watch?v=DSU2tX7LArM (accessed 3 March 2015)

Postop Algorithm: Haemorrhage/Hypovolemia: https://www.youtube.com/watch?v=CO7WTzNLpyY (accessed 3 March 2015)

Postoperative Bleeding: https://www.youtube.com/watch?v=HDH8Np-gaGU (accessed 3 March 2015)

79. Managing Postoperative Nausea and Vomiting

References

Apfel CC, Läärä E, Koivuranta M, Greim CA and Roewer N (1999) A Simplified Risk Score for Predicting Postoperative Nausea and Vomiting. *Anesthesiology Journal* **91**: 693–700.

Chandrakantan A and Glass PSA (2011) Multimodal Therapies for Postoperative Nausea and Vomiting, and Pain. *British Journal of Anaesthesia* **107** (Suppl. 1): i27–i40. Available at http://bja.oxfordjournals.org/content/107/suppl_1/i27.full (accessed 4 March 2015)

Chatterjee S, Rudra A and Sengupta S (2011) Current Concepts in the Management of Postoperative Nausea and Vomiting. *Anesthesiology Research and Practice Journal* 2011: 748031. Available at http://www.hindawi.com/journals/arp/2011/748031/ (accessed 4 March 2015)

Chung F and Mezei F (1999) Factors Contributing to a Prolonged Stay after Ambulatory Surgery. *Anesthesia and Analgesia* **89**: 1352–1359.

Hill RP, Soppitt AJ and Gan TJ (2000) The Effectiveness of Rescue Antiemetics in Patients Who Received a Prophylactic Antiemetic. *Anesthesia and Analgesia Journal* **90**: S8.

Kovac AL (2000) Prevention and Treatment of Postoperative Nausea and Vomiting. *Drugs* (Journal) **59**: 213–243.

Lewis SJ, Salem G and Khater M (2015) Recent Advances in the Management of Postoperative Nausea and Vomiting. *Journal of Operating Department Practitioners* **3** (2): 62–65.

Magner JJ, McCaul C, Carton E, Gardiner J and Buggy D (2004) Effect of Intravenous Crystalloid Infusion on Postoperative Nausea and Vomiting after Gynaecological Laparoscopy: Comparison of 30 and 10 ml kg. *British Journal of Anaesthesia* **93**: 381–385.

Miniche S, Ramsing J, Dahl JB and Tramer MR (2003) Nonsteroidal Anti-inflammatory Drugs and the Risk of Operative Site Bleeding after Tonsillectomy: A Quantitative Systematic Review. *Anesthesia and Analgesia Journal* **96**: 68–77.

Pierre S and Whelan R (2013) Nausea and Vomiting After Surgery. *Continuing Education Anaesthetic Critical Care and Pain Journal* **13** (1): 28–32. Available at http://www.medscape.com/viewarticle/782388 (accessed 4 March 2015)

Smith HS, Smith EJ and Smith BR (2012) Postoperative Nausea and Vomiting. *Annals of Palliative Medicine* **1** (2). Available at http://www.amepc.org/apm/article/view/1035/1261 (accessed 5 March 2015)

Wilhelm SM, Dehoorne-Smith ML and Kale-Pradhan PB (2007) Prevention of Postoperative Nausea and Vomiting. *Annals of Pharmacotherapy Journal* **41**: 68–78.

Further Reading

Jokinen J, Smith AF, Roewer N, Eberhart LH and Kranke P (2012) Management of Postoperative Nausea and Vomiting: How to Deal with Refractory PONV. *Anesthesiology Clinics* **30** (3): 481–493.

Tramer MR (2003) Treatment of Postoperative Nausea and Vomiting. *British Medical Journal* **327**: 762.

Rosenblatt MA (2009) *Management of Postoperative Nausea and Vomiting*. The American Society of Anesthesiologists. Philadelphia, Lippincott Williams and Wilkins. Available at http://rileyanesthesia.org/links/documents/medical_students/4th_year_articles/Management%20of%20PONV.pdf (accessed 4 March 2015)

Websites

Consensus Guidelines for Managing Postoperative Nausea and Vomiting (2003): http://clinicaldepartments.musc.edu/anesthesia/education/medicalstudent/outline/ponv%20consensus.pdf (accessed 4 March 2015)

Consensus Guidelines for the Management of Postoperative Nausea and Vomiting (2014): http://www.anzca.edu.au/resources/endorsed-guidelines/related-documents/2014-consensus-guidelines-for-the-management-of-ponv.pdf (accessed 4 March 2015)

How to Prevent and Manage Postoperative Nausea and Vomiting: http://www.pharmaceutical-journal.com/learning/learning-article/how-to-prevent-and-manage-postoperative-nausea-and-vomiting/11096163.article (accessed 4 March 2015)

Videos

Physiology of Vomiting: http://www.youtube.com/watch?v=L92VzBWfSEw (accessed 5 March 2015)

Nausea Vomiting Antiemetics: http://www.youtube.com/watch?v=ztc4JQqk8TY (accessed 5 March 2015)

Risk Factors for PONV: http://www.youtube.com/watch?v=ft58EsCi1bg (accessed 5 March 2015)

Treatment for Postoperative Nausea and Vomiting: https://www.youtube.com/watch?v=bcbJCYFtJIYandlist=PL_SZKXlIExkE19L3vY8N8p-_TbpUuqV-C (accessed 5 March 2015)

80. Critical Issues in Postoperative Care

References

Association of Surgeons of Great Britain and Ireland (ASGBI) (2012) Consensus Statements. London, ASGBI. Available at http://asgbi.org.uk/en/publications/consensus_statements.cfm (accessed 7 March 2015)

Department of Health (2009) Competencies for Recognising and Responding to Acutely Ill Patients in Hospital. Available at http://webarchive.nationalarchives.gov.uk/20130107105354/http:/www.dh.gov.uk/prod_consum_dh/groups/dh_digitalassets/documents/digitalasset/dh_096988.pdf (accessed 8 March 2015)

Gawande AA, Kwaan MR and Regenbogen SE (2007) An Apgar Score for Surgery. *Journal of the American College of Surgeons* **204**: 201–208.

Hatfield A (2014) *The Complete Recovery Book*, 5th ed. Oxford, Oxford University Press.

Intensive Care Society (2009) *Levels of Critical Care for Adult Patients*. Standards and Guidelines. London, Intensive Care Society.

Jhanji S, Thomas B, Ely A, Watson D, Hinds CJ and Pearse RM (2008) Mortality and Utilisation of Critical Care Resources amongst High-Risk Surgical Patients in a Large NHS Trust. *Anaesthesia* **63** (7): 695–700.

NICE (2007) Acutely Ill Patients in Hospital: Recognition of and Response to Acute Illness in Adults in Hospital. Available at https://www.nice.org.uk/guidance/cg50/evidence/cg50-acutely-ill-patients-in-hospital-full-guideline3 (accessed 8 March 2015)

Peden CJ (2009) *Improving Outcome in High Risk Surgical Patients*. Practicum for Masters in Public Health (Clinical Effectiveness). Boston, Harvard School of Public Health.

Further Reading

Gwinnutt C and Smith G (2010) Recognition and Management of the Acutely Ill Surgical Patient. Available at http://www.frca.co.uk/Documents/170%20Recognition%20and%20management%20of%20the%20acutely%20ill%20surgical%20patient.pdf (accessed 9 March 2015)

Loftus I (2010) *Care of the Critically Ill Surgical Patient*. Boca Raton, CRC Press.

Royal College of Surgeons of England and Department of Health (2011) The Higher Risk General Surgical Patient. Available at http://www.rcseng.ac.uk/publications/docs/higher-risk-surgical-patient/@@download/pdffile/higher_risk_surgical_patient_2011_web.pdf (accessed 9 March 2015)

Websites

Acutely Ill Patients in Hospital: Recognition of and Response to Acute Illness in Adults in Hospital. Available at http://www.nice.org.uk/guidance/cg50 (accessed 9 March 2015)

Competencies for Recognising and Responding to Acutely Ill Patients in Hospital.

Available at http://webarchive.nationalarchives.gov.uk/20130107105354/http:/www.dh.gov.uk/prod_consum_dh/groups/dh_digitalassets/documents/digitalasset/dh_096988.pdf (accessed 9 March 2015)

Post-operative Critical Care Management of Patients Undergoing Cytoreductive Surgery and Heated Intraperitoneal Chemotherapy (HIPEC).

Available at http://www.wjso.com/content/9/1/169 (accessed 9 March 2015)

Videos

Critically Ill Patient: https://www.youtube.com/watch?v=sXeTppCcuuo (accessed 9 March 2015)

Fluid Responsiveness in the Critically Ill Patient: https://www.youtube.com/watch?v=ew0H6eTrt90 (accessed 9 March 2015)

Nutrition Support for the Critically Ill and Injured Patient: https://www.youtube.com/watch?v=c13TIOLlqUQ (accessed 9 March 2015)

Recognising the Critically Ill Patient: https://www.youtube.com/watch?v=uqQVGHihjpI (accessed 9 March 2015)

81. Enhanced Recovery

References

Archer S, Montague J and Bali A (2014) Exploring the Experience of an Enhanced Recovery Programme for Gynaecological Cancer Patients: A Qualitative Study. *Perioperative Medicine Journal* **3** (1): 2. Available at http://www.perioperativemedicinejournal.com/content/3/1/2 (accessed 10 March 2015)

Bernard H (2014) The Importance of Patient Warming for Enhanced Recovery. *Journal of Operating Department Practitioners* **2** (4): 166–172.

Cottle S (2013) Patient Involvement in Enhanced Recovery. *Nursing Times* **109**: 13, 24–25. Available at http://www.nursingtimes.net/home/specialisms/infection-control/patient-involvement-in-enhanced-recovery/5056813.article (accessed 10 March 2015)

Department of Health (DoH) (2010) *Delivering Enhanced Recovery*. London, NHS Enhanced Recovery Partnership Programme. Available at http://webarchive.nationalarchives.gov.uk/20130107105354/http://www.dh.gov.uk/prod_consum_dh/groups/dh_digitalassets/@dh/@en/@ps/documents/digitalasset/dh_115156.pdf (accessed 9 March 2015)

Hollins L and Mavrommatis S (2012) How Enhanced Recovery Can Improve Elective Surgery Experiences and Outcomes. *Health Service Journal*. Available at http://www.hsj.co.uk/resource-centre/best-practice/referral-management-admissions-and-discharge-resources/how-enhanced-recovery-can-improve-elective-surgery-experiences-and-outcomes/5043550.article#.VP74jPmsV8E (accessed 10 March 2015)

Royal College of Anaesthetists (2012) Guidelines for Patients Undergoing Surgery as Part of an Enhanced Recovery Programme (ERP). Available at http://www.rcoa.ac.uk/system/files/CSQ-ERP-Guide2012.pdf (accessed 9 March 2015)

Further Reading

Oxford University Hospitals (2015) Enhanced Recovery After Surgery. Available at http://www.ouh.nhs.uk/patient-guide/leaflets/files%5C10086Perasbowelsurgery.pdf (accessed 10 March 2015)

Wrightington, Wigan and Leigh NHS Foundation Trust (2015) Enhanced Recovery after Breast Surgery. Available at https://www.wwl.nhs.uk/Library/All_New_PI_Docs/Audio_Leaflets/Surgical/Enhanced_Recovery_Breast/Enhanced_Recovery_after_Breast_Surgery.pdf (accessed 10 March 2015)

Websites

Enhanced Recovery Care Pathway: http://www.nhsiq.nhs.uk/8846.aspx (accessed 10 March 2015)

How Enhanced Recovery Can Boost Patient Outcomes: http://www.nursingtimes.net/how-enhanced-recovery-can-boost-patient-outcomes/5043753.article (accessed 10 March 2015)

Risks of Anaesthesia: http://www.rcoa.ac.uk/patients-and-relatives/risks (accessed 9 March 2015)

Videos

Enhanced Recovery after Liver Surgery (ERAS) in Liver Surgery: https://www.youtube.com/watch?v=r413DDy-KcY (accessed 10 March 2015)

Enhanced Recovery after Surgery in Forth Valley: https://www.youtube.com/watch?v=xdx30Eup7iQ (accessed 10 March 2015)

Introduction to Enhanced Recovery after Surgery: https://www.youtube.com/watch?v=GMs1g-TqFyY (accessed 10 March 2015)

Pathway to Enhanced Recovery after Colon and Rectal Surgery: https://www.youtube.com/watch?v=vHRD1JLhKyk (accessed 10 March 2015)

SECTION 7

Perioperative Critical Care

Paul Wicker

82 Critical Care Nurses and Practitioners Roles

Patients with life-threatening problems need nurses or operating department practitioners (ODPs) to deal with their problems effectively and quickly. Nurses and ODPs can undergo training in critical care and are therefore responsible for supporting critically ill patients, and their families or friends, so the patient receives the best possible care.

Critically ill patients have life-threatening health problems that leave them in a vulnerable state, becoming unstable and having complex problems that need sorting in an emergency (McConnachie 2014). Patients in this state therefore need intensive and consistent patient care.

Critical care nurses often spend most of their time in an intensive care unit (ICU) (Aitken *et al.* 2013). However, practitioners and nurses who train in critical care can also work in places like emergency departments, cardiac care units, cardiac catheter labs, trauma units, operating departments and recovery rooms. Practitioners and nurses can also work in organisations or departments outside hospitals, such as outpatient departments or clinics (Photo 10).

Critical care practitioners can therefore work in operating departments including anaesthetic rooms, operating rooms and recovery rooms. In these rooms, critically ill patients need a detailed assessment as well as high-quality therapies, managed by continuous observation and monitoring (McConnachie 2014). Critical care practitioners and nurses therefore need high-quality knowledge, skills and experience to support critically ill patients, and to care for them suitably and effectively (Aitken *et al.* 2015).

Examples of the roles undertaken by critical care practitioners working in operating rooms or recovery rooms may include (McConnachie 2014):

- If patients cannot speak or listen, take immediate actions if they are critically ill.
- Observe, monitor and record the care the patient receives.
- Communicate effectively with the patient, the family and other healthcare professionals who are involved with caring for the patient.
- Respect and support the patient.
- Take actions to support patients when they are suffering from health problems.
- Support the patient to ensure they receive suitable care.
- Respect the patient with dignity.
- Provide information or knowledge to the patient to help them make their own decisions.
- Support the choices the patient makes about their critical illness (McConnachie 2014).

The roles of critical care nurses

Critical care nurses work in a wide variety of settings compared with ODPs, who usually work in the operating department. Critical care nurses fulfil several different roles such as educators, researchers, clinical nurse specialists and so on. Because of the ageing population and increase in diseases and illnesses, critical care nurses care for seriously ill patients in wards. In years gone past, patients would have passed away because of the lack of knowledge and clinical skills.

Rapid Perioperative Care, First Edition. Paul Wicker and Sara Dalby.

There are also increasing numbers of advanced practice nurses who have received advanced education at either the master's or doctoral level and are normally clinical nurse specialists (CNSs). A CNS is an expert clinician who is responsible for improving the care of critically ill patients, which includes the identification, intervention and management of clinical problems. The CNS also provides direct patient care, which includes assessing, diagnosing, planning and prescribing pharmacological and non-pharmacological treatment (Salisbury *et al.* 2010). Encouraging the patient to exercise also helps to improve their recovery (Burtin *et al.* 2009).

The role of critical care practitioners (commonly used in the icu)

OCPs and recovery nurses with critical care skills are provided with clinical skills training and education to care for critically ill patients during surgery and in the recovery room. Patients may also remain in recovery or transfer to an intensive care unit. Critically ill patients in recovery need care by suitably trained and educated practitioners (McConnachie 2014). Examples of equipment used in the operating room or recovery room may include:

- *Monitors*: Monitors measure breathing, pulse rate and rhythm, temperature and so on. Monitors have alarms which alert the anaesthetist or practitioner when figures are higher or lower than normal levels (Aitken *et al.* 2015).
- *Catheters, drains and tubes*: Intravenous catheters are inserted into patients' veins to dispense fluids, blood, medicine or nutrition. A nasogastric tube may also help to provide food, water or drugs for the patient. Urinary catheters may also be used to help drain urine from the bladder.
- *Respirators*: These are mechanical ventilators which help patients to breathe through an endotracheal tube (ETT) which inserts into the trachea. The ETT connects to the ventilator to enable normal breathing patterns (Aitken *et al.* 2015).

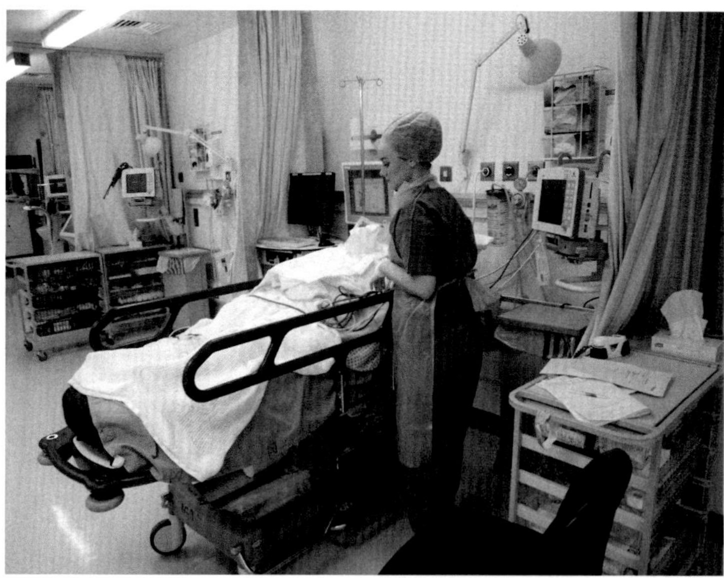

Photo 10 Monitoring the critical care patient. Courtesy of Aintree Hospital, Liverpool

Critically ill patients also have several disorders that will need treatment in the operating room or the recovery room (McConnachie 2014). These patients need urgent treatment and support to prevent morbidity or mortality. Examples of disorders that are possible can include:

- Smoking related to lung disorders such as emphysema or bronchitis.
- *Sepsis*: Sepsis is a potentially life-threatening complication caused by infection. Sepsis often occurs when medicines released into the bloodstream to fight infection trigger inflammatory responses throughout the body. Inflammation creates a myriad of changes that can lead to damage of organs in the body (Aitken *et al.* 2015).
- *Asthma*: Asthma causes obstruction of the airways resulting in difficulty breathing, wheezing, chest tightness and coughing.
- *Pneumonia*: This is often a result of infection inside the lungs which is likely to cause interference with breathing (McConnachie 2014).
- *Chronic obstructive pulmonary disease (COPD)*: COPD can prevent the patient from breathing out, leading to acute airway problems. COPD may be a result of the patient smoking, inhaling pollution or developing asthma.
- *Acute respiratory distress syndrome (ARDS)*: ARDS happens when there is severe lung failure which then needs the use of a ventilator to enable the patient to breathe effectively. ARDS can occur because of illnesses such as infections or serious injuries to the chest or lungs (McConnachie 2014).
- Trauma involves severe injuries, for example car crashes, falling off bridges and limbs trapped in machines. Patients undergoing trauma would almost always need surgery to repair bones, tissues, muscles and so on.

Conclusion

Patient care has become more complex because of the changes and advances in medicine, equipment and devices. Therefore, nurses and practitioners who are delivering care to critically ill patients need specialised knowledge and skills to provide effective support for the patient, including continuous monitoring and treatment (McConnachie 2014).

Patients who are transferred to ICU immediately after surgery may be vulnerable because of their postoperative state, the use of sedatives, their reactions to anaesthetic drugs and the complexity of surgery (Kaplow 2013). The patient may also feel unstable and unsafe. ICU nurses and practitioners need to have knowledge and understanding of the anaesthetic agents that the anaesthetist delivers to patients during anaesthesia and surgery, and any drugs that have been used throughout the entire procedure. They must also know about potential complications caused by anaesthesia or surgery, so they can optimise patient outcomes and prevent the patient from suffering from morbidity or mortality (Kaplow 2013).

As the NHS progresses and changes, the use of technology has helped to keep more people out of hospitals. However, seriously ill patients who are in critical care units, ICUs or operating departments need much more care and attention (Salisbury *et al.* 2010). Critical care practitioners therefore need to keep up to date with current information and develop new skills to manage modern treatment methods and technologies. Critical care staff will therefore need to be more knowledgeable and develop new clinical skills as patient care is becoming even more complex while new technologies and treatments are introduced.

83 Management of the Critically Ill Surgical Patient

Introduction to critical illness

Undertaking critical care is a speciality, often within nursing, which aims to reduce life-threatening problems in seriously ill patients. A critical care practitioner is responsible for ensuring that critically ill patients and their families receive the best care possible. Critical care practitioners work in various departments where critically ill patients are located, such as intensive care units, cardiac care units, emergency departments, operating departments and recovery rooms.

Critically ill patients have a high risk of life-threatening health problems depending on the condition of the patient. Critically ill patients are highly vulnerable and unstable, and they need complex support by requiring intense and regular patient care (Smith and Yeung 2010, Bancroft 2013). Patients who have life-threatening illnesses, or are critically ill, therefore usually need intensive care to survive. Critically ill patients may be cared for in recovery, but it is also likely that they will be sent to the intensive care unit (ICU) which can provide higher quality care because of the presence of anaesthetists and well-trained and educated ICU nurses (McConachie 2014).

The presence of multiple medical conditions can influence the patient's outcome. For example, patients may have a combination of diseases such as ischaemic heart disease, diabetes, peripheral vascular disease or obstructive airways (Smith and Yeung 2010). Old age can also lead to further problems. Total care of critically ill patients, including monitoring, assessment and managing ethical issues (Bancroft 2013), is therefore essential to support their health and provide positive outcomes.

Infection

When the patient acquires severe infection, it can lead to many other problems or illnesses, including circulatory, respiratory and organ failure (McConachie 2014). Infection can also cause sepsis and septic shock leading to mortality, even though patients will receive antibiotics and intensive life support (Smith and Yeung 2010). Those who survive sepsis will need prolonged hospitalisation because of problems due to sepsis, including organ dysfunction and inflammation throughout the body (Ranieri *et al.* 2012).

The most common organisms involved in sepsis include *Staphylococcus aureus*, *Staphylococcus epidermidis*, *Streptococcus pneumoniae*, *Streptococcus pyogenes*, various enterococci and Gram-negative bacilli (Ranieri *et al.* 2012). When sepsis is suspected, the abdomen and lungs are the two most likely sites, although intravascular catheters can also lead to sepsis if they have been inserted (Smith and Yeung 2010).

The best agent to overcome sepsis is drotrecogin alfa, which is a recombinant human activated protein C. This is highly expensive and may cause severe side effects, but it often helps to reduce mortality in patients who have severe sepsis (Ranieri *et al.* 2012). Drotrecogin alfa has anti-thrombotic, anti-inflammatory and profibrinolytic properties.

Rapid Perioperative Care, First Edition. Paul Wicker and Sara Dalby.

Fluid balance

A critically ill patient needing fluids must be dealt with promptly to treat hypovolaemia in order to maintain circulating blood volume, organ and tissue functions. The choice of fluids for acute resuscitation includes crystalloids such as 0.9% sodium chloride or Hartmann's solution, and colloids such as 4% albumin or polygeline, which is a polymer of urea and polypeptides derived from degraded gelatine (NICE 2007). Polygeline is a blood plasma expansion drug which helps maintain the blood plasma level. Hypertonic saline (3%) and blood products can also be used (NICE 2007).

When blood flow is restored to an acceptable level and cardiac filling pressures are maximised, then fluid infusion is complete. If the patient remains hypovolaemic due to poor infusion techniques, then inotrope therapy will help repair cardiac filling pressures, and vasopressor therapy may be needed to re-establish blood pressure levels (NPSA 2007). Haemodynamic monitoring is essential to identify that normal fluid levels have been achieved and remain at the appropriate level.

Organ dysfunction and failure

Multiple organ dysfunction syndrome (MODS) can vary depending on the patient's surgery and their health status. Organ dysfunction rarely happens in simple surgery; however, it can happen in major surgery such as trauma, or when incidents occur such as haemorrhage, sepsis, necrosis or shock (Smith and Yeung 2010). All organs and tissues of the body may be affected depending on the state of the patient. Blood can also be affected leading to disseminated intravascular coagulation. This can also lead to leakage in capillaries, interstitial oedema and haemorrhage (McConachie 2014).

The clinical results of organ dysfunction can result in:

- *Systemic inflammatory response*: This may affect the whole body.
- *Hyperdynamic circulatory state*: Increased circulatory volume
- *Hypermetabolic state*: Increased rate of metabolic activity
- *Respiratory dysfunction*: Within 48 h
- *Liver and kidney dysfunction*: Within 1 week
- *Infection*: For example, respiratory, urinary and wound infection (Smith and Yeung 2010, McConachie 2014).

MODS often progresses over a 3-week period, which can lead to at least half the patients dying. MODS is reversible, although treatment of MODS can be complex and expensive, leading to prolonged treatment. Rehabilitation following MODS can also take up to 1 year before the patient is restored to better health.

Actions for the critically ill

Caring for and managing the critically ill patient can be complex and sophisticated, depending on the state of the patient (Smith and Yeung 2010). Actions that may need to be taken for critically ill patients can include:

- Maintain optimal blood volume; ensuring an adequate circulatory state is a continuous task.
- Treat respiratory failure, using mechanical ventilation to provide respiratory support.
- Undertake early diagnosis (following poor circulation or respiratory issues), and offer specific therapy if required.
- Urgent treatment of initial sepsis and other infections.
- Provide essential metabolic support by providing nutrition, which is needed for tissues repairs (Martindale *et al.* 2009).
- Monitor and assess renal problems, and provide support for renal replacement therapy.

- Provide psychosocial support for the patient and the family. This may include analgesia, comfort and dignity for the patient, and the family will need access to the patient along with information and support.
- Provide continuous patient management by the highly skilled multidisciplinary team in a specialised environment (NICE 2007, NPSA 2007, Smith and Yeung 2010).

Conclusion

Advances in healthcare and technology have contributed to keeping more people out of the hospital and allowed them to get treatment in the community. However, patients in critical care units may be more ill than ever, because of the interaction between people from different parts of the country and different parts of the world. Critically ill patients may no longer be placed in a critical care unit and instead may be treated at home. Hospitals in the future, however, will provide extended critical care units to allow more patients to enter their department. Patients who have minor illnesses or conditions may be provided alternative locations or given treatment at home. Critical care practitioners need to understand and keep in line with the latest information, as well as develop skills to manage all the new treatment methods and technologies that are being developed. Issues relating to patient care are becoming more complex, and as new technologies and treatments are introduced, critical care practitioners and nurses will need to develop further in their knowledge and skills (Bancroft 2013).

84 Malignant Hyperthermia

Introduction

Patients who develop malignant hyperthermia (MH) do so because it is a rare, inherited condition that has the potential to be fatal to the patient. MH happens because of exposure to anaesthetic drugs or muscle relaxants, and it may happen during anaesthesia or soon after surgery is complete (Lay 2014). However, MH occurs because of a reaction in muscles caused by the anaesthetic drugs which then leads to activation of the muscles, leading to temperature rises (AAGBI 2011, Lay 2014). This results in the patient developing a high body temperature and the breakdown of muscle tissue caused by the high temperatures. When monitoring of the patient's temperature occurs repeatedly, anaesthetists can detect malignant hyperthermia and treat it urgently. Patients are likely to get malignant hyperthermia if their family members have had it previously or the patient has a disease that affects the muscles (Goodman and Spry 2014). Patients can undergo genetic testing or a muscle biopsy if they are aware they may succumb to malignant hyperthermia. When the anaesthetist understands the patient may suffer from hyperthermia, reducing the chances of this condition developing can occur by choosing anaesthetic drugs that do not trigger malignant hyperthermia (Jevon *et al.* 2012).

Causes of malignant hyperthermia

MH happens because of a severe reaction to anaesthetic drugs which occurs because of a rare, inherited muscle abnormality (Lay 2014). If a patient undergoes extreme exercise, such as running or workouts, or suffers from heat stroke because of high temperatures, malignant hyperthermia may develop if the person has a muscle abnormality, such as multiminicore myopathy or central core disease (autosomal dominant) (MedlinePlus 2015). When patients have a muscle abnormality, it occurs because muscle cells have an abnormal protein on their surfaces. Under normal circumstances, the protein will not affect muscle function, unless the muscles are exposed to a drug that can start a reaction. Examples of drugs which can cause MH include volatile anaesthetic agents and succinylcholine (a neuromuscular blocking agent) (Stoppler 2015).

When these anaesthetic drugs are in use, calcium which is stored in muscle cells is released, causing the muscles to contract and stiffen, and leading to an increase in body temperature leading to MH (AAGBI 2011). Although MH often occurs because of anaesthesia or following surgery, it can also occur in other places if anaesthetic medications have been used, such as in emergency rooms, dental offices, surgeon's offices and intensive care units. Normally, symptoms of MH will occur within an hour of delivering the medications. However, sometimes MH can have a delayed onset of 12 h. MH occurs mostly in young children and adults who are younger than 30 years old (Jevon *et al.* 2012, Stoppler 2015).

Muscle abnormality leading to malignant hyperthermia can be caused by genetic mutations in genes such as CACNA1S (a gene which produces calcium channels) and RYR1 (a ryanodine receptor 1 gene which serves as a calcium release channel) which make proteins in muscles used for movement (Stoppler 2015). An adult with this mutation has a

Rapid Perioperative Care, First Edition. Paul Wicker and Sara Dalby.

50% chance of passing the abnormal gene on to his or her baby on conception (Stoppler 2015). Reactions can differ within families, leading to mild or severe reactions. Sometimes a patient may take medications on several occasions before developing MH. MH may also occur in patients who have muscular dystrophy or other muscle diseases which associate with genetic mutations (MedlinePlus 2015).

Symptoms of MH

The various symptoms of malignant hyperthermia may include:

- A quick rise in body temperature, 105 °F (40.5 °C) or higher
- Rigid or painful muscles
- Flushed skin
- Sweating
- A rapid or irregular heartbeat
- Rapid or uncomfortable breathing
- Dark brown urine
- Low blood pressure (leading to shock)
- Confusion
- Muscle weakness or swelling after the event (Stoppler 2015).

Diagnosis

Patients are usually not diagnosed for MH until they react to general anaesthetic agents. Anaesthetists will recognise MH if the patient develops high fever and rigid muscles because of receiving anaesthetic drugs (Goodman and Spry 2014). Blood tests can show changes in the body's biochemistry which may suggest MH is developing. Examples include high levels of the creatinine phosphokinase and changes in electrolytes; kidney failure may also be recognised (Stoppler 2015). It is essential that MH is identified soon and acted on quickly; otherwise, the patient's heart may fail during surgery, leading to morbidity. Once severe reactions to MH develop, several other complications may also develop, including respiratory or kidney failure (Goodman and Spry 2014). Such complications may not restore for several days or weeks, and sometimes damage may be permanent.

Prevention of MH

Doctors do not usually test patients for MH before surgery unless the patient lets the anaesthetist or surgeon know of issues they have. This could include having a family history of malignant hyperthermia, having hyperthermia following heatstroke or exercise or having muscle abnormalities (Goodman and Spry 2014). Patients who do not have a previous episode of MH may still develop MH during anaesthesia or surgery which may not be preventable and may lead to continuing health problems.

Following diagnosis of the patient with MH, it is likely that anaesthetists and surgeons will avoid using drugs or surgery which may cause MH. It is therefore important that any patient with previous MH should tell the GP, anaesthetist or surgeon about the likelihood of developing MH during surgery. Once the anaesthetist knows of this risk, he or she will avoid the use of succinylcholine or high-risk anaesthetic volatile gases (Goodman and Spry 2014).

Patients with MH, however, do not have to avoid surgery or anaesthesia, as they may use other safe anaesthetic drugs. For example, local or regional anaesthesia may be used for minor cases. Patients susceptible to MH should wear a medical alert tag so professional staff members can identify the risk associated with the patient, especially during an emergency situation.

A useful website is the British Malignant Hypothermia Association which can be found at www.bmha.co.uk. This website offers support and information to patients which may be of their benefit.

Treatment

Malignant hyperthermia can happen whenever susceptible patients receive anaesthetic drugs or gases. Anaesthetists must act quickly to treat the condition and prevent serious complications from occurring. Without prompt treatment, the complications of MH can be life-threatening (Goodman and Spry 2014). The first action to take would involve stopping medication that is causing the MH and, if possible, stopping surgery from progressing. Surgery may not always be able to stop, but if it is in the early stages it is better to prevent surgery from leading to even more serious problems. Anaesthetists will then administer dantrolene, which is a muscle relaxant and helps to reduce the critical increase in muscle metabolism (Lay 2014, MedlinePlus 2015).

Dantrolene is usually given intravenously until the MH has reduced in the patient and the patient's health has stabilised (Lay 2014). Dantrolene may then be administered as a pill for up to three days to prevent MH from returning. Other actions that can be taken include:

- Lowering body temperature with:
  - Cool mist and fans
  - Cooling blankets
  - Cooled intravenous fluids
- Administering oxygen
- Using medications to:
  - Control the heartbeat
  - Stabilise blood pressure
- Constant monitoring in recovery or an intensive care unit (Jevon *et al.* 2012).

Conclusion

Malignant hyperthermia can cause major problems for patients and staff and also be life-threatening. However, if anaesthetists or practitioners detect early signs of MH and commence treatment urgently and quickly, then the patient may recovery fairly quickly and be able to undergo surgery later. If the patient develops MH, then this should be recorded in their notes for future use in the event of further anaesthesia or surgery being needed. Future prevention of MH can be stopped by avoiding known drug agents that lead to MH.

85 Inadvertent Hypothermia

Patients in the operating room sometimes develop inadvertent hypothermia because of low temperatures in the operating room and also because of exposure of the body or internal organs during surgery (Singh 2013). This can result in serious cardiac problems, coagulation of blood, and wound-healing complications either during surgery or in the postoperative recovery room. Sometimes patients do not have their temperatures monitored, and therefore the perioperative team is not aware that their temperatures are falling (PPSA 2008). To ensure patients maintain normal temperatures levels, it is important to monitor the patient's temperature constantly throughout surgery, and if necessary use warming measures, such as heated blankets, Bair Huggers and warm IV fluids (Burger and Fitzpatrick 2009, Singh 2013).

Avoiding hypothermia during surgery is therefore a major challenge, given the low room temperatures, the effects of anaesthetic drugs on thermoregulatory responses in the body, and the possibility of the patient losing heat due to convection or evaporation in the operating room environment (PPSA 2008, Singh 2014). Other problems that can lead to hypothermia include:

- Lack of covers on the patient when the OR has a low temperature and humidity
- Administration of cold IV fluids, for example if they are taken out of a fridge and given to the patient (PPSA 2008)
- Evaporation from surgical sites, for example if the wound is wide open
- Administration of cold irrigation fluid (e.g. into the abdomen)
- Evaporation of skin-cleaning solutions can lead to loss of heat from the skin surface.

Hypothermia occurs when temperatures drop to 36 °C (96.8 °F) or lower. Inadvertent perioperative hypothermia produces serious complications involving poor circulation of blood, coagulation within bloodstreams, poor wound healing and decreased drug metabolism (PPSA 2008).

Elderly patients and children are often at high risk from hypothermia. Elderly patients who are suffering from hypothermia have less subcutaneous tissue and may not start shivering or vasoconstricting, with or without anaesthesia, because of their physiological state (PPSA 2008). Young children and neonates are also likely to develop hypothermia because of their large heads, the thin bone surrounding their skulls, and small amounts of hair which enable heat to leave the brain and the head. Children and neonates also have a larger surface area compared to body mass, small amounts of fat and poor muscle activity, making them more likely to lose heat and reduce their body temperatures. Other potential problems in patients can include patients with burns, small body mass, damaged muscles, problems with circulation or thyroid disease (Arndt 1999).

Physiology of thermoregulation

Humans normally try to preserve normal temperatures regardless of the environment, even if it is too cold or too hot. Under normal circumstances, body temperature is maintained around 37 °C, plus or minus 0.2 °C. This helps to provide the normal rate of metabolism,

Rapid Perioperative Care, First Edition. Paul Wicker and Sara Dalby.

maintains nervous system conduction and allows muscles to relax and contract as needed (Insler and Sesler 2006). To preserve normal temperatures, the brain produces positive and negative feedback to ensure normal values and thresholds for core temperatures. The hypothalamus is the main thermoregulatory control centre and acts as a thermostat to ensure temperature remains within normal parameters. However, thermoregulation is also affected by signals from other parts of the body, such as the midbrain, medulla, spinal cord, cortex and deep abdominal and thoracic structures (Insler and Sessler 2006). If the patient's temperature reduces below 36 °C, then this will induce vasoconstriction and shivering. If the temperature rises above 37 °C, the heat response will lead to vasodilation and sweating (Sessler 2005).

Managing temperature during anaesthesia

Patients entering the anaesthetic room, before anaesthesia, will not usually become hypothermic because their bodies will react to cold by producing shivering and peripheral vasoconstriction which will help to maintain core body temperature. If the patient is cold, he or she will tell the anaesthetist or anaesthetic practitioner, who may then give them additional coverings to keep them warm (Burger and Fitzpatrick 2009). However, when anaesthetic induction starts, there is a decrease in core body temperature (Singh 2013). The first action of the anaesthetic drugs is to cause peripheral vasodilation which enables redistribution of heat from the core to the periphery, leading to convection, conduction or radiation of heat from the body (Burger and Fitzpatrick 2009, Singh 2013). This happens because anaesthetic drugs inhibit vasoconstriction and encourage vasodilation; however, under normal situations, vasoconstriction helps to preserve core body temperature (Matsukawa *et al.* 1995). Once the heat is redistributed to the peripheries, the patient's core temperature will decrease slowly, mainly because there is little metabolic heat production due to the patient being unconscious. As the patient's temperature falls, the anaesthetist and anaesthetic practitioners will take actions to warm the patient (Singh 2014). After three to four hours, the core temperature will remain stable during surgery if the patient is being kept warm and well insulated (Burger and Fitzpatrick 2009).

As well as general anaesthesia, epidural, spinal and regional anaesthesia also decreases the patient's temperature as there will be little or no thermoregulatory responses for vasoconstriction or shivering. Regional anaesthesia in particular decreases thermoregulatory responses of vasoconstriction and shivering. This is because analgesics and sedatives are used alongside regional anaesthesia, and these drugs will also undermine thermoregulatory responses, leading to decreases in the patient's temperature (Sessler 2005).

Complications associated with inadvertent hypothermia

Inadvertent hypothermia during surgery can result in serious problems arising throughout the patient's body. The main issues are in regard to the cardiovascular system, coagulation, wound infection and healing, and drug metabolism (PPSA 2008, Singh 2014).

Cardiovascular events

- Vasoconstriction, which increases arterial blood pressure
- Increased oxygen consumption, which may cause hypoxaemia and myocardial ischaemia
- Depressed myocardial contraction which slows conduction of blood through the heart
- Atrial or ventricular fibrillation, especially when temperatures drop below 30 °C.

Monitoring for signs of hypothermia and keeping patients warm during surgery will decrease the risks of cardiac morbidity (Insler and Sessler 2006).

Coagulation

The onset of hypothermia undermines the coagulation system because it affects the platelet function, the coagulation cascade and fibrinolysis (Burger and Fitzpatrick 2009). Main issues include:

- Platelet function is impaired because hypothermia inhibits the formation of the platelet plug.
- Enzymes used in the coagulation cascade are inhibited by hypothermia, and their actions are slowed down.
- Fibrinolysis (the enzymatic breakdown of the fibrin in blood clots) is increased by hypothermia, which leads to breakdown of clot formation (Burger and Fitzpatrick 2009).

Hypothermia, either mild or severe, also increases blood loss leading to the need for blood transfusions, to preserve the circulatory system and to prevent hypovolaemia and hypoxia from developing (Rajagopalan *et al.* 2008).

Wound infection and healing

Following surgery, surgical wounds may become infected if patients become hypothermic and drop their temperatures by 2 °C or more (Kurz *et al.* 1996). This is caused by reducing immune function and also because of vasoconstriction which has the effect of reducing blood flow and oxygen delivery to peripheral tissues (Hopf *et al.* 1997). Hypothermia also affects macrophage function which prevents the destruction of bacteria or viruses, and also the decrease in tissue perfusion which increases the likelihood of infection starting (Rajagopalan *et al.* 2008). Patients with hypothermia are therefore likely to stay in hospital longer than patients with normothermia (Kurz *et al.* 1996).

Pharmacokinetics and pharmacodynamics

The metabolism of drugs is affected by inadvertent hypothermia in perioperative patients (PPSA 2008). Enzymes in the body are temperature sensitive, and so hypothermia can lead to slowing down the metabolism of the anaesthetic drugs and also affecting organ functions. Most muscle relaxants can be prolonged by hypothermia; however, vecuronium is usually not affected unless the patient has severe hypothermia. Propofol and atracurium can both be affected by mild hypothermia, prolonging the duration of their actions.

The pharmacodynamics of volatile anaesthetic gases are greatly altered by hypothermia, which increases the solubility of the gases, leading to greater increase in the content of anaesthetic gases within the body. This leads to the patient recovering slowly from muscle relaxants and anaesthetic gases, leading to delayed recovery times, following general anaesthesia (PPSA 2008).

Temperature measurements

Patients who are undergoing inadvertent hypothermia need temperature measurements throughout surgery and postoperatively (Photo 11) (Burger and Fitzpatrick 2009). Intraoperatively, the following methods for monitoring core temperatures may include:

- *Pulmonary artery catheters*: These measure central blood temperatures.
- *Distal oesophageal temperature*: This measures core body temperature.
- *Nasopharyngeal temperature*: Measured with an oesophageal probe which can measure the brain temperature and core body temperature.
- *Tympanic membrane temperature monitoring*: This monitor is close to the carotid artery and hypothalamus and measures core body temperature.
- *Urinary catheter*: This can contain a temperature transducer which measures bladder temperature.

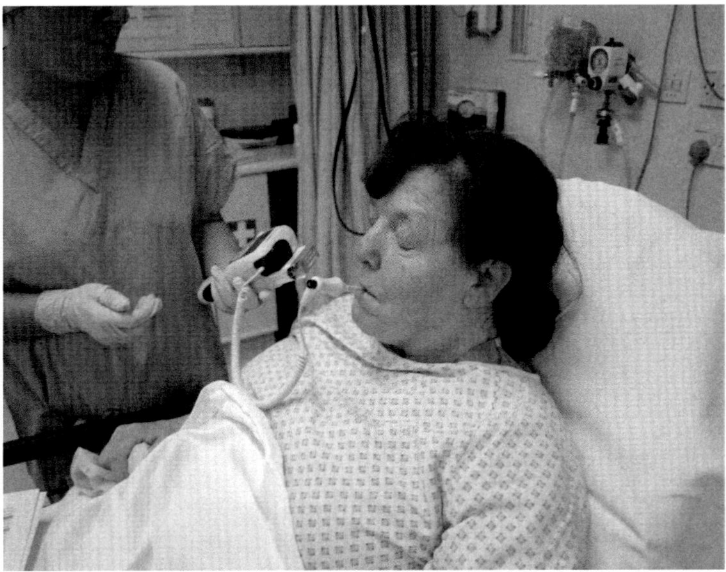

Photo 11 Monitoring the patient's temperature. Courtesy of Liverpool Women's Hospital

- *Rectal temperature*: This measures core body temperature but may be affected by the contents of the bowels, leading to false temperature results.
- *Axillary temperature*: This can help to identify core body temperature (Sessler 2005, Singh 2014).

The patient's temperature should be routinely measured during long periods of surgery in case of the development of inadvertent hypothermia (PPSA 2008). However, the temperature of the patient may not be accurate because of vasoconstriction and the effect on skin temperature. Temperature probes that are used inside the body would be more accurate (Sessler 2005).

Postoperative care

Postoperatively, the hypothermic patient will need constant assessment of their condition (Burger and Fitzpatrick 2009, Singh 2014). This may include:

- Measure the hypothermic patient's temperature on admission to Recovery, every 30 min, until the patient becomes normothermic (PPSA 2008).
- Assess the patient's comfort every 30 min; for example, if the patient is shivering or shaking, this needs to be addressed.
- Assess for further signs and symptoms of hypothermia, for example poor circulation.

Interventions that need to be taken for hypothermic patients can include:

- Initiate warming measures; for example, deliver warm IV fluids and warmed and humidified oxygen, give the patient warm blankets, ensure the patient is fully covered and so on (Sessler 2005).
- Assess temperature every 30 min until the patient becomes normothermic.

- Ensure the recovery room has an average temperature of 20 to 24 °C (PPSA 2008).
- Record the patient's assessment and evaluation, and the plan of care.
- Ensure the patient is normothermic on discharge from the recovery room.

Conclusion

Monitoring the patient's temperature perioperatively and ensuring that his or her temperature is maintained around 37 °C will improve patient outcomes, in terms of the problems that can arise during surgery and postoperatively (Singh 2013, 2014). However, when patients have not been preoperatively assessed for the risk of hypothermia, or their temperature is not routinely measured during anaesthesia or surgery, this can result in severe postoperative complications. Nowadays, patients usually have their temperatures monitored routinely, especially when surgery can take a long time, thus preventing the risk of inadvertent hypothermia.

86 Congestive Heart Failure

Introduction

The heart works as a pump for sending blood around all parts of the body (Figure 86.1). The heart consists of four chambers – two atria and two ventricles:

- The right atrium and ventricle receive blood from the inferior and superior vena cavae, which connect to veins in the body.
- The right ventricle pumps the blood towards the lungs via the pulmonary arteries, where carbon dioxide is released into the lungs, and oxygen is passed through the alveoli into the blood.
- The blood leaves the lungs and enters the left atrium and left ventricle, and it is then pumped into the aorta towards the arteries of the body, which circulates blood and oxygen to the organs and body tissues.
- The left ventricle is larger than the right ventricle because it has to pump blood throughout the entire body.

Cardiac failure reduces the amount of blood and oxygen in the tissues of the body (Hosenpud and Greenberg 2006). However, because of improved surgery and medications, patients with heart failure can recover faster and live longer. Heart failure occurs when the action of the heart becomes less powerful, reducing the circulation of the blood. This increases pressure in the blood vessels and forces fluid to leave the blood vessels and move into body tissues (Hosenpud and Greenberg 2006). Effects include:

- *Pulmonary congestion*: The left ventricle starts to fail and fluid collects in the lungs, leading to oedema. Oedema reduces the patient's chances of breathing properly, leading to hypoxia.
- *Oedema in the lower legs*: This occurs when the right ventricle starts to fail and oedema develops in the lower legs.
- *Ascites*: As the right ventricle continues to reduce its ability to pump blood, oedema travels up the legs and fluid collects in the abdomen. The patient gains weight because of the extra fluid being retained in the abdomen and legs (ESC 2009).

Heart failure is a serious medical condition, and the patient can acquire many problems as a result. Heart failure may develop slowly, or quickly after a heart attack or heart disease. Congestive heart failure (CHF) occurs because of systolic or diastolic heart failure and is more common in elderly people (Smith and Yeung 2010).

Systolic heart failure: When the pumping action of the heart is weak, systolic heart failure occurs. The blood which is ejected out of the left ventricle is measured, and the amount of blood left in the left ventricle is also measured using medical devices. Normally, at least 55% or more of the blood is ejected from the left ventricle, but systolic heart failure is identified if the amount ejected is lower than 55% (Hosenpud and Greenberg 2006).

Rapid Perioperative Care, First Edition. Paul Wicker and Sara Dalby.

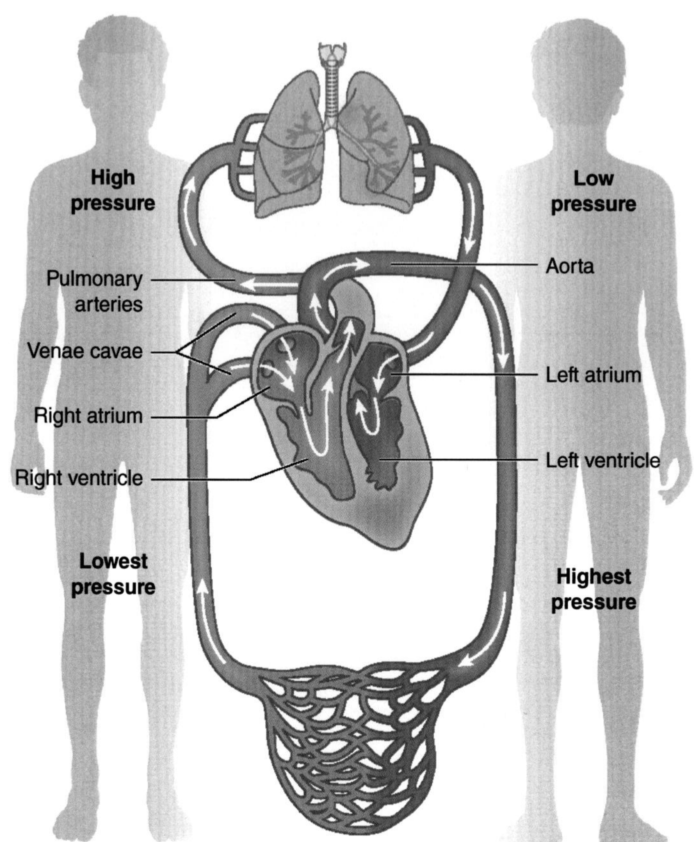

Figure 86.1 Circulation of the blood throughout the body

Diastolic heart failure: When the two ventricles are stiff and cannot expand, the heart cannot fill with blood, and so much of the blood stays in the lungs, and symptoms of heart failure may commence. Old patients, especially women over 75 years, and those with high blood pressure develop diastolic heart failure (Sear and Higham 2002).

Heart failure affects about 2% of the adult population, and about at least half of the patients develop CHF and die within five years (Hosenpud and Greenberg 2006). However, the health of the patient depends on their diagnosis and response to therapy; for example, being active may help to reduce CHF.

Congestive cardiac failure

CHF is a condition that is brought about by heart or blood vessel problems, and other issues such as:

- *Cardiomyopathy*: Weak heart muscles
- *Damaged heart valves*: Leading to changes in the bloodstream

- *Ischaemia*: normally Caused by blocked blood vessels
- *Infections*
- *High blood pressure*: This effect causes ventricular hypertrophy which is thickening of the left ventricle muscles (Smith and Yeung 2010).

Many other issues can lead to CHF, including chemotherapy, endocrine problems, toxic effects (caused by illegal drugs), thyroid disorders and excess alcohol. CHF may also develop because of lifestyle habits such as smoking, obesity, lack of exercise, high salt intake and problems with medications or therapies.

The heart can be damaged because of muscles, valves, blood vessels and so on caused by various physiological problems (Hosenpud and Greenberg 2006), which can include:

- *Cardiomyopathy*: The heart muscle becomes weak, which may be caused by damage or disease leading to poor blood circulation.
- *Muscle damage*: Muscles can be damaged when the coronary blood supply is blocked, resulting in myocardial infarction, leading to cardiac arrest or damage to the left ventricle. This can result in cardiac arrest and morbidity. Emergency medical support would be needed in this situation.
- *Hypertension*: High blood pressure forces the left ventricle to push blood into the circulatory system. High workloads can damage the heart, leading to left ventricular failure. Reducing high blood pressure is essential to prevent damage to the heart.
- *Heart valves*: Damage to heart valves impedes the flow of blood in both directions, leading to collection of blood in the heart, or lack of blood entering the heart (Hosenpud and Greenberg 2006). There are two major problems associated with valves:
  - A valve that cannot close causes blood to flow backward, forcing the heart to work harder to enable its output towards the lungs and circulatory systems. This can lead to weakening of heart muscles.
  - A stenotic valve (which doesn't open) blocks blood flow, leading to increased workload on the heart and possibly leading to heart failure (Smith and Yeung 2010).
- *Abnormal rhythm*: Abnormal heart rhythms, which may be slow, fast or irregular, reduce the pumping action of the heart. The heart has a higher workload to push blood out of the heart, and this again can lead over time to weakening of the heart and heart failure.

Congestive heart symptoms and signs

People with CHF do not always have symptoms that they suspect are associated with their heart. However, there are various conditions which can arise because of CHF (Hosenpud and Greenberg 2006, ESC 2009), and these can include:

Early Symptoms

- Shortness of breath and coughing
- A patient may consider that they have a cold, flu or bronchitis without considering the chance of CHF.
- These conditions may occur along with CHF.

Major Symptoms

- Exercise intolerance
  - The patient may be unable to exercise because of the need for oxygen and nutrients during physical activity, which cannot be provided due to CHF.
  - The patient may feel tired or have shortness of breath, and not be able to undertake exercises.

- Shortness of breath
  - The patient may have difficulty breathing when he or she is active.
  - Fluid can collect in the lungs and reduce oxygen transferring into blood. This leads to dyspnoea and shortness of breath. The patient may also cough up a frothy, pink liquid as the condition becomes more serious.
- Fluid retention and oedema
  - Oedema may develop in the legs, feet and ankles by the end of the day, due to sitting or walking.
  - Oedema may also eventually happen in the hips, scrotum, abdominal wall and abdominal cavity.
  - Daily weight checks should be taken by patients to reflect the amount of weight gain and the resultant increasing shortness of breath (Hosenpud and Greenberg 2006, ESC 2009).

Diagnosis of congestive heart failure

Undertaking a definitive diagnosis of CHF can sometimes be confusing, because of the possibility of other illnesses such as bronchitis or asthma also affecting the patient. Physical exams and tests are undertaken in hospitals to ensure the illness is properly identified (ESC 2009). Examples of tests that need to be taken include:

- *Chest x-ray*: This can identify the build-up of fluid in the lungs and also the enlargement of the heart.
- *Electrocardiogram (ECG)*: The ECG can reveal heart problems (such as rhythm disorders and strain on the heart) that lead to heart failure.
- *Blood tests*: These may include:
  - Low blood cell counts
  - Abnormal electrolyte levels
  - B-type natriuretic peptide (BNP), which is a hormone that increases as the heart muscles deteriorate.
- *Echocardiogram*: The echocardiogram is an ultrasound device which displays the heart beats and cardiac structures. It identifies problems with the anatomy of the heart, and it can measure the ability of the heart to pump blood in and out of the heart.
- *Stress testing*: A stress test helps to evaluate the cause of heart failure, especially if the patient has coronary artery disease (WHCPCC 2002). The stress test is combined with other tests to provide accurate results.
- *Magnetic resonance imaging (MRI)*: The MRI provides images of the heart and its ability to pump blood to the body as well as information about inflammation, injury and blood flow in the heart.
- *Cardiac catheterisation*: A catheter is inserted into an artery in the leg or arm and then moved to the heart to measure pressure inside the heart, look for blockages and diagnose certain disorders of the heart valves (Hosenpud and Higham 2002, ESC 2009, Smith and Yeung 2010).

Congestive heart failure treatment

Treating CHF relies on the cause of the illness. However, the patient's symptoms can be eased by removing excess fluid from the body, improving blood flow, improving heart muscle function and increasing delivery of oxygen to the body tissues. If CHF cannot be cured by surgery or catheterisation procedures, then medical treatment is offered which leads to lifestyle changes and medications (Sear and Higham 2002, Hosenpud and Greenberg 2006). This can be achieved by the actions discussed in this section.

Lifestyle changes

In some cases, treatment at home may help reduce the symptoms of CHF and increase patients' chances of a longer, healthier life (WHCPCC 2002). Patients at home can:

- Increase their comfort.
- Undertake an active role in managing heart failure.
- Elevate the feet and legs if they are swollen.
- Eat a reduced-salt diet.
- Avoid prescribed medications (unless they are essential).
- Avoid smoking.
- Avoid alcohol.
- Avoid excessive emotional stress.
- Stay active, for example by walking or aerobic exercises.
- Measure blood pressure (BP) daily (systolic BP should normally be below 140 mmHg) (WHCPCC 2002).

Medications

Patients are given medications by doctors to lessen heart failure symptoms and to help rectify any heart problems.

Diuretics

- To reduce fluids and salt in the body
- To improve the ability to breathe and reduce oedema
- Diuretics may include frusemide, bumetanide, hydrochlorothiazide, spironolactone and metolazone.

Digoxin: Digoxin is a mild inotrope which can reduce heart failure symptoms. Digoxin can also stop atrial fibrillation and flutter.

Vasodilators: Vasodilators enlarge small arteries or arterioles to relieve the systolic workload of the left ventricle which results in lower blood pressure. Vasodilators include angiotensin-converting-enzyme (ACE) inhibitors which block the production of angiotensin II which can cause vasoconstriction and may improve heart muscle function. ACE inhibitors include captopril, benazepril and ramipril.

Nitroglycerin: This drug is a nitrate preparation that can be given for treatment of acute chest pain or angina.

Beta blockers: These drugs reduce heart rate, lower blood pressure and strengthen heart muscle. Examples include metoprolol, atenolol and propranolol. They work by preventing norepinephrine from binding to beta receptors in the heart muscle and arterial walls.

Inotropes: IV inotropes are stimulants, such as dobutamine and milrinone, which increase the pumping ability of the heart by supporting the ventricles and muscles of the heart (Hosenpud and Greenberg 2006, ESC 2009).

These medications have been shown to be effective in treatment of patients with systolic CHF. Several other types of medications may also be used. Other surgical procedures may also be offered, depending on the severity of the heart failure. Examples of this include:

Angioplasty: This is used to unblock the coronary artery that supplies the left ventricle with blood.

Pacemaker: This controls and sustains the rate of the heartbeat.

Temporary cardiac support: Following a heart attack, an intra-aortic balloon pump is inserted to support left ventricle function. It is removed once the heart has recovered.

Conclusion

The increasing acceleration in ageing of the population will have a major impact on perioperative patient management (Sear and Higham 2002). Elderly people need surgery four times more than the rest of the population (ESC 2009). Although mortality from cardiac disease is decreasing in the general population, the prevalence of congestive heart failure and cardiovascular risk factors, especially diabetes, is increasing. Age, however, is responsible for only a small increase in the risk of complications; greater cardiac risks are associated with significant cardiac, pulmonary and renal diseases (Sear and Higham 2002). The number of affected individuals is likely to be higher in countries with high cardiovascular disease mortality, particularly those in Central and Eastern Europe. These conditions should, therefore, have a greater impact on evaluating patient risk than age alone (ESC 2009).

87 Venous Thromboembolism

Introduction

Venous thromboembolism (VTE) can occur often in patients and may result in major issues such as pulmonary hypertension and thrombosis in blood vessels leading to damage to nearby tissues. The main features of VTE can include deep vein thrombosis (DVT) and pulmonary embolism (PE) (Narani 2010). VTE can develop by risk factors in patients through blood coagulating which leads to thrombosis occurring. Thrombosis may occur because of issues such as venous stasis, vessel wall damage and activation of clotting factors (Bates *et al.* 2012).

Venous thrombi develop with red blood cells, platelets and leukocytes which combine with fibrin. Venous thrombi form because of blood vessel damage and slow or stagnant blood flow in the deep veins of the calf or thigh (De Martino *et al.* 2012). Thrombi may remain in the peripheral veins, or they may separate and travel through the blood vessels to the pulmonary arteries, causing PE.

VTE often occurs after acute coronary syndrome and stroke, and it can also be caused by smoking, hypertension, diabetes and high cholesterol levels (NICE 2011).

Deep venous thrombosis (DVT)

DVTs usually develop in the lower legs or thighs, but they can also develop in the mesenteric veins, pelvic veins and cerebral veins (Kucher 2011). If the DVT occurs in the lower body, there is a risk of PE occurring, and also for thrombi to migrate to the popliteal vein or above. However, because the lungs are close to the upper extremities, it is more likely for PE to occur when thrombi form in the upper part of the body (Narani 2010, Kucher 2011).

Pulmonary embolism

PEs obstruct the pulmonary arteries, leading to:

- Increased rate of breathing
- Hypoxaemia because of alveoli preventing the exchange of gases
- Atelectasis, in which one or more areas of the lungs collapse or don't inflate properly.

Also, vasoconstriction occurs because of the release of serotonin and thromboxane which cause the blood vessels to constrict (Stein *et al.* 2007).

PE can also cause decreased output of blood in the right ventricle (RV), leading to hypotension. The RV can evict a thrombus by increasing the pressure of the heart muscles which generates higher systolic pressures and pulmonary artery pressures (NICE 2011). However, in the right side of the heart, because the ventricle cannot generate high pressures, the result is right-sided heart failure.

Rapid Perioperative Care, First Edition. Paul Wicker and Sara Dalby.

Signs and symptoms of DVT and PE

Deep Venous Thrombosis

- Pain, tenderness and swelling in limbs
- Increased warmth in the body
- Oedema – in various parts of the body
- Erythema – the skin becomes red in patches because of injury or irritation, leading to dilatation of the blood capillaries.
- Dilated veins on the chest wall or leg
- Limb swelling, hypertension, ischaemia and gangrene occur – if the thrombus is not treated urgently and occludes venous outflow (Heit 2005, NICE 2011, De Martino *et al.* 2012).

Pulmonary Embolism

- Dyspnoea – difficult and laboured breathing
- Tachypnoea – rapid breathing
- Pleuritic chest pain – a sharp and stabbing chest pain
- Anxiety
- Coughing
- Tachycardia – a fast heart rate
- Fever
- Leg erythema – redness of the skin due to congestion of the capillaries (Stein *et al.* 2007, Narani 2010, NICE 2011).

Risk factors for DVT

Examples include (Heit 2005, NICE 2011):

- Medical illness (e.g. heart failure or chronic obstructive pulmonary disease)
- Surgery
- Air travel
- BMI >30
- Pregnancy, oral contraceptives or hormone replacement therapy
- Previous episode of VTE
- Cancer or certain cancer treatments
- Immobilisation
- Central venous catheters or pacemakers inside the patient
- Cardiovascular risk factors (e.g. smoking, hypertension, hyperlipidaemia and diabetes mellitus)
- Heparin-induced thrombocytopenia
- Acquired risk factors
- Inflammatory bowel disease
- Trauma
- DVT
- Antithrombin deficiency
- Prothrombin gene mutation.

Diagnostic tests for DVTs

Various diagnostic tests can be used to help identify and diagnose DVTs (Heit 2005, Dentali *et al.* 2007). These may include:

Duplex ultrasonography: Duplex ultrasonography is a device that uses ultrasound to visualise the structure or architecture of the body part. However, no motion or blood flow can be assessed accurately. Duplex ultrasonography is useful to diagnose DVTs, and it is less invasive and costs less than other procedures. Duplex ultrasonography is sensitive and specific for detecting DVT in patients. There are problems associated with distinguishing between acute and chronic DVT, and it is also difficult to use in obese patients. Duplex ultrasonography can also identify venous distention, absent or decreased spontaneous flow and abnormal Doppler signals.

Contrast venography: Venography is an x-ray test that provides an image of the leg veins after injecting a contrast dye into the patient's blood vessel. Venography is an invasive diagnostic test that provides images of leg veins on a fluoroscope screen. Venography can also identify the location, extent and degree of attachment of thrombi which enables the condition of the deep leg veins to be assessed. It is useful when doctors suspect DVT, but non-invasive tests often fail to identify the disease.

Other diagnostic tests: Other tests used to detect DVT include magnetic resonance venography (MRV) imaging and computed axial tomography venography (Dentali *et al.* 2007, Bates *et al.* 2012).

Risk factors for PE

Examples include:

- Clinical signs and symptoms of DVT
- Heart rate above 100 bpm
- Immobilisation following 3 days or surgery in the previous week
- Previous problems with PE or DVT
- Haemoptysis – coughing up blood from the respiratory tract
- Malignancy – a descriptive term for conditions that threaten life or well-being.

Diagnostic tests for PE

Several devices can be used to diagnose PEs (Narani 2010, NICE 2011). These may include:

D-dimer testing for PEs: D-dimer tests are used to help exclude, diagnose and monitor diseases and conditions that cause hypercoagulability, a tendency to clot inappropriately. Patients who have a high pre-test probability score with a negative D-dimer require further diagnostic testing to exclude PEs.

Electrocardiography: The ECG machine may be used to diagnose PE and to assess heart problems such as myocardial infarction (MI). Examples of problems seen on the ECG include sinus tachycardia, atrial fibrillation and right bundle-branch block.

Chest radiography: Chest radiography may help to diagnose PE and may also identify pleural effusion and atelectasis.

Arterial blood gas determination: Pulmonary embolism can result in significant hypoxia, which can be identified with assessment of the arterial blood gas. Urgent action is needed if hypoxia is considered.

Computed tomographic pulmonary angiography (CTPA): The CTPA device is useful for diagnosing PE, as it can visualise small or large thrombi directly. The CTPA takes direct imaging of the inferior vena cava and the pelvic and leg veins. However, this machine is expensive and also exposes the patient to radiation. The CTPA can also identify right ventricle enlargement which can indicate the possibility of adverse clinical events.

Echocardiography: The echocardiography monitor can identify several issues, including diastolic left ventricular injury, pulmonary artery hypertension, lack of inspiratory collapse of the inferior vena cava and direct visualisation of the thrombus. Following this, it may be possible to address the issue of PE (Stein *et al.* 2007, Narani 2010, NICE 2011).

Several other machines and monitors can also be used to identify PEs or DVTs, depending on their availability and costs.

Treatment

Medications are the primary way to reduce or remove thrombi. This may include unfractionated heparin (UFH), low-molecular-weight heparin (LMWH) or an oral anticoagulant (vitamin K antagonist [VKA]) (NICE 2011). However, if the patient is haemodynamically unstable, thrombolysis or pulmonary embolectomy should be considered as an alternative. Examples of drugs used include the following examples (NICE 2011, Bates *et al.* 2012, De Martino *et al.* 2012).

Unfractionated heparin

UFH achieves a therapeutic activated partial thromboplastin time (aPTT) more rapidly than other drugs. However, the aPTT should not be followed in patients with antithrombin deficiency or patients who are pregnant. In these situations, other drugs should be used. UFH is also administered subcutaneously using a dose of 17,500 units twice daily.

Low-molecular-weight heparin

LMWH is administered as a weight-based subcutaneous injection. In the current ACCP guidelines, LMWH is recommended over UFH for the early treatment of DVT or PE. Agents available include enoxaparin, dalteparin and tinzaparin. LMWH is advised in patients with renal insufficiency, or in obese, paediatric or pregnant patients. Monitoring is needed to ensure that drug treatment is working effectively.

Warfarin

Warfarin is one of the major medicines for long-term treatment of VTE, and it is in use for a minimum of 5 days. Doctors assess whether patients need low, intermediate or high doses of warfarin, in case of complications arising by giving too much or too little of the drug, leading to thrombosis or bleeding. Warfarin needs monitoring every 12 weeks to ensure it is not affecting the patient too much because of anticoagulation (Dentali *et al.* 2007).

New oral anticoagulants

There are several new anticoagulants that have been developed, including:

Dabigatran: This drug is an oral anticoagulant from the class of the direct thrombin inhibitors. However, there is no way available to reverse the anticoagulant effect of dabigatran in the event of a major bleeding event.

Rivaroxaban: This supports the treatment of VTE, and may be used for surgery on the hip or knee, as well as for treatment of DVT or PE. The drug is given orally once daily and is contraindicated in patients with renal insufficiency. The major side effect observed with rivaroxaban is bleeding, which is similar to other anticoagulants.

Thrombolytic therapy

Thrombolytic therapy for DVT using streptokinase (used to dissolve blood clots) may be beneficial for patients; it can be administered systemically or preferably by infusion using a catheter. However, there is a higher risk of haemorrhage compared to normal anticoagulants. Streptokinase is given to the patient as a 250,000 IU loading dose followed by 100,000 IU/h for 24 h; this is followed by tissue plasminogen activator (rtPA) given as a 100 mg infusion over 2 h. Bleeding remains the most serious complication of thrombolytic therapy, and the risk of intracranial bleeding is 1% to 2% (NICE 2011, Bates *et al.* 2012, De Martino *et al.* 2012).

Surgical interventions

Pulmonary embolectomy

Pulmonary embolectomy is usually only taken if the patient has a massive PE and shock, and anticoagulants fail to reduce the thrombosis (Narani 2010). Other actions could include embolectomy procedures based on catheters that use aspiration and fragmentation (breaking up the thrombus), and rheolytic therapy may also be used. This involves pumping saline into the thrombus from the tip of a catheter using an AngioJet, and then sucking the saline and clot particles back into the catheter.

Compression stockings

Following DVT, there may be damage to venous valves, leading to venous hypertension and resulting in situations such as oedema, skin pigmentation, pain and ulceration (NICE 2011). Compression stockings are able to reduce the chance of post-thrombotic syndrome happening, if they are in use for up to 1 year following thrombus formation, DVT or PE.

Conclusion

Following the diagnosis of VTE, a long period of treatment may increase the risk of recurrence. The chances of recurrence may include more DVTs or PEs, and the development of further coagulation. Other risk factors could include further coagulation factors following discontinuation of warfarin, old age, male sex and increased body mass index. Doctors must therefore assess the risk of bleeding against the risk of new thrombosis.

Patients undergoing surgery, especially those with previous cardiovascular problems and those undergoing long surgical procedures, are at high risk of developing VTE, which may result in DVT and PE (NICE 2011). Over 25,000 patients each year in the United Kingdom die because of VTE, and around 20% of patients undergoing major surgery suffer from DVT. Orthopaedic surgery can lead to even higher rates (40%) of DVT if thromboprophylaxis, which is any measure taken to prevent thrombosis, is not put in place (Narani 2010, NICE 2011).

88 Latex Allergy

Introduction

Latex allergy occurs in patients who have a reaction to latex protein or chemicals used when touching latex materials. When members of staff or patients are exposed to latex frequently, this may result in latex allergy developing. If the staff member or patient develops adverse reactions following contact with latex, or products that contain latex, then they may recognise that they have a latex allergy. Under normal circumstances following allergic reactions, patients may develop swelling of the lips and tongue if latex materials are placed in their mouths, and staff may have a rash or swelling after contacting latex gloves (Mercurio 2011). The patient or staff member will be diagnosed by the doctor and may undergo allergy testing.

In the operating department, there is sometimes difficulty in preparing latex allergy guidelines as the sensitivity to latex varies between patients and between staff. Most patients can tolerate skin contact with latex; however, other patients may have an allergy due to latex powder in a ward or contact with latex materials in the operating room (Dianne 2005). Therefore, hospital guidelines are useful, but they may not prevent serious reactions in patients or staff.

Definition of latex allergies

Latex allergies affect patients in different ways – and staff too. The following gives a list of three types of latex reactions:

Known latex allergy: Patients with known latex allergy normally have confirmation from their GP, or evidence of latex allergy test results such as a serum latex antibody test or skin prick. Most latex allergy patients would also have a past history of latex allergy following contact with latex products.

Latex alert: A high-risk patient has a latex alert within their documents, implying that they are at a high risk of developing latex allergy (Dianne 2005). This will include patients on the ward, and in operating rooms where they will need surgical operations or catheterisation which may involve the use of latex chemicals or equipment. A patient with spina bifida or other congenital anomalies is at high risk of gaining a latex allergy which will lead to serious problems (Mercurio 2011).

Increased risk: Staff and patients who have hand eczema are likely to be at risk from latex allergy. Also, certain foods also contain latex, because of cross-reactive plant proteins, which can lead to latex allergy because of food-allergic patients. Foods that contain latex include banana, papaya, kiwi fruit, avocado, chestnut and peaches (DHHS 2012).

Assessment of latex allergy

Screening for patients with latex allergy will normally be undertaken before the admission of elective patients, or when non-elective patients are admitted. If the patient has a known latex allergy or a high-risk latex allergy, then this needs to be recorded on medication charts,

Rapid Perioperative Care, First Edition. Paul Wicker and Sara Dalby.

prescriptions and admission forms so that all staff know of the patient's allergies (Mercurio 2011). The patient may also be known to have a latex allergy if a latex allergy test is taken or the patient reacts to latex powder, a latex glove, food containing latex or a device containing latex (Beckford-Ball 2005).

Management of latex allergy patients

In some hospitals, patients with latex allergy have a red identification band which identifies their latex allergy when they are admitted. Patients with latex allergy should be cared for in a single room, as there is a higher chance that there will be no latex in the room, which will create a safe environment for the patient.

Latex-allergic patients should also have information about their condition sent to the consultant on admission. A patient who may be identified as having a latex allergy, or with an uncertain diagnosis, should also be referred to a medical consultant (Brown 1999).

When a patient with latex allergy is admitted to the hospital, all staff must be informed of their condition, so there is no contact with latex by the patient. Information given to staff includes:

- Medical
- Nursing
- Allied health
- Domestic services
- Volunteer staff
- Anybody else contacting the patient.

Preventing contact with latex

Preventing exposure of the patient to latex in any form is the most effective prevention strategy. All patients who have a latex allergy need to be managed suitably to ensure they do not touch latex which will minimise the risk of sensitivity.

Taking precautions against latex allergies includes removing latex gloves from the area and replacing them with sterile latex-free or vinyl gloves, and non-sterile gloves for cleaning the operating room (DHHS 2012). Latex-free boxes are normally available in the operating department (and so should be checked before the patient enters the operating room), and suitable items can be used that are latex-free (Mercurio 2011).

It is essential that all items containing latex are removed from the anaesthetic room and operating room, as well as the recovery room or area where the patient undergoes recovery (DHHS 2005). Ideally, signs would be placed in the rooms where the patient is located which indicate the patient's susceptibility to latex allergy. Normally, these signs may be found in the latex-free boxes, or alternatively they may be written and printed. Before the patient enters the anaesthetic or operating rooms, all item of equipment which are going to be used must be checked for any latex content and removed from the area if they do contain latex (Brown 1999). It is also essential that equipment and drugs are available in case the patient develops an acute allergic reaction, so immediate action can be undertaken.

Minimising contact with latex

Latex allergies can develop in any department or area in a hospital. Specific clinical areas are most likely to have latex gloves or equipment containing latex; therefore, it is important that any latex-sensitive patient is protected. Examples of four areas include:

- Accident and Emergency Department (A&E)
- Operating Department
- Outpatients Department
- Home.

Accident and emergency department

Trauma patients who enter the A&E may declare they have latex allergy. If so, they must be treated carefully to ensure they are not connected to latex gloves, powder, equipment or the like. In some cases, there may be a bay available which is latex free and appointed for patients with latex allergies (Beckford-Ball 2005). If this is not available, then all staff should be aware of the need for a latex-free environment for the patient.

Operating department

Nursing staff in wards need to tell operating department staff of the preoperative patients who have latex allergies. The patient will need to be prepared for being latex free and have notices available which inform all members of theatre staff about the need for lack of latex products (Mercurio 2011). Normally, latex-allergic patients will be placed first on the operating list so that latex from previous cases does not result in allergic reactions. Alternatively, a separate operating room may be used which has been cleaned and had all latex products removed at least 2 or 3 hours in advance, including gloves, latex powder, equipment containing latex and so on (Mercurio 2011). If this is not possible, a clean operating theatre should be utilised with all latex products, for example latex gloves should be removed from the area before the patient arrives. Other actions to take include (Mercurio 2011):

- The operating list must provide notice of the patient's latex allergy.
- Place 'latex-free' signs within the operating theatre.
- Ensure all products are latex free, for example oropharyngeal airways, endotracheal tubes, anaesthetic circuits, oxygen masks and so on.
- Ensure members of the perioperative team have cleaned their hands and changed their theatre attire before entering the operating theatre.
- Ensure staff remain within the operating room once surgery has started to make sure it is a latex-free zone. Other members of theatre staff can collect and deliver any extra equipment to the theatre if it is needed, without entering the operating theatre. External staff should not wear the latex gloves or come into contact with any latex products during collection and delivery of equipment or items.
- Do not allow external staff to enter the operating room during surgery.
- Patients with latex allergy should undergo recovery in a latex-free area. Recovery staff need to be aware of the need to keep latex away from the patient.
- On discharge of the patient from the recovery room and transfer to the ward, all staff need to be latex free, including ward nurses. The ward nurse must know the risks associated with latex allergy and the need to keep the patient free of latex in the ward.

Outpatient department

Patients who attend outpatient departments, such as clinics or pathology labs, must tell the staff of their latex allergy. They should then be protected from latex allergy by ensuring they are managed in an area that is latex free. Staff need to be aware of the patient's condition, risks for latex, latex prevention and management of the patient.

Home

On return home, patients with latex allergy need to have it well documented on their notes about the risk of latex allergy. This is so any nurses or practitioners who care for the patient at home are aware of the risks involved. Any healthcare practitioners caring for the patient at home must have latex-free equipment and devices, so the patient is kept safe (ASA 2005).

Conclusion

Latex is extracted from rubber trees and is composed of natural proteins (ASA 2005). Many staff, as well as patients, develop latex allergies because of the regular and frequent use of latex gloves, or other devices used in the operating department that contain latex. Managers should support the reduction of latex wherever possible, as long as it does not interfere with safe patient care. Informing and training staff in the safe use of latex products, and risk assessments, should minimise the dangers and risks to health (Mercurio 2011). The operating environment needs to be safe if a patient has a latex allergy; this can be achieved by using a specific and individualised risk action plan or hospital policies (Brown 1999). When a patient develops a latex allergy, this should be reported to the manager as soon as possible. A member of staff with latex allergy will also need to go to the occupational health service for support and treatment options.

89 Pressure Ulcers

Perioperative practitioners assist in preventing skin injury during surgery because of the length of time that patients remain immobile. This is caused by poor circulation due to anaesthetic drugs, and also the pre-existing condition the patient may have before surgery. The operating table has a mattress which helps to prevent pressure ulcers, and also pillows and gel pads may be used to prevent pressure on skin. However, given the long time for some operations, practitioners need to be aware of the need to protect the patient from pressure ulcers (Neighbors *et al.* 2006). Patients developing skin injuries may need an extended period of time in the hospital, which will lead to increased costs and possibly other problems such as infection, pain and other issues. The length of hospital stay will depend on the surgery being performed. An example could be an increase of 3.5 days to 5 days, or as much as 16 days, if a pressure ulcer develops (Allman *et al.* 1999).

Other complications often arise in patients with pressure ulcers, leading to further problems (Edlich *et al.* 2004) which could include:

- *Osteomyelitis*: Inflammation of bone or bone marrow, usually due to infection
- *Amyloidosis*: A disorder marked by deposition of amyloid (an abnormal protein that is produced in bone marrow) in the body
- *Sepsis*: Sepsis occurs when chemicals are released into the bloodstream to fight the infection and then trigger inflammatory responses throughout the body, leading to multiple organ failure.
- *Sinus tract formation*: A channel that connects with an abscess or suppurating area
- *Bacteraemia*: The presence of bacteria in the blood
- *Squamous cell carcinoma*: Skin cancer that develops in the thin, flat squamous cells that make up the outer layer of the skin
- *Pyarthroses*: The formation or presence of pus within a joint, due to pressure on the joint (Allman *et al.* 1999, Edlich *et al.* 2004).

Surgical patients who develop pressure ulcers may come under much stress because of the pain and inability to be active. This can affect the patient emotionally and physically. Following development of pressure ulcers, patients may suffer from pain and disfigurement, require additional treatment and suffer from an increased hospital stay.

Intraoperative pressure ulcers

Surgical patients are more likely to develop pressure ulcers than patients in wards. The reason for this is there is a risk of developing pressure ulcers because of the surgical patient being unable to move and also being susceptible to pressure due to faulty body positioning or other factors. The chance of surgical patients developing pressure ulcers can be as high as 66% (Sanders and Allen 2006) on some occasions, depending on their positioning and the length of surgery. The type of procedure being performed can also lead to pressure ulcers; for example, if high pressure is put on an area of the patient's body, then this may lead to developing ulcers (Neighbors *et al.* 2006). The patient cannot move during surgery because of general anaesthesia; therefore, due to the time taken for surgery, the incidence

Rapid Perioperative Care, First Edition. Paul Wicker and Sara Dalby.

of pressure ulcers increases greatly. For example, surgery taking up to 6 hours can lead to a 10% chance of developing ulcers (Price *et al.* 2005). Because of the impact of pressure ulcers on patients, practitioners need to support and assist the patient to preventing pressure ulcers from developing. Practitioners therefore need to understand and recognise the risk factors and mechanisms which develop pressure ulcers in patients and take action if necessary.

Risk factors for the development of pressure ulcers

Pressure ulcers can be prevented if risk assessments are carried out on the patient both before surgery and during surgery, as long as actions are taken to prevent the risk of pressure ulcers. During the perioperative period, there are high levels of risk factors leading to pressure ulcers developing. Table 89.1 identifies some of the risks associated with pressure ulcers during the intraoperative and postoperative periods.

Formation of pressure ulcers

Pressure ulcers can develop because of vascular occlusion, ischaemia or intense pressure on the area of the body that is being affected (Brillhart 2006). When the arteries, veins and lymphatic system are occluded due to pressure over a long time, the tissues lack oxygen and nutrients (leading to ischaemia), and waste products build up because they cannot exit the area (Sanders and Allen 2006). The blood vessels will collapse and lead to thrombosis if the pressure is sustained over a long period of time. Occlusion of the blood flow results in ulceration because of tissue breakdown, which may continue even when pressure has been relieved. The tissue damage can occur because of low pressures over a long period of time, or high pressures over a short period of time (Brillhart 2006).

During general anaesthesia and surgery, the patient is unconscious, and therefore he or she feels no pain and is unable to move. Factors such as anaesthetic drugs, surgical trauma, patient age and other pre-existing conditions that the patient has (e.g. low blood pressure or poor circulation) will cause changes in the patient's metabolism and circulation (Neighbours *et al.* 2006). This will result in the weight of the patient's body pressing on bones and joints and creating pressure ulcers due to pressure on tissues.

Pressure Ulcer Development

1. Pressure on tissues – occludes capillaries
2. Reduces or eliminates blood supply to tissues
3. Tissues become ischaemic.
4. Tissue cells become necrotic and die.
5. Necrosis spreads throughout the tissue because of spreading of waste materials from the cells.
6. Eventually, ulceration occurs (Price *et al.* 2005).

The above sequence indicates the development of pressure ulcers, which may appear a few hours after surgery, or within 2 or 3 days following surgery, depending on the extent of the damage (Price *et al.* 2005).

In addition to pressure on tissues, other factors can also lead to the development of ulcers, such as shearing of skin, high pressure affecting the tissues, high temperature and the length of time spent not moving. Shearing of the skin may reduce pressure as the patient is moved, but it may still result in skin and tissue damage, because of the long period of ischaemia when the tissues were being compressed (Edlich *et al.* 2004). Using supports, straps, tourniquets and other devices may stop the patient from moving and cause further tissue damage. High temperature in patients can also lead to hypoxia because of the increased oxygen consumption by tissue cells; this may also increase ischaemia and lead to serious complications (Pearce 1996). As the length of time and intensity of pressure

Table 89.1 Risk factors (Pearce 1996, Brillhart 2006, Neighbors *et al.* 2006)

Intraoperative	Postoperative
Patient morbidity – due to loss of blood, fluids, infection, pain etc.	The patient will arrive hypothermic and will need some time to become normothermic. Warm blankets, warmed IV fluids, Bair Huggers etc. need to be used.
Type of surgical procedure – for example, placing the patient in a lithotomy position for a long time may result in pressure ulcers on the hips, legs, buttocks, elbows etc.	Patient positioning – this has to be considered to ensure that pressure is not put on joints, skin, muscles etc. Using an inflatable mattress may be the best option.
Hypothermia – leads to loss of circulation and damage to tissues. The patient needs warming blankets (and other warming devices) to encourage maintaining normothermia.	Activity – Moving the patient from side to side will help to reduce the chances of pressure ulcers. Mobility is essential to reduce pain from pressure ulcers.
Anaesthetic agents – such as sedatives, muscle relaxants and vasodilators; these can lead to tissues damage.	Reduce pressure on the surgical area – this may need the patient to be supported on pillows, gel pads, inflatable mattresses etc.
Haemodynamics – loss of blood results in hypotension, low blood pressure, low perfusion of tissues and reduced peripheral blood flow. This can cause tissue damage that leads to pressure ulcers.	Skin cleansing – keeping skin clean and free from bacteria or viruses will help to reduce infection.
Excess time spent on the operating table can reduce blood flow to parts of the body, leading to pressure ulcers.	Sitting patient upright – this would involve raising the top of the bed and allowing the patient to sit upright. Surgery needs to be taken into account.
Body positioning during surgery – poor positioning can produce pressure on parts of the body, leading to tissue damage.	Environmental risk factors – for example, temperature of the recovery room, humidity, lighting, noise etc. need to be taken into consideration to keep the patient comfortable and reduce anxiety.
Skin friction and/or shear – this can be caused by pulling the patient up the operating table, or pushing limbs. This leads to skin damage and possible postoperative pain.	
Wet skin can be caused by incontinence or pooling of prep solutions. Alcoholic prep solutions may also lead to burns if diathermy is in use.	

and shearing forces on tissues are prolonged during surgery, there is a greater likelihood of pressure ulcers forming.

Preventing pressure ulcers

Perioperative practitioners need to understand the risks associated with pressure ulcers and how to prevent them from happening. This can be achieved by attending study sessions to gain information and understanding of the need to prevent pressure ulcers from occurring. Practitioners must also understand the need to assess patients who have potential issues with pressure ulcers, before anaesthesia or surgery.

Actions to take may include (Pearce 1996, Sanders and Allen 2006):

- Developing a plan to monitor the incidence of pressure ulcers during the perioperative period

- Providing education and training regarding:
  - Developing a patient-centred care plan
  - Assessing the patient to prevent pressure ulcers, before anaesthesia or surgery
- Reassessing the patient consistently before and after a surgical procedure – preoperatively, intraoperatively and postoperatively.

Preoperative strategies (Price *et al.* 2005, Neighbours *et al.* 2006)

These can include:

- Collect information on devices to be used during surgery. This may include:
  - Positioning or using gel pads
  - Identifying settings used during the procedures, for example dates of prep solutions, electrodes and electrode gels and serial numbers for equipment.
- Complete a risk assessment to identify the possibility of pressure ulcers developing.
- Assess contributing factors and measures to be taken to prevent pressure ulcers and improve nutritional status.
- Maintain normothermia, and develop a strategy including regular monitoring of temperature.
- Ensure skin is dry following skin prepping before the surgical procedure.
- Assess and reduce pressure situations affecting the patient.
- Prevent friction and shearing of the skin of the patient.
- Assess bony prominences, and defend them against pressure.

Intraoperative strategies (Pearce 1996, Price *et al.* 2005, Neighbours *et al.* 2006)

- Protect the patient, and position them correctly and safely.
- Protect areas likely to develop pressure ulcers when the patient is placed in a prone, supine or lateral position (Figure 89.1). For example, use cushions, pillows, gel pads and other protective devices.
- Assess the peripheral tissue perfusion in areas which are under pressure, and take action if perfusion is decreased.
- Reduce the chances of exposure of skin to fluids intraoperatively.
- Ensure the patient is comfortable by smoothing the materials beneath the patient while on the operating table.
- Maintain a patient's normothermia by regular assessment and monitoring of their temperature (Pearce 1996).
- Protect the patient's bony prominences from excess pressure caused by the weight of the patient or increased pressure by the surgical team.

Postoperative strategies (Neighbours *et al.* 2006, Hatfield 2014)

Postoperatively, the patient is likely to develop pressure ulcers due to pressure on the tissues during surgery. Several actions may need to be taken, including:

- Monitor and record any changes or abnormalities.
- Mobilise the patient as soon as possible after the surgical procedure – this may only be possible on return to the ward.
- Prevent patients from lying on their trochanters, and ensure they are comfortable.

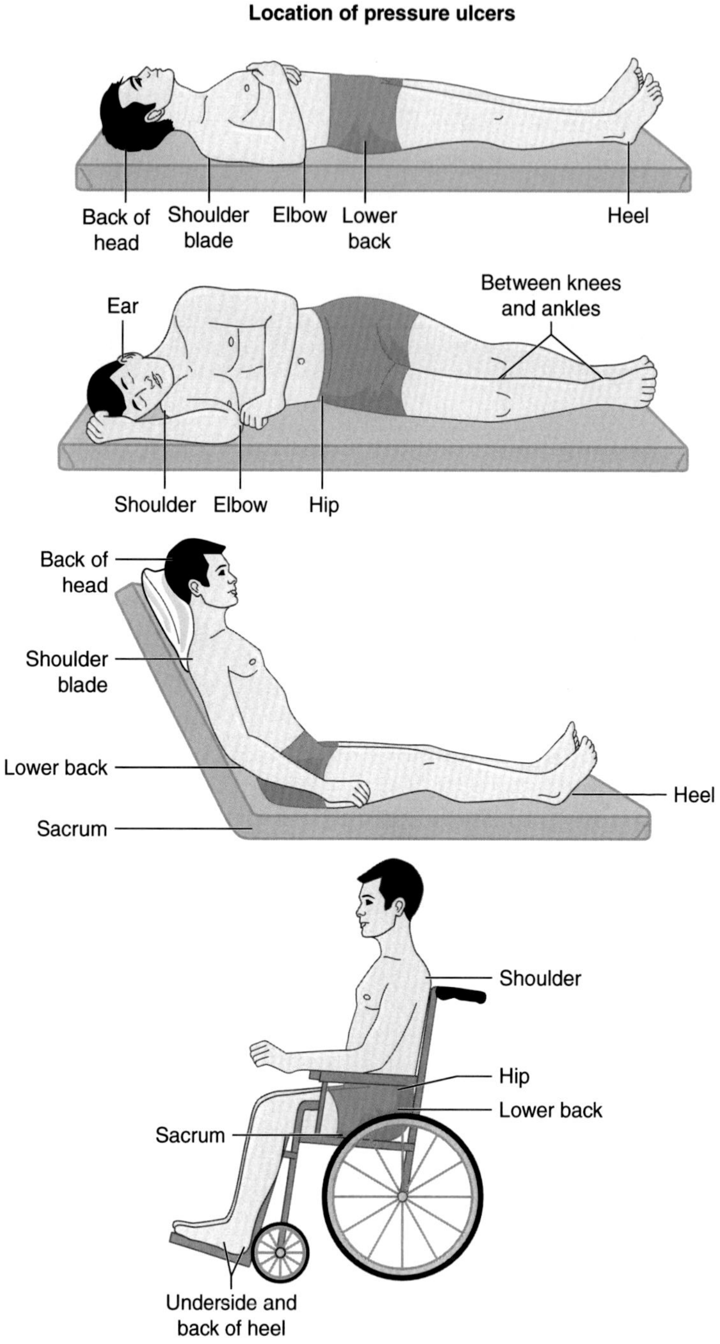

Location of pressure ulcers

Back of head
Shoulder blade
Elbow
Lower back
Heel

Ear
Between knees and ankles
Shoulder
Elbow
Hip

Back of head
Shoulder blade
Lower back
Sacrum
Heel

Shoulder
Hip
Lower back
Sacrum
Underside and back of heel

Figure 89.1 Main areas where pressure ulcers can occur.

- Consistently reposition patients recovering from anaesthesia every hour, to reduce pressure on tissue areas.
- Relieve pressure from areas that appear to have been placed under pressure during surgery.
- Use pressure-relieving devices to help areas that have been under pressure during extended surgery times, or if the patient has vascular disease or diabetes.
- Use devices, such as gel pads, to prevent contact with bony prominences, such as elbows, hips, knees and so on.
- Ensure skin that is soiled is kept clean on a regular basis.
- Keep the bed flat if possible, as raising the head of the bed will put pressure on the patient's lower extremities.
- Ensure the patient remains warm, comfortable and pain free during recovery.

Conclusion

Pressure ulcers occur because of the breakdown of skin and underlying tissues caused by high pressure during surgery, when the patient cannot move or change position. Pressure ulcers are also known as *bedsores* or *pressure sores*, depending on their causes or the choice of the healthcare practitioners.

Pressure ulcers can result in minor patches of discoloured skin (when pressure is low and the surgery occurs within minutes) and also open wounds that can expose the underlying bone or muscle, following high pressures and long surgical times. Pressure ulcers happen often in surgical patients because of the length of surgery and the extended period of time that pressure is impacting on bony prominences. Medical staff and healthcare practitioners must understand the problems that patients face following excessive pressure on areas of their body.

Therefore, staff need to understand the need to assess and action areas that are likely to suffer from pressure ulcers, to prevent them from occurring. When plans are developed and staff are aware of the risks of pressure ulcers, the surgical patient may avoid the risks of developing pressure ulcers.

90 Managing Diabetes in Perioperative Patients

Introduction

Diabetes affects around 4–5% of people in the United Kingdom and creates a serious metabolic disorder in these patients (Dhatariya *et al.* 2011). Because of the ready-made food provided by supermarkets, which contains much sugar and fat, there has been a rise in obesity which is likely to increase diabetes even further. This will have a high impact on patient care, especially during anaesthesia and surgery. Following perioperative care, many diabetic patients develop increased morbidity and remain in the hospital longer, which increases costs for the NHS. There are various reasons for morbidity to develop, and these can include:

- Hypo or hyperglycaemia – caused by too much or too little dextrose infusions
- Complications with blood vessels, especially capillaries
- Misuse of insulin
- Inappropriate use of intravenous insulin infusion
- Perioperative infection (Dhatariya *et al.* 2011).

Due to the increase in elderly patients, there is now a high-risk surgical population who have various medical conditions that need major surgery. Examples of such diseases and illnesses include diabetes, cardiovascular problems, ischaemia, respiratory disease and renal problems (Rubino *et al.* 2009). Patients who have similar diseases or illnesses may result in a poor outcome after surgery.

Diabetes can also result in a huge increase in cardiovascular diseases, leading to high blood pressure, coronary artery disease and strokes (Dhatariya *et al.* 2011). Patients who have an impaired cardiac function or kidney problems are likely to have a risk of fluid overload, which may lead to cardiac arrhythmias intraoperatively or postoperatively. It is also possible that perioperative patients have low levels of fluid replacement and hypotension which can lead to renal failure in elderly patients who have kidney problems or preoperative hypotension (NPSA 2009). Errors such as these occur for several reasons, including:

- Lack of a care plan, for patients who are at high risk of morbidity
- Communication failure between team members
- Inadequate experience and knowledge in the perioperative team
- Lack of understanding of the need to involve the diabetes specialist team (Dhatariya *et al.* 2011).

Preoperative assessment

To manage a surgical patient who has diabetes, it is important that they are not fasted for longer than 6 h before surgery. Usually, the patient will continue to eat and drink until 2

Rapid Perioperative Care, First Edition. Paul Wicker and Sara Dalby.

or 3 h before the start of anaesthesia and surgery which will help to minimise starvation and hypovolaemia. Patients with diabetes are therefore normally sent to surgery early in the morning so they can recover and have lunch or an evening meal once they have recovered from anaesthesia. It is therefore advisable not to have diabetic patients undertaking surgery in the evening as this may result in glucose levels falling after taking medication for anaesthesia (Dhatariya *et al.* 2011).

Supporting diabetic patients before anaesthesia is essential, and the main actions could include:

- Manage control of the patient's glycaemic level before surgery.
- Develop a diabetic management plan with the patient, to help manage diabetes before and during surgery.
- Assess the patient to identify any illnesses or diseases that can be supported or treated before admission.
- Ensure a plan is in place to manage critical care patients during their intraoperative phase, including the use of medications such as warfarin, heparin, insulin and so on (Plodkowski and Edelman 2001, Dhatariya *et al.* 2011).

Preoperative action plan

Devising an action plan will help support the patient and inform the staff of actions they need to take. These will include:

- Diabetic patients must attend a preoperative assessment clinic. Staff should:
  - Assess adequacy of glycaemic control.
  - Consider referral to the diabetes specialist team.
  - Identify any other issues apart from diabetes.
  - Plan admission, for example time of admission, wards number, time of surgery, medications required and so on.
  - Discuss the availability of insulin that the patient normally uses.
- Develop a plan for enhanced recovery to improve the patient's recovery.
- Discuss the plan with the patient to ensure all actions are suitable for the patient.
- Teach the patient about medication changes before admission.
- Discuss and plan preoperative management of diabetes with the patient.
- Do not place the patient on an evening or late list so there are no prolonged fasting times.
- If the patient has a risk of venous thromboembolism, risk-assess and identify actions that need to be taken, such as the use of anti-embolism stockings.
- Discuss duration of stay and discharge arrangements.
- Tell ward staff of the plans for activation on day of admission.
- Discuss the need for support at home following discharge from the hospital (NPSA 2009, Dhatariya *et al.* 2011, Banasch and McConachie 2014).

Intraoperative care

During intraoperative care, the team must work together and liaise about the plans and guidelines for caring for diabetic patients. This is likely to be covered during the World Health Organization (WHO) checklist, especially during the team gathering before the patient arrives. One of the main elements of the plan would be to assess the patient's blood glucose levels and deliver action if needed. The main elements of the plan needed during intraoperative care may include:

- Monitor and control appropriate levels of glycaemia during surgery.
- Assess and manage normal electrolyte concentrations in the patient's bloodstream.
- Monitor and optimise cardiovascular and renal functions.

- Assess the patient's need for analgesia and anti-emetics to maintain the health of the patient.
- Avoid pressure ulcers from developing during surgery (Dagogo-Jack and Alberti 2002, Banasch and Mcconachie 2014).

Intraoperative action plan

The intraoperative action plan would be aimed at maintaining the patient's health during surgery and defending the patient against hypoglycaemia and other problems that may arise. Actions could include:

- Implement the WHO surgical safety checklist, and discuss the perioperative care plan.
- Assess and consistently monitor the patient's blood glucose; the average range is 4–12 mmol/L.
- Assess and monitor the capillary blood glucose level before induction of anaesthesia.
- Treat a high blood glucose level by using insulin.
- Deliver intravenous fluids as needed.
- Document all actions during surgery.
- Prepare the patient for a critical care ward if needed.
- Use anaesthetic drugs (e.g. ondansetron) to reduce the incidence of postoperative nausea and vomiting (PONV) (NPSA 2009, Dhatariya *et al.* 2011, Banasch and McConachie 2014).

The anaesthetist must record all actions taken during intraoperative care, including glucose levels, fluids and drugs (including insulin) and so on. Constant monitoring of capillary blood glucose level will depend on the condition of the patient. Blood glucose levels are normally monitored every 30 min if the levels are unstable, or every hour if blood glucose levels are stable (Plodkowski and Edelman 2001).

Postoperative care

Managing the patient's glycaemic levels during surgery is very difficult and may lead to hyperglycaemia because of neuroendocrine stress leading to insulin resistance. Following long periods of surgery, the patient may become hypoglycaemic because of lack of nutrition (Hatfield 2014). Management of glucose levels is therefore the responsibility of the anaesthetist to ensure good control of glycaemia both during and after surgery.

The use of insulin is essential for the patient, but it must be used safely and correctly or the patient may become increasingly morbid (NPSA 2009). Examples of errors may include using the wrong kind of insulin, giving the wrong dosage, using it at the wrong time and not giving the patient insulin when it is required (NPSA 2009). A 'never-event' in regards to insulin can result in death or severe harm to the patient.

Postoperatively, patients can be at high risk because of diabetes, and so a specialist diabetic team may be required to monitor and manage the patient. Other reasons why the patient's glycaemic levels change are because of emergency surgery, catabolic stress and infection, and in all cases the patient needs to be closely monitored (Hatfield 2014). The main aims of caring for diabetic patients postoperatively can include:

- Maintain glycaemic control, fluids and electrolyte balance.
- Manage control of pain.
- Encourage the patient to eat and drink as soon as the patient has recovered to help stabilise their diabetic condition.
- Follow the principles of the enhanced recovery.
- Avoid any injuries due to drugs, infection, pressure damage and so on (Hatfield 2014).

Postoperative action plan

Developing an action plan is essential for postoperative diabetic patients. Various actions that should be considered may include:

- Use staff with skills in diabetes management to monitor and care for the patient.
- Following recovery from anaesthesia, patients should be able to manage their diabetes if they have the skills and knowledge about their condition.
- Ensure the anaesthetist has provided instructions on the use of intravenous fluids and insulin.
- Prescribe and administer insulin as required.
- Monitor the capillary blood glucose level and ensure it stays within 4–12 mmol/L.
- Monitor and record levels of electrolytes and fluid balance, and check with the anaesthetist if problems arise.
- Monitor and observe for signs of postoperative nausea and vomiting, and treat if necessary using drugs. This will help the patient to start eating food once they have recovered.
- Monitor and assess for infection.
- Check the patient for high-pressure areas, and move the patient regularly to prevent the development of pressure ulcers (NPSA 2009, Dhatariya *et al.* 2011, Banasch and McConachie 2014, Hatfield 2014).

Conclusion

Diabetes is a serious condition that requires urgent care of the patient during the surgical procedure and may also lead to the chance of morbidity and mortality postoperatively (Rubino *et al.* 2009). The patient may become stressed during surgery because of the surgical actions being taken, which can lead to effects such as hyperglycaemia and osmotic diuresis. Lack of insulin can also cause ketoacidosis or hyperosmolar syndrome which leads to very high blood glucose levels. Hyperglycaemia will lead to damage of leukocyte function and may also prevent effective wound healing. Managing the care of the diabetic patient is therefore important and may include monitoring and assessment of body fluids and electrolytes, the level of calories and the careful use of insulin.

91 Smoking, Alcohol and Drug Abuse

Smoking, alcohol and drug abuse, taken hours or even days before surgery, can have a massive impact on patients undergoing anaesthesia and surgical procedures, because of the interaction with anaesthetic drugs and the effects of surgery. This may lead to critical illness and may result in mental disorders following surgery (Evans 2014).

It is also likely that students or young adults are more likely to drink, smoke and take drugs than the older population in general. This is because peer pressure (from other students or friends), student bars (offering cheap beer) and living away from home (for the first time) contribute to the actions that young adults undertake. Most students or young adults are not aware of the dangers associated with smoking, drinking and taking drugs, and the impact it may have on their health. So finding out more about the unhealthy use of smoking, drugs and alcohol can help students think twice about the way they live their lives and its impact on their health (Bourhenne 2007).

People drinking alcohol

People from the age of 18 upwards live a life that may revolve around alcohol, especially students who have student bars and local pubs which are often part of the university campus. Drinking in moderation is acceptable and has little impact on individuals; however, getting drunk every day can lead to serious physical, social and academic effects (Evans 2014). Drinking alcohol excessively at a particular event can also lead to accidents, headaches, confusion and other problems.

Drinking too much can undermine work performance because it affects concentration and makes people more likely to misunderstand what is needed in their work time, for example writing in the incorrect way, arguing with their colleagues and so on. Students may also miss classes, hand in work late and do badly in exams, leading to expulsion from their programme (Evans 2014).

Drinking alcohol may also put people at risk of serious harm, ranging from date rape (men who are drunk are more likely to rape women), car crashes if they happen to be driving home, or walking in the middle of a road. Drunk people are also likely to be attacked, and drunk women may be raped which can lead to sexually transmitted infections and also the possibility of unplanned pregnancy (Bourhenne 2007).

Over years, people who drink alcohol on a regular daily basis may develop liver disease, cardiac problems, weight gain and possibly cancer (Evans 2014). Because the use of alcohol has increased because of stress and anxiety in modern times, health problems are now occurring at younger ages and may lead to serious problems. People who have had a heavy drinking session should remain alcohol-free for a full 48 h to give their body time to recover. Research (Vizcaychipi 2013) has also shown that magnesium can defend people's tissues, organs and brain against damage by alcohol. The use of magnesium also prevents elderly people from becoming demented following the use of anaesthetic drugs (Vizcaychipi 2013).

Rapid Perioperative Care, First Edition. Paul Wicker and Sara Dalby.

The effect of drinking depends on both the strength of alcohol being taken and the health and fitness of the individual (Evans 2014). The way alcohol affects people can depend on:

- Previous drinking episodes of alcohol
- The quantity of alcohol in the drink
- The speed at which alcohol is consumed
- The rate at which alcohol is absorbed
- The person's body weight – thin people cannot handle alcohol in the same way as overweight people
- The physiological response to alcohol
- Motivation for drinking (such as a party or social meeting) (Evans 2014).

Alcohol is absorbed into the bloodstream and carried to the brain and spinal cord, leading to physical and psychological effects. Alcohol acts as a sedative, tranquilliser, depressant and sometimes stimulant. Alcohol also induces mood changes by depressing the part of the brain which sends nerve impulses out to the body (Evans 2014). This results in poor motor coordination, leading to staggering as the person walks.

Drinkaware.co.uk (Drinkaware 2015) recommends that men should not regularly drink more than three to four units a day and women should not regularly drink more than two to three units a day to preserve a healthy state.

People smoking

Students are often under pressure to smoke, especially in social gatherings or parties. People who smoke have a high risk of lung cancer (caused by tar substances in tobacco) and heart disease because of the smoke being inhaled into their lungs and because of the various drugs associated with tobacco (Bourhenne 2007). Smoking also ages the skin, leading to wrinkles and a greyish, wasted appearance. Smoking or living in a smoky environment dries the skin's surface and constricts blood vessels. This reduces blood flow to the skin because of the constricted blood vessels and depletes the skin of oxygen and essential nutrients. Smoking can also cause impotence and reduced sperm count in men, as well as reduced fertility in women. Cigarette smokers tend to die at least 10 years sooner than non-smokers because of damage to the heart and lungs, and because of cerebrovascular disease (Bourhenne 2007).

Smoking can also cause chronic bronchitis and emphysema which will result in chronic obstructive lung disease (Bourhenne 2007). Emphysema is a condition in which the air sacs (alveoli) of the lungs are damaged and enlarged, causing breathlessness. People with emphysema may therefore struggle to breathe at normal rates.

Smoking doesn't necessarily reduce stress or calm people down during stressful experiences, such as exams or work problems. However, smoking can sometimes calm people because the craving for nicotine, when the person is not allowed to smoke, can make him or her feel stressed and anxious until they actually start smoking, and then they become calm temporarily (Evans 2014). People, however, would feel less stressed once they stop smoking and no longer have cravings for the nicotine and other drugs present in tobacco. Stopping smoking is an advantage for anybody, as it could lead to a healthier life and better chance of not acquiring issues such as lung cancer.

People taking drugs

Taking illegal or unnecessary drugs can affect a person's health easily. For example, in Liverpool, buying a small metal cylinder (about 2 inches long with a snap-off top) which contains nitrous oxide is not seen as illegal, but it can definitely affect a person's health. Cannabis, however, is probably the most common illegal drug in the United Kingdom. However, it appears the use of cannabis has fallen in the age group of 16–59 year olds from 10.6% in 2003–04 to 6.6% in 2013–14 (NHS Choices 2015).

The effects of cannabis can vary between people, but may result in good feelings such as:

- Feeling relaxed and happy
- Becoming more talkative
- Developing hunger pangs
- Experiencing intensified colours and the sound of music
- Feeling a slowing down of time.

However, negative effects of cannabis can include:

- Feeling faint or sick
- Feeling sleepy and lethargic
- Effects on people's memory, for example friend's names or the location of their home
- Feeling confusion, anxiety or paranoia, panic attacks and hallucinations (Bourhenne 2007, NHS Choices 2015).

Using cannabis regularly can demotivate people and make them less interested in education, work or doing other activities in their life. It can also reduce their capacity to remember facts and to concentrate on particular matters (NHS Choices 2015).

Other examples of illegal drugs include heroin, cocaine, crack, ecstasy, ketamine and LSD. Addiction to drugs such as these will have a serious effect on health and the person's ability to live a good life. Dangerous drugs are therefore made illegal to improve the health of the population. People taking illegal drugs are likely to be fined or sent to prison; for example, taking cocaine can lead to 7 years in prison. Also, if people take illegal drugs, their workplace or university would probably ban them from the campus and expel them from the programme they are undertaking. Many universities would ban students from campus or drop them from their programme. The best way to minimise the risk from drugs is to confirm with your GP and find out as much information as you can about the drugs that you are using.

Conclusion

Smoking, drinking alcohol excessively and taking illegal drugs can severely affect a patient's health, especially if they are undertaking major surgery and becoming critically ill. Post-operatively, there can be serious complications which may result in the patient's death or, alternatively, keeping them in hospital for several weeks or months until they recover. Reducing or prohibiting smoking, alcohol and the use of drugs is therefore an important element to consider several weeks or months before surgery, and the patient must be fully informed of the need to avoid this by the GP, anaesthetist or surgeon.

92 Perioperative Care of Elderly Patients

The number of elderly people in the United Kingdom is steadily increasing over the years, possibly due to the 'baby boom' in the 1960s. Elderly patients who are undergoing anaesthesia and surgery therefore have a high risk of morbidity and mortality. Optimising care for elderly patients is therefore essential to ensure they are cared for effectively and efficiently, which also includes the generation of individualised care pathways. Elderly patients have several different conditions, for example diabetes, osteoporosis, cardiovascular problems and so on (Shippee-Rice *et al.* 2012). Following surgery, enhanced recovery techniques are also better for elderly patients which can help them to recover quicker and preserve their state of health.

The UK population in 2009 had 16% of people aged 65 years or older, and by 2034, it is expected the number of elderly people will rise to 23%. There were 1.4 million people who were aged 85 or older in 2009, and by 2034 this is likely to increase to 3.5 million in the United Kingdom (ONS 2012).

Elective surgery

Elderly patients who undergo elective surgery need best care following surgery as they are often limited in their ability to care for themselves. This needs practitioners to follow the clinical care pathway that was developed for them. Before surgery, it is likely the GP will list the various conditions the patient has and the actions needed to be taken. These could include reviewing the use of medication (in case it interacts with anaesthetic medication), dietary advice regarding food and fluids, and also advising the patient not to smoke, drink alcohol or take illegal drugs (AAGBI 2014). The pre-assessment of the patient is normally discussed or passed on to the anaesthetist and surgeon so they are fully aware of the patient's condition.

Within hospitals and the ward, nurses and practitioners will discuss the issues with elderly patients and put measures in place to improve the care pathway before undergoing surgery. Changes to the care pathway would include the assessment of the patient's health, the level of illnesses the patient has and the ability of the patient to walk or move around safely (Shippee-Rice *et al.* 2012). Before surgery, it is likely the surgeon and anaesthetist, and maybe perioperative staff, will become involved in developing the pathway, which could involve elements such as interprofessional discussions, preoperative care required and a thorough assessment of the patient's health and fitness. Developing this clinical pathway will provide clear improvements for the patient and reduce the length of stay in the hospital.

Undertaking pre-assessment of the patient by ward staff and perioperative staff occurs before the patient arriving for surgery. Normally this will be listed in a care plan and will identify any issues that may need to be sorted. This will encourage staff to care better for the elderly patient and ensure the patient is supported in all areas (AAGBI 2014).

Rapid Perioperative Care, First Edition. Paul Wicker and Sara Dalby.

Emergency surgery

Elderly patients may undergo emergency surgery because of falls, accidents or cardiovascular problems, and this carries a high risk for the patient compared to elective surgery. Elderly patients may develop serious illness or even death following emergency surgery, because of their poor state on admission to the hospital and the lack of time for assessing the patient and developing suitable care pathways (Shippee-Rice *et al.* 2012).

To build a care pathway, it is important that elderly patients are assessed rapidly before surgery. An evaluation needs to be undertaken by a surgeon or anaesthetist about how the patients can be supported before surgery for minimising pain, providing fluid therapy, preventing bleeding and so on (Shippee-Rice *et al.* 2012). The patient may also need other actions taken such as providing nutrition, medicines, infusions and the like (AAGBI 2014). This will be undertaken by nurses or practitioners via the care pathway, and further information will be passed on to the operating room admissions team and recovery department. Again, enhanced recovery needs to be implemented in elderly patients who are seriously ill, which may also include the use of critical care practitioners, surgeons and anaesthetists.

Care pathways for elderly patients

Nurses and practitioners need to know the core principles for care pathways for elderly patients both in day-care and when patients are kept in hospital for long periods of time. Patient outcomes are therefore optimised by using main principles of support, and they are usually applicable for all elderly patients in elective and emergency surgery (Shippee-Rice *et al.* 2012). Managing postoperative elderly patients using the *enhanced recovery* pathways will also greatly benefit patients and hopefully would help them to fully recover from their surgery.

Potential actions that need to be included in perioperative patient care pathways may include the following examples:

- Preoperative assessment of cognitive dysfunction
- Receive patient information about their health status.
- Preoperative assessment of postoperative delirium or cognitive dysfunction, to support the patient postoperatively
- Use perioperative staff who have the skills to treat elderly patients:
  - Assessment of cognitive dysfunction
  - Understanding of enhanced recovery principles
  - Clinical skills for applying enhanced recovery
- Assess the patient's physical status and level of frailty.
- Improve the rapid mobilisation of the patient postoperatively if suitable.
- Ensure the use of anaesthetic drugs and drugs used during the perioperative phases are suitable:
  - Correct use of anaesthetic agents that provide rapid recovery and minimal side effects
  - Monitor the depth of anaesthesia during surgery and minimise use of anaesthetic agents.
  - Ensure satisfactory fluid management.
  - Provide pain management and support early mobilisation.
- *Provide monitoring during anaesthesia and surgery, and postoperatively, to ensure the patient is keeping satisfactory health levels. This may include pulse, oxygen level, blood pressure, temperature, depth of anaesthesia, circulation and so on* (Shippee-Rice *et al.* 2012, Dodds *et al.* 2013, AAGBI 2014).

Postoperative delirium

Elderly patients who undergo major surgery are often at risk of delirium postoperatively, and they need early identification of delirium for referral and treatment using psychiatrists or psychiatric nurses (Sharma *et al.* 2005). Once delirium has been identified, there needs to be a management plan carried out to optimise patient care, involving doctors, nurses and/or practitioners who can carry out further assessment and support, as well as providing guidance for the recovery and ward staff (AAGBI 2014).

Most elderly patients develop delirium because of the use of anaesthetic drugs, such as sedatives or induction agents, and possibly because of the effects of surgery. Postoperative delirium can occur immediately after waking up in recovery and can last for days, weeks or months (Sharma *et al.* 2005). Delirium can also occur when patients undergo regional or local anaesthesia, but are also given sedatives to calm them down. It is important to be aware that delirium also occurs where sedation is used in regional or local anaesthesia (Sieber *et al.* 2010). Delirium can result in longer lengths of stay in hospitals leading to increased costs, and also serious consequences for the patient leading to, for example, death or permanent dementia (Dodds *et al.* 2013).

Vizcaychipi (2013) states the use of magnesium helps to preserve the body's homeostasis and prevents avoidable complications during the perioperative period by reducing the incidence of critical events, as well as improving the patient's recovery after surgery. Magnesium stabilises cells in the tissues and organs of the body. In particular, magnesium can be used during anaesthesia to reduce the quantity of anaesthetic drugs being used and protects the brain from developing delirium in older patients (Vizcaychipi 2013).

Postoperative pain

Elderly patients often suffer pain at high levels, compared with younger people, possibly because they have stiff joints, sore wounds and chronic pain syndromes, for example because of osteoarthritis or osteoporosis leading to nerve damage or painful bones (Shippee-Rice *et al.* 2012, Malcolm 2015). Pain assessment is therefore essential and will require the elderly patient to describe the pain and perhaps use a pain scale to identify the level of pain. However, the patient, if suffering from delirium, may not be able to describe or discuss the level of pain, making the opportunity for pain relief more challenging. Recovery practitioners therefore have to be careful when delivering analgesics to elderly patients to ensure that pain relief is carefully controlled (Sharma *et al.* 2005, Malcolm 2015).

Assessing and effectively managing acute pain in elderly patients throughout the perioperative period are therefore essential to maintain their health status. This would therefore include pain assessment, pharmacological management of pain, using drugs such as paracetamol, NSAIDS, codeine, opioids and local anaesthetics and so on (Malcolm 2015). Pain relief will help the elderly patient to be more comfortable and may also avoid adverse outcomes following anaesthesia and surgery (Malcolm 2015).

Discharge of elderly patients

Elderly patients who have undergone serious surgery are often at risk of problems with their physical or mental functioning, and they may require longer periods of time in the hospital. Effective discharge management planning for elderly patients is therefore essential to ensure their level of health is maintained as much as possible; otherwise, they may need to be readmitted or they may need long-term care in their own home or in nursing homes (Shippee-Rice *et al.* 2012, AAGBI 2014).

Conclusions

The elderly surgical patient needs the best care during preoperative, intraoperative and postoperative periods, to ensure they preserve their state of health as much as possible and to enable them to return home. It is therefore essential that elderly people are cared for at a high level and that practitioners, and doctors, are fully aware of the need to care for elderly people at the best level possible. Possible actions that may be taken throughout the patient's stay in hospital include:

- Effective preoperative assessment and optimisation of health issues
- Surgical management about the physical and mental state of the patient
- Minimal use of anaesthetic agents, analgesics, sedatives and so on to reduce the chances of delirium or poor health
- Use of techniques to maximise rapid recovery
- Providing assessment in recovery about pain, delirium, normothermia, fluid balance, oxygenation, circulation, blood pressure and so on (Shippee-Rice *et al.* 2012, Dodds *et al.* 2013, AAGBI 2014).

The care of the elderly patient is therefore essential during the perioperative period to ensure their health is maintained and their recovery is rapid and effective.

93 Anaemia, Coagulopathy and Bleeding

Anaemia can occur because of a nutritional shortage, loss of red blood cells (RBCs) caused by bleeding, lack of production of RBCs in bone marrow, increased destruction of RBCs caused by infection, and the short life of RBCs (Cave 2014). Patients in hospital may also develop anaemia because of nutritional deficiencies, medical drugs suppressing the production of RBCs, inflammation, phlebotomy (opening a blood vessel using a needle and syringe to extract blood) and chronic or acute bleeding (Cave 2014).

Anaemia can therefore affect many elderly patients, and when this occurs in the operating room it may lead to morbidity or mortality (Shippee-Rice *et al.* 2012). Anaemia can be resolved following the transfusion of RBCs, which is a common treatment for anaemia. Patients in hospital often develop anaemia because of iron deficiency (Goodnough 2012), trauma, phlebotomy, coagulopathy (impaired coagulation of blood) and adverse effects and reactions to medications (Cave 2014).

Anaemia is a haemoglobin level which is less than 13 g/dL in men and below 12 g/dL in women (Goodnough 2012). Most patients who develop anaemia also include those with kidney disease, cancer, heart disease, bowel disease, rheumatoid arthritis and HIV (Nissenson *et al.* 2005).

Nutritional deficiency anaemia

Critically ill patients of any age may suffer from iron deficiency, although one-third of elderly patients aged 65 years or older have nutritional deficiency anaemia, so critically ill adults usually have a high rate of anaemia (Woodman *et al.* 2005, Shippee-Rice *et al.* 2012).

Healthy patients have an inverse relationship between haemoglobin and erythropoietin, which is a hormone that stimulates production of RBCs. When the patient has hypoxaemia because of low haemoglobin levels, erythropoietin stimulates an increase in RBCs. However, if the patient has low iron levels, then this does not occur because of low levels of haemoglobin (Shippee-Rice *et al.* 2012). Patients with iron deficiency can be treated with oral iron tablets or intravenous iron solutions (Goodnough 2012, Okam *et al.* 2012). Intravenous iron therapy is the preferred choice because of abdominal problems following oral iron tablets in many elderly patients (Shippee-Rice *et al.* 2012).

Phlebotomy

The surgical opening or puncture of a vein (called *phlebotomy*) can also lead to blood loss, leading to anaemia on the ward or in the operating room. Under normal circumstances, people produce around 0.5 L of blood per week; however, phlebotomies can lead to a daily loss of around 70 ml or more of blood every day (Corwin *et al.* 1995). In most cases, this amount of blood loss cannot be replaced in critically ill patients, therefore leading to an increased likelihood of anaemia developing (Cave 2014). Reducing blood sampling (to prevent anaemia) can include using low-volume phlebotomy tubes (e.g. paediatric tubes); it

Rapid Perioperative Care, First Edition. Paul Wicker and Sara Dalby.

may also be possible to use closed-loop systems which return blood to the patient. Assessing the patient after phlebotomy and on a regular basis using pulse oximetry will help to identify blood loss or circulation issues (Cave 2014).

Drug reactions

Patients who take drugs may have negative effects that lead to anaemia by causing haemolytic anaemia or by suppressing the release of erythropoietin in the kidneys. Haemolytic anaemia is caused by destroying erythrocytes which are damaged by antibiotic drugs such as piperacillin, cefotetan and ceftriaxone, and then destroyed by macrophages in the spleen and liver (Hayden *et al.* 2012). These drugs need to be stopped if the antibodies activate the macrophages.

If the patient develops haemolytic anaemia, drugs such as corticosteroids and rituximab (an antibody) can be used to reduce the macrophages, which are responsible for haemolysis. Drugs such as angiotensin-converting enzyme inhibitors and angiotensin-receptor blockers (for treatment of high blood pressure), calcium channel blockers, theophylline, and β-adrenergic blockers reactions can also cause anaemia in patients by suppressing erythropoietin, which is a hormone that increases the production of RBCs (Hayden *et al.* 2012).

Bleeding complications

Bleeding complications during surgery and postoperatively are common in many patients. Patients may develop coagulation abnormalities and mucosal lesions caused by induced stress, which are high-risk factors for significant bleeding in patients (Murphy 2010). In patients with coagulopathy, retroperitoneal bleeding can increase morbidity and mortality, and leads to an extended stay in the hospital because of the need for blood transfusion and the need to stop the bleeding (Murphy 2010). Detection of bleeding during surgery can help to reduce these risks.

Coagulation abnormalities

Critically ill patients sometimes have coagulation issues such as thrombocytopenia or disseminated intravascular coagulation (DIC) (Cave 2014). Thrombocytopenia, which is a deficiency of platelets in the blood that can cause bleeding in the tissues, bruising and slow blood clotting after injury, is often the main issue for critically ill patients, who have low platelet counts (Murphy 2010). Thrombocytopenia can occur because of several different clinical events such as:

- Haemodilution caused by increased fluids in blood from intravenous transfusions
- Low platelet levels because of major trauma or bleeding
- Platelet destruction, possibly because of sepsis
- Liver disease leading to reduced platelet production
- Defective bone marrow or viral infection leading to non-production of platelets (Murphy 2010, Cave 2014).

Medicines used for patients can also lead to thrombocytopenia.

DIC is far less common in most patients; however, it can be severe in patients with sepsis. DIC has a low platelet count caused by coagulation and destruction of platelets over a long period of time (Murphy 2010).

Although DIC is rarely seen in patients, it can lead to severe bleeding and possibility of mortality. As well as bleeding, organ damage can occur because of microvascular thrombosis, and this can be even more severe, leading to morbidity and mortality (Cave 2014).

Like thrombocytopenia, DIC is common in patients with sepsis and trauma, which can lead to systemic inflammation or infection (Murphy 2010). DIC can be prevented and treated by avoiding haemodilution, hypothermia and acidosis, and also by delivering blood components such as RBCs, fresh frozen plasma and platelets (Murphy 2010).

Blood transfusion

The best method of increasing haemoglobin levels in blood is via RBC transfusions (Thomas *et al.* 2010). Patients with low haemoglobin levels will receive at least one or two units of RBCs (Chant *et al.* 2006, Cave 2014). Postoperatively, patients with bleeding problems or low haemoglobin levels may stay in hospital for more than a week, also leading to more regular RBC transfusions (Cave 2014).

RBC transfusion is expensive, costing at least £140 per unit, and it is also associated with risks including morbidity and mortality over weeks or months.

Research by Marik and Corwin (2008) shows that RBC transfusions can often produce poor results in critically ill patients. Examples of issues include mortality, infections, organ dysfunction and acute respiratory distress syndrome (Marik and Corwin 2008). In 42 of the 45 studies reviewed, the risks of transfusion outweighed the benefits of treating anaemia with transfusion (Marik and Corwin 2008). Examples of issues that can be raised during RBC transfusions include lung injury, circulatory overload, nosocomial infections and increased chances of cancer forming (Marik and Corwin 2008). Further transfusions of RBCs can also lead to iron overload, resulting in organ damage. Blood transfusions therefore have to be carefully evaluated before delivery to ensure they are for the patient's benefit (Thomas *et al.* 2010).

Conclusion

Critically ill patients who develop anaemia, coagulopathy (impairment of blood's ability to clot), thrombocytopenia (deficiency of platelets) and internal bleeding have serious clinical issues leading to the need for clinical resources and usually poorer outcomes for patients (Murphy 2010). The cause of anaemia can be for several different reasons, including nutritional problems, drug reactions, chronic disease or coagulopathies, and will need specialised treatment.

Blood transfusion is usually given to patients with anaemia, although it may cause severe problems such as infection, iron overload or high levels of fluid in the blood, especially in critically ill patients (Thomas *et al.* 2010, Cave 2014). An alternative to blood transfusion in anaemic patients can include using intravenous iron therapy (Okam *et al.* 2012), using small-volume phlebotomy tubes and assessing haemoglobin levels using non-invasive techniques.

Monitoring blood levels in critically ill patients with anaemia is therefore a complex issue that needs careful treatment to avoid further complications. Caring for the anaemic critically ill patient is therefore a major requirement in the perioperative period.

94 Care of Morbidly Obese Patients

Obesity is increasing in most countries because of the increase in sugar, fat, oil and so on in food eaten by individuals, leading to increased obesity in patients undergoing surgery. Morbidly obese patients are at significant risk because of their weight, normally over 150 kg, and the fat in their body which can cause problems in their cardiovascular system. The patient also needs special considerations while being positioned and kept safe during surgery, and needs additional equipment and safe handling (Al-Benna 2011). Patients who are not obese, or are slightly obese, provide fewer risks in perioperative management. Anaesthetists, surgeons and theatre practitioners need to deal with obese patients who are submitting themselves for bariatric surgery, emergency surgery or, in the case of women, obstetric surgery (Singh *et al.* 2014).

When an obese patient is admitted into the operating department, the availability of specialised equipment needs to be arranged in advance. Obese patients also need preoperative assessment and care, anaesthetic techniques, careful patient positioning (Dybec 2004) and appropriate postoperative care (Cobbold and Lord 2012).

Caring for obese patients

Obese patients need safe treatment which needs effective organisation of patient care, safe protocols put in place, and expertise within the staff. Patients undergoing bariatric surgery are usually treated well by all staff, but occasionally an obese patient may be admitted to a non-bariatric hospital because of car accidents or trauma (Cobbold and Lord 2012).

The specific needs of obese patients therefore need to be addressed, including for example psychological and personal needs, counselling and appropriate information (Al-Benna 2011). Hospitals who admit obese patients must have suitable processes in place to ensure best care of the patient. These can include the following.

Staff training

Staff training is important to provide the care and support needed for obese patients (Al-Benna 2011). This would include:

- Consultant anaesthetist or surgeon will ensure all suitable equipment is in place.
- Theatre teams should be trained and educated for the care of obese patients.
- Additional staff may be required to transfer the patient safely from their bed to the operating table and to ensure the patient is secure (Singh *et al.* 2014).
- All staff must have undergone appropriate manual handling training on a regular basis (e.g. once per year) to reduce the risks for the patient.

Rapid Perioperative Care, First Edition. Paul Wicker and Sara Dalby.

Risk reduction

Obese patients are at high risk during anaesthesia and surgery, and therefore strategies need to be in place to protect them from harm. Strategies can include guidelines or checklists which identify the stages of perioperative care that the obese patient is at (Al-Benna 2011, Brette 2015). Examples of key points may include:

- Policies and protocols should be in place for morbidly obese patients (Brette 2015).
- Waiting list management – including identifying time of operation, clinical area, availability of the anaesthetist and surgeon and so on (Smedley 2014).
- Obese patients should be risk-assessed pre, intra and postoperatively, and suitable care given throughout their perioperative pathway.
- Preoperative advice – for example, stopping smoking, taking alcohol, identifying drugs being used, and diet (Green *et al.* 2003).
- Case selection – a detailed analysis of the patient from a medical, psychological and social point of view.
- Preoperative assessment of the status of the patient, including cardiovascular status, respiratory status, neurological status and so on (Singh *et al.* 2014).
- Planning for postoperative care – including analgesia, prevention of nausea and vomiting, respiratory status, fluids and electrolytes and so on (Green *et al.* 2003).
- Thromboprophylaxis – a measure taken to prevent the development of a thrombus or a coronary thrombosis (Cobbold and Lord 2012).
- Discharge planning – taking into account the status of the patient and his or her ability to manage their health.

Specialised equipment

Specialised equipment may be needed because standard equipment such as beds or operating tables may not support the weight of morbidly obese patients (Cobbold and Lord 2012). Operating departments who accept morbidly obese patients therefore need to ensure they have specialised equipment and critical care beds to care for these patients safely (Garza 2004). Actions to be taken may include:

- Label operating tables, trolleys and beds with its maximum weight allowed.
- Secure the patient when placed on beds or operating tables (Brette 2015).
- Assess and monitor pressure areas and apply gel pads, pillows and so on if required.
- Ensure the width of the operating table is acceptable for the patient to prevent parts of the body from overhanging.
- Ensure manual handling equipment is available for obese patients, for example hoists, prone turners and sliding sheets.
- Ensure enlarged items such as gowns, TED stockings, blood pressure cuffs and so on are available.
- Use electrically operated equipment such as beds, trolleys or hoists where possible.
- Encourage patients to keep moving whenever possible pre and postoperatively.
- Obese patients should be placed in a semi-recumbent posture with support for legs, buttocks and head; this is more effective than placing the patient in the lateral or prone position which can lead to poor breathing, pressure sores, pain and so on (Dybec 2004, Garza 2004, Al-Benna 2011, Brette 2015).

Preoperative assessment

Obese patients must undertake preoperative assessment before surgery to identify those patients who are at high risk during anaesthesia and surgery (Cobbold and Lord 2012). The main examples of areas to assess may include:

- Record the patient's height, weight and body mass index (BMI).
- Pre-assess patients for conditions such as echocardiography, stress testing, spirometry arterial blood gas analysis and so on (Garza 2004).

- Provide advice from consultant anaesthetists and surgeons.
- Assess any illnesses or diseases the patient has, such as cardiac, respiratory and metabolic diseases, which can put the patient at high risk (Smedley 2014).
- Assess the history of the patient.
- Radiographs or imaging techniques, such as computed tomography (CT) or magnetic resonance imaging (MRI), may not be possible in morbidly obese patients, because of their size (Garza 2004).
- Undertake interventions that have been identified after assessment of the patient. This may include losing weight, exercising and engaging in activities.

Respiratory system

Obese patients do not breathe easily and often have trouble with their airways. Problems can include airway closure when the patient is placed in the supine position, and often intubation is difficult when the patient is supine (Singh *et al.* 2014). Intubation is difficult because of fat being deposited into the back of the neck or into the soft tissues of the neck. Patients with this condition may also suffer from acid reflux, in which case antacids should be given to the patient (Cobbold and Lord 2012).

Sleep apnoea (interruption of breathing when the patient is asleep) and hypoventilation are common in patients with morbid obesity. CPAP (continuous positive airway pressure) and BiPAP (bi-level positive airway pressure) may be used for patients affected by breathing difficulties (Garza 2004).

Morbidly obese patients who suffer from asthma or chronic obstructive pulmonary disease (COPD) are at a greater risk of respiratory complications during the perioperative period. However, wheezing may be due to airway closure rather than asthma, in which case bronchodilator therapy may be used (Singh *et al.* 2014).

Cardiac disease

Cardiovascular disease in obese patients can include hypertension, hyperlipidaemia (too much lipid in the blood), ischaemic heart disease and heart failure (Smedley 2014). Pre-assessment of the patient may help to reveal signs and symptoms of cardiac disease. It may also be impossible to measure and record the patient's blood pressure using an upper arm cuff; therefore, areas such as the forearm or leg may need to be used, or alternatively intravenous arterial blood pressure measurement may be used before and during surgery (Al-Benna 2011).

Metabolic disease

Diabetes occurs in most patients who are morbidly obese; therefore, they need to be assessed to ensure their glucose levels are appropriate (Green *et al.* 2003). For example, glucose levels increase within haemoglobin if diabetes mellitus is not controlled, leading to glycosylated haemoglobin. Diabetes can also lead to other issues such as cardiac disease, renal disease and autonomic dysfunction (i.e. problems with the autonomic nervous system). The patient therefore needs glucose control and dietary advice perioperatively which will help to reduce issues such as infection or ketoacidosis (caused by lack of insulin in the body). Regardless of the weight of morbidly obese patients, they may still have an inadequate nutritional status, because of lack of food, so this may have to be addressed before and after surgery (Cobbold and Lord 2012).

Thromboprophylaxis

Obese patients have a high risk of venous and pulmonary thromboembolism because of the high levels of fat in their bodies, which can affect the blood circulation. Thromboprophylaxis (the prevention of development of a thrombus) is therefore essential for all obese patients; however, the appropriate dose of low-molecular-weight heparin needs to be assessed, according to the state of the patient (Al-Benna 2011).

Preoperative assessment will also help to plan for surgery and for early discharge, and it provides an opportunity to discuss any specific risks related to anaesthesia. Based on the issues which may occur during anaesthesia and surgery, the patient has the right to decide whether or not to proceed with surgery (Smedley 2014).

Intraoperative care

Intraoperative care of obese patients needs careful consideration because of the state of the patient's health. Problems that may arise can include cardiovascular problems, airway problems, bleeding problems, development of thrombi and so on (Al-Benna 2011). These patients therefore need specific care that considers all their body dimensions, and also associated comorbidities and factors related to surgical and anaesthetic risks (Cobbold and Lord 2012). The two main areas to consider are airway management and regional anaesthesia.

Airway management

- The chances of gastro-oesophageal reflux happening should be assessed preoperatively, and antacids prescribed if required.
- The anaesthetist may need a second anaesthetist and at least one anaesthetic practitioner.
- The anaesthetic assistant must understand the need for airway equipment and have it available before induction.
- If the patient has undergone anaesthesia in previous times, the anaesthetist should check for previous airway problems.
- Several practitioners should be available in the operating room to turn the patient in an emergency situation.
- Pre-oxygenation is needed for the obese patient before induction of anaesthesia, because of possible issues with the airway.
- The use of a tracheostomy may not be possible in a morbidly obese patient because of the size of the neck and the technical difficulties in accessing the trachea (Garza 2004, Cobbold and Lord 2012, Smedley 2014).

Regional anaesthesia

Regional anaesthesia for the morbidly obese patient is better to use where possible, compared to general anaesthesia. However, the use of regional anaesthesia may not be possible because of the size and weight of the patient. Therefore, preoperative assessment of the patient, followed by discussion with the patient, is essential to make sure the patient is aware of issues that might arise (Cobbold and Lord 2012).

An experienced anaesthetist is needed to provide suitable resuscitation and regional anaesthesia equipment, which would include longer regional block needles and may also need higher amounts of regional anaesthetic drugs (Green *et al.* 2003).

Spinal anaesthesia is a good option for surgery on the lower limbs. Obese patients need to sit up so the midline of their back can be easily identified and the spinal needle is placed appropriately. Spinal anaesthesia may be used more often in day case surgery with low dosage of drugs (Garza 2004). However, there is still a chance of potential difficulties, and aortocaval compression (compression of the abdominal aorta and inferior vena cava when the patient is in the supine position) may occur (Smedley 2014).

Conclusion

Morbidly obese patients may need further care after leaving hospital. This would be assessed on discharge, and rehabilitation, long-term care, or care at home may be arranged. Recovery practitioners and ward staff need to work with the patient and doctor to identify the patient's needs, including medical drugs, equipment and any services the patient needs when arriving home (Al-Benna 2011). During their hospital stay, morbidly obese patients need assessment and special care to meet their needs and problems that can occur (Smedley 2014). This will help to minimise complications and ensure the patient remains safe and secure, and hopefully undergoes the surgery and anaesthesia safely and quickly.

References and Further Reading

82. Critical Care Nurses and Practitioners Roles

References

Aitken LM and Marshall AP (2015) Monitoring and Optimising Outcomes of Survivors of Critical Illness. *Intensive and Critical Care Nursing Journal* **31**: 1–9.

Aitken LM, Rattray J, Hull A, Kenardy JA, Le Brocque R and Ullman AJ (2013) The Use of Diaries in Psychological Recovery from Intensive Care. *Critical Care Journal* **17** (6): 253.

Burtin C, Clerckx B, Robbeets C, Ferdinande P, Langer D, Troosters T *et al.* (2009) Early Exercise in Critically Ill Patients Enhances Short-Term Functional Recovery. *Critical Care Medicine* **37** (9): 2499–2505.

Kaplow R (2013) Safety of Patients Transferred From the Operating Room to the Intensive Care Unit. *Critical Care Nurse Journal* **33** (1): 68–70.

McConachie I (2014) *Anesthesia and Perioperative Care of the High Risk Patient*, 3rd ed. Cambridge, Cambridge University Press.

Salisbury LG, Merriweather J and Walsh TS (2010) Rehabilitation after Critical Illness: Could a Ward-Based Generic Rehabilitation Assistant Promote Recovery? *Nursing in Critical Care Journal* **15** (2): 57–65.

Further Reading

Allou N, Allyn J, Snauwaert A, Welsch C, Lucet J, Kortbaoui R *et al.* (2015) Postoperative Pneumonia following Cardiac Surgery in Non-ventilated Patients versus Mechanically Ventilated Patients: Is There Any Difference? *Critical Care Journal* **19**: 116. Available at http://ccforum.com/content/pdf/s13054-015-0845-5.pdf (accessed 11 March 2015)

Lane-Fall MB, Beidas RS, Pascual JL, Collard ML, Peifer HG, Chavez TJ *et al.* (2014) Handoffs and Transitions in Critical Care (HATRICC): Protocol for a Mixed Methods Study of Operating Room to Intensive Care Unit Handoffs. *BMC Surgery Journal* **14** (96). Available at http://www.ncbi.nlm.nih.gov/pmc/articles/PMC4255652/ (accessed 11 March 2015)

Websites

Improving Recovery with Critical Care Rehabilitation: http://www.nursingtimes.net/nursing-practice/specialisms/critical-care/improving-recovery-with-critical-care-rehabilitation/5060409.article (accessed 11 March 2015)

Intensive Care – Recovery: http://www.nhs.uk/Conditions/Intensive-care/Pages/Recovery.aspx (accessed 11 March 2015)

Recovery from Intensive Care: http://www.ncbi.nlm.nih.gov/pmc/articles/PMC1127042/ (accessed 11 March 2015)

Videos

Cardiac Surgery Intensive Care Unit: https://www.youtube.com/watch?v=xfC1Nl8ZMEk (accessed 11 March 2015)

Critical Care Nursing: https://www.youtube.com/watch?v=G9C-4i3RNs8andlist=PLs0CmusRpQA4TP89w_LG-JfEDBAmuk-7z (accessed 11 March 2015)

Critical Care Nursing Procedures and Skills: https://www.youtube.com/watch?v=5l6kBs2nvRsandlist=PL9xvj8AY46C1aRfxqQ2xGXGm6KjmaJpNc (accessed 11 March 2015)

Surgical Critical Care: https://www.youtube.com/watch?v=iPsZ_XuiSesandlist=PL1B7758B7D08A221E (accessed 11 March 2015)

Rapid Perioperative Care, First Edition. Paul Wicker and Sara Dalby.

83. Management of the Critically Ill Surgical Patient

References

Bancroft D (2013) Caring for the Critically Ill Patient: The Ethical Issues. *Journal of Operating Department Practitioners* **1** (2): 91–94.

Martindale RG, McClave SA, Vanek VW, McCarthy M, Roberts P, Taylor B *et al.* (2009) Guidelines for the Provision and Assessment of Nutrition Support Therapy in the Adult Critically Ill Patient. *American College of Critical Care Medicine* **37** (5): 1–30.

McConachie I (2014) *Anesthesia and Perioperative Care of the High-Risk Patient*, 3rd ed. Cambridge, Cambridge University Press.

National Institute of Health and Care Excellence (NICE) (2007) *Acutely Ill Patients in Hospital*. Manchester, NICE.

National Patient Safety Agency (2007) *Recognising and Responding Appropriately to Early Signs of Deterioration in Hospitalised Patients*. London, National Patient Safety Agency.

Ranieri VM, Thompson BT, Barie PS, Dhainau JF, Douglas MD, Finfer S *et al.* (2012). Drotrecogin Alfa (Activated) in Adults with Septic Shock. *New England Journal of Medicine* **366**: 2055–2064.

Smith FG and Yeung J (2010) *Core Topics in Critical Care Medicine*. Cambridge, Cambridge University Press.

Further Reading

Kaplow R (2013) Safety of Patients Transferred from the Operating Room to the Intensive Care Unit. *Critical Care Nurse Journal* **33** (1): 68–70.

McArthur-Rouse F and Prosser S (2007) *Assessing and Managing the Acutely Ill Adult Surgical Patient*. Oxford, Wiley-Blackwell.

Robertson LC and Al-Haddad M (2013) Recognizing the Critically Ill Patient. *Anaesthesia and Intensive Care Medicine Journal* **14** (1): 11–14.

Websites

About Critical Care Nursing: http://www.aacn.org/wd/publishing/content/pressroom/aboutcriticalcarenursing.pcms?menu (accessed 29 March 2015)

Care of the Critically Ill Patient: http://www.slideshare.net/JocelynSladeAnderson/care-of-the-critically-ill-patient-student (accessed 29 March 2015)

Critical Care Nursing Concept: http://www.slideshare.net/nilobanluta/critical-care-nursing-concept?qid=49a45b0a-3727-41f4-b2c5-e27f4eaf32a3andv=qf1andb=andfrom_search=6 (accessed 29 March 2015)

Monitoring the Critically Ill Patient: http://www.rcsed.ac.uk/RCSEDBackIssues/journal/vol44_6/4460032.htm (accessed 29 March 2015)

Presentation on Management of Critically Ill Patient: http://www.authorstream.com/Presentation/malonimurugaiyan-1670963-presentation-management-critically-ill-patient/ (accessed 30 March 2015)

Videos

Critically Ill Patient: https://www.youtube.com/watch?v=sXeTppCcuuo (accessed 30 March 2015)

Fluid Responsiveness in the Critically Ill Patient: https://www.youtube.com/watch?v=ew0H6eTrt90 (accessed 30 March 2015)

Nutritional Support in Critically Ill Patients: https://www.youtube.com/watch?v=nTuk_dp5edM (accessed 30 March 2015)

Recognising the Critically Ill Patient: https://www.youtube.com/watch?v=uqQVGHihjpI (accessed 30 March 2015)

84. Malignant Hyperthermia

References

Association of Anaesthetists of Great Britain and Ireland (AAGBI) (2011) *Malignant Hyperthermia Crisis*. London, AAGBI. Available at http://www.aagbi.org/sites/default/files/MH_paediatric_laminate_2013_for_members.pdf (accessed 12 March 2015)

Goodman T and Spry C (2014) *Essentials of Perioperative Nursing*. Burlington MA, Jones and Bartlett Learning.
Jevon P, Ewens B and Pooni JS (2012) *Monitoring the Critically Ill Patient*, 3rd ed. Chichester, John Wiley and Sons.
Lay R (2014) Recognising and Managing Malignant Hyperthermia. *Journal of Operating Department Practitioners* **2** (1): 19–23.
MedlinePlus (2015) *Malignant Hyperthermia*. Available at http://www.nlm.nih.gov/medlineplus/ency/article/001315.htm (accessed 13 March 2015)
Stoppler MC (2015) *Malignant Hyperthermia*. Available at http://www.medicinenet.com/malignant_hyperthermia/article.htm (accessed 13 March 2015)

Further Reading

Dinarello CA and Porat R (2008) Fever and Hyperthermia. In Kasper DL, Braunwald E, Fauci AS, Hauser SL, Longo DL, Jameson JL and Loscalzo J (eds) *Harrison's Principles of Internal Medicine*, 17th ed. New York, McGraw-Hill.
Genetics Home Reference (2015) Malignant Hyperthermia. Available at http://ghr.nlm.nih.gov/condition/malignant-hyperthermia (accessed 13 March 2015)
Lay R (2014) Recognising and Managing Malignant Hyperthermia. *Journal of Operating Department Practitioners* **2** (1): 19–23.

Websites

British Malignant Hypothermia Association: www.bmha.co.uk (accessed 12 March 2015)
Harrison's Principles of Internal Medicine (18th ed.): http://accessmedicine.mhmedical.com/book.aspx?bookid=331 (accessed 12 March 2015)
Malignant Hyperthermia: http://www.nlm.nih.gov/medlineplus/ency/article/001315.htm (accessed 12 March 2015)
Malignant Hyperthermia: http://www.patient.co.uk/doctor/malignant-hyperthermia (accessed 12 March 2015)
Malignant Hyperthermia Association of the United States: www.mhaus.org (accessed 13 March 2015)

Videos

Malignant Hyperthermia: https://www.youtube.com/watch?v=F_fo9lbcMNs (accessed 12 March 2015)
Malignant Hyperthermia Presentation: https://www.youtube.com/watch?v=nppeo1ugEl8 (accessed 12 March 2015)
Malignant Hyperthermia: Intraoperative Video – Case Report: https://www.youtube.com/watch?v=Q0FighAlizQ (accessed 12 March 2015)
Understanding Malignant Hyperthermia: https://www.youtube.com/watch?v=iPDYWZdhDp0andlist=PL7C8FLXOA2t_8mZCHqNOdLC1YXSnC7cQd (accessed 12 March 2015)

85. Inadvertent Hypothermia

References

Arndt K (1999) Inadvertent Hypothermia in the OR. *AORN Journal* **70** (2): 204–206, 208–214.
Burger L and Fitzpatrick J (2009) Prevention of Inadvertent Perioperative Hypothermia. *British Journal of Nursing* **18** (18): 1114–1119.
Hopf HW, Hunt TK, West JM, Blomquist P, Goodson WH and Jensen A (1997) Wound Tissue Oxygen Tension Predicts the Risk of Wound Infection in Surgical Patients. *Archives of Surgery* **132** (9): 997–1004.
Insler SR and Sessler DI (2006) Perioperative Thermoregulation and Temperature Monitoring. *Anesthesiology Clinics Journal* **24** (4): 823–837.
Kurz A, Sessler DI and Lenhart R (1996) Perioperative Normothermia to Reduce the Incidence of Surgical-Wound Infection and Shorten Hospitalization. *New England Journal of Medicine* **334** (19): 1209–1215.
Matsukawa T, Sessler DI, Sessler AM, Schroeder M, Ozaki M and Kurz A (1995) Heat Flow and Distribution during Induction of General Anesthesia. *Anesthesiology Journal* **82** (3): 662–673.
Pennsylvania Patient Safety Advisory (2008) Prevention of Inadvertent Hypothermia. *Pennsylvania Patient safety Advisory Journal* **5** (2): 44–52. Available at http://patientsafetyauthority.org/ADVISORIES/AdvisoryLibrary/2008/Jun5%282%29/Pages/44.aspx (accessed 14 March 2015)
Rajagopalan S, Mascha E, Na J *et al.* (2008) The Effects of Mild Perioperative Hypothermia on Blood Loss and Transfusion Requirement. *Anesthesiology Journal* **108** (1): 71–77.

Sessler DI (2005) Temperature Monitoring. In Miller RD (ed) *Miller's Anesthesia*, 6th ed. Philadelphia, Elsevier, pp. 1571–1579.

Singh A (2013) Preoperative Patient Warming in the Prevention of Hypothermia. *Journal of Operating Department Practitioners* **1** (1): 8–14.

Singh A (2014) Strategies for the Management and Avoidance of Hypothermia in the Perioperative Environment. *Journal of Perioperative Practice* **24** (4): 75–78.

Further Reading

Bernard H (2014) The Importance of Warming for Enhanced Recovery. *Journal of Operating Department Practitioners* **2** (4): 166–172.

Cooper S (2006) The Effect of Preoperative Warming on Patient's Postoperative Temperatures. *AORN Journal* **83** (5):1073–1076, 1079–1088.

Knaepel A (2012) Inadvertent Perioperative Hypothermia. *Journal of Perioperative Practice* **22** (3): 86–90.

Mulry D and Mooney B (2012) Prevention of Perioperative Hypothermia. *World of Irish Nursing* **20** (2): 26–27.

National Institute for Health and Clinical Excellence (NICE) (2008) *Inadvertent Perioperative Hypothermia*. London, NICE.

Websites

Effect of Hypothermia and Shivering on Standard PACU Monitoring of Patients: http://www.aana.com/newsandjournal/Documents/p47-53.pdf (accessed 15 March 2015)

Inadvertent Perioperative Hypothermia: https://www.nice.org.uk/guidance/cg65 (accessed 15 March 2015)

Normothermia Clinical Guideline: http://www.aspan.org/Clinical-Practice/Clinical-Guidelines/Normothermia (accessed 15 March 2015)

Risk Factors for Inadvertent Hypothermia: http://www.ncbi.nlm.nih.gov/books/NBK53804/ (accessed 15 March 2015)

Videos

Inadvertent Hypothermia Education (4 Videos): https://www.youtube.com/watch?v=KylnUv5hfKlandlist=PLA8D4BC24FB21CCB0 (accessed 15 March 2015)

Inadvertent Perioperative Hypothermia: https://www.youtube.com/watch?v=I_-ITYHn2Ag (accessed 15 March 2015)

Intraoperative Normothermia: Improving Outcomes and Decreasing Costs: https://www.youtube.com/watch?v=LyV8kn5w2GA (accessed 15 March 2015)

Patient Warming (8 Videos): https://www.youtube.com/watch?v=N7Mlhek5_pEandlist=PLC42D327659D0F3F9 (accessed 15 March 2015)

86. Congestive Heart Failure

References

European Society of Cardiology (ESC) (2009) Guidelines for Pre-operative Cardiac Risk Assessment and Perioperative Cardiac Management in Non-cardiac Surgery. *European Heart Journal* **30**: 2769–2812. Available at http://eurheartj.oxfordjournals.org/content/30/22/2769.full.pdf (accessed 17 March 2015)

Hosenpud JD and Greenberg BH (2006) *Congestive Heart Failure*, 3rd ed. Philadelphia, Lippincott Williams and Wilkins.

Sear JW and Higham H (2002) Issues in the Perioperative Management of the Elderly Patient with Cardiovascular Disease. *Journal of Drugs and Aging* **19** (6): 429–451.

Smith GS and Yeung J (2010) *Core Topics in Critical Care Medicine*. Cambridge, Cambridge University Press.

The Washington Home Center for Palliative Care Studies (2002) Living with Advanced Congestive Heart Failure: A Guide for Family Caregivers. Available at http://www.medicaring.org/educate/download/chfbookfinal.pdf (accessed 17 March 2015)

Further Reading

Mant J, Al-Mohammad A, Swain S and Laramee P (2011) Guideline Development Group. Management of Chronic Heart Failure in Adults: Synopsis of the National Institute for Health and Clinical Excellence guideline. *Annals of Internal Medicine Journal* **155** (4): 252–259.

Emanuel LL and Bonow RO (2011) Care of Patients with End-Stage Heart Disease. In Bonow RO, Mann DL, Zipes DP and Libby P (eds) *Braunwald's Heart Disease: A Textbook of Cardiovascular Medicine*, 9th ed. Philadelphia, Saunders Elsevier.

Mann DL (2011) Management of Heart Failure Patients with Reduced Ejection Fraction. In Bonow RO, Mann DL, Zipes DP and Libby P (eds) *Braunwald's Heart Disease: A Textbook of Cardiovascular Medicine*, 9th ed. Philadelphia, Saunders Elsevier.

Websites

American Heart Association: http://www.heart.org/HEARTORG/Conditions/HeartFailure/Heart-Failure_UCM_002019_SubHomePage.jsp (accessed 17 March 2015)

Congestive Heart Failure: http://www.healthline.com/health/congestive-heart-failure#Overview1 (accessed 17 March 2015)

Heart Disease and Congestive Heart Failure: http://www.webmd.com/heart-disease/guide-heart-failure (accessed 17 March 2015)

Videos

Congestive Heart Failure: https://www.youtube.com/watch?v=pPDPpAepUtM (accessed 17 March 2015)

Congestive Heart Failure (CHF) Explained: https://www.youtube.com/watch?v=zy_fK1P2odM (accessed 17 March 2015)

Heart Disease and Heart Attacks: http://www.youtube.com/watch?v=vYnreB1duro (accessed 17 March 2015)

Reducing Perioperative Cardiac Risk: Does Revascularization Work?: http://www.youtube.com/watch?v=h5xiaSns4jw (accessed 17 March 2015)

87. Venous Thromboembolism

References

Bates SM, Greer IA, Middeldorp S, Veenstra DL, Prabulos AM and Vandvik PO (2012) VTE, Thrombophilia, Antithrombotic Therapy, and Pregnancy: Antithrombotic Therapy and Prevention of Thrombosis, 9th Ed: American College of Chest Physicians Evidence-Based Clinical Practice Guidelines. *Chest Journal* **141** (2 Suppl.): e691S–736S.

De Martino RR, Wallaert JB, Rossi AP, Zbehlik AJ, Suckow B and Walsh DB (2012) A Meta-analysis of Anticoagulation for Calf Deep Venous Thrombosis. *Journal of Vascular Surgery* **56** (1): 228–237.

Dentali F, Douketis JD, Gianni M, Lim W, Crowther MA (2007) Meta-analysis: Anticoagulant Prophylaxis to Prevent Symptomatic Venous Thromboembolism in Hospitalized Medical Patients. *Annals of Internal Medicine* **146** (4): 278–288.

Heit JA (2005) Venous Thromboembolism: Disease Burden, Outcomes and Risk Factors. *Journal of Thrombosis and Haemostasis* **3** (8): 1611–1617.

Kucher N (2011) Clinical Practice. Deep-Vein Thrombosis of the Upper Extremities. *New England Journal of Medicine*. **364**: 861–869

Narani KK (2010) Deep Vein Thrombosis and Pulmonary Embolism – Prevention, Management, and Anaesthetic Considerations. *Indian Journal of Anaesthesia* **54** (1) 8–17. Available at http://www.ncbi.nlm.nih.gov/pmc/articles/PMC2876903/ (accessed 20 March 2015)

National Institute for Health and Care Excellence (NICE) (2011) Venous Thromboembolism: Reducing the Risk of Venous Thromboembolism (Deep Vein Thrombosis and Pulmonary Embolism) in Patients Undergoing Surgery. London, NICE. Available at http://guidance.nice.org.uk/CG92 (accessed 20 March 2015)

Stein PD, Beemath A, Matta F, Weg JG, Yusen RD, Hales CA *et al.* (2007) Clinical Characteristics of Patients with Acute Pulmonary Embolism. *American Journal of Medicine* **120** (10): 871–879.

Further Reading

Ageno W, Becattini C, Brighton T, Selby R and Kamphuisen PW (2008) Cardiovascular Risk Factors and Venous Thromboembolism: A Meta-Analysis. *Circulation* **117** (1): 93–102.

Becattini C, Agnelli G, Schenone A, Eichinger S, Bucherini E, Silingardi M *et al.* (2012) Aspirin for Preventing the Recurrence of Venous Thromboembolism. *New England Journal of Medicine* **366** (21): 1959–1967.

National Institute for Health and Care Excellence (NICE) (2010) Venous Thromboembolism Prevention and Quality Standard. Available at https://www.nice.org.uk/guidance/qs3 (accessed 20 March 2015)

Websites

Deep Venous Thrombosis: www.oocities.org/sheraz1978us/dvt.ppt (accessed 20 March 2015)

Venous Thromboembolism: http://www.clevelandclinicmeded.com/medicalpubs/diseasemanagement/cardiology/venous-thromboembolism/ (accessed 20 March 2015)

VTE Risk Assessments: http://www.rcn.org.uk/development/practice/cpd_online_learning/nice_care_preventing_venousthromboembolism/vte_risk_assessments (accessed 20 March 2015)

Videos

Deep Vein Thrombosis (DVT) and Pulmonary Embolism (PE): http://www.youtube.com/watch?v=0PEhvACEROI (accessed 20 March 2015)

How Deep Vein Thrombosis (DVT) Forms: https://www.youtube.com/watch?v=0QEo9QAqA3k (accessed 20 March 2015)

A Look at Deep Vein Thrombosis and Pulmonary Embolism: http://www.youtube.com/watch?v=2K0WskqBWdw (accessed 20 March 2015)

Preventing Venous Thromboembolism: https://www.youtube.com/watch?v=CZuknY8D2-A (accessed 20 March 2015)

88. Latex Allergy

References

American Society of Anesthesiologists (2005) Natural Rubber Latex Allergy. Available at http://ecommerce.asahq.org/publicationsAndServices/latexallergy.pdf (accessed 21 March 2015)

Beckford-Ball J (2005) Tackling Latex Allergies in Patients and Nursing Staff. *Nursing Times* **101**: 24, 26–27. Available at http://www.nursingtimes.net/Journals/2013/03/15/p/g/f/050614Tackling-latex-allergies-in--patients-and-nursing-staff.pdf (accessed 20 March 2015)

Brown K (1999) Care of the Latex Sensitive Patient in Theatre. *British Journal of Theatre Nursing* **9** (4): 170–173.

Department of Health and Human Services (2012) How to Prevent Latex Allergies. Available at http://www.cdc.gov/niosh/docs/2012-119/pdfs/2012-119.pdf (accessed 21 March 2015)

Dianne R (2005) Latex Sensitivity Awareness in Preoperative Assessment. *British Journal of Perioperative Nursing* **15** (1): 27–32.

Mercurio J (2011) Creating a Latex Perioperative Environment. *OR Nurse* **5** (6): 18–25. Available at http://www.nursingcenter.com/lnc/pdf?AID=1253787andan=01271211-201111000-00006andJournal_ID=682710andIssue_ID=1253733 (accessed 23 March 2015)

Further Reading

Binkley HM, Schroyer T and Catalfano J (2003) Latex Allergies: A Review of Recognition, Evaluation, Management, Prevention, Education, and Alternative Product Use. *Journal of Athletic Training* **38** (2): 133–140.

Bowler G (2006) Safer Surgical Gloves: Evaluation and Implementation. *Journal of Perioperative Practice* **16** (2): 67–70.

Duger C, Kol IO, Kaygusuz K, Gursoy S, Ersan I and Mimaroglu C (2012) A Perioperative Anaphylactic Reaction Caused by Latex in a Patient with No History of Allergy. *Anaesthesia Pain and Intensive Care* **16** (1): 71–73. Available at http://www.apicareonline.com/?p=1118 (accessed 23 March 2015)

Websites

Latex Allergies: http://www.webmd.com/allergies/latex-allergies (accessed 23 March 2015)

Operating Suite Guidelines for Latex Allergic Patients: http://www.allergy.org.au/health-professionals/papers/management-of-latex-allergic-patients/operating-suite (accessed 23 March 2015)
Rubber Latex Allergy: https://www.allergyuk.org/rubber-latex-allergy/rubber-latex-allergy (accessed 23 March 2015)

Videos

Latex Allergies: https://www.youtube.com/watch?v=1PjbCWa64ew (accessed 23 March 2015)
Latex Allergies: What You Need to Know:
http://www.youtube.com/watch?v=R9GJ-FixkuM (accessed 23 March 2015)
Latex Allergy: http://www.youtube.com/watch?v=4RQE4mMgqgl (accessed 23 March 2015)
Latex Allergy 101 Webinar with Kevin Kelly, MD: https://www.youtube.com/watch?v=PyLz5gwtlzc (accessed 23 March 2015)

89. Pressure Ulcers

References

Allman RM, Goode PS, Burst N, Bartolucci AA and Thomas DR (1999) Pressure Ulcers, Hospital Complications, and Disease Severity: Impact on Hospital Costs and Length of Stay. *Advances in Wound Care Journal* **12** (1): 22–30.
Brillhart B (2006) Preventive Skin Care for Older Adults. *Geriatrics Aging Journal* **9** (5): 334–339.
Edlich RF, Winters KL, Woodard CR, Buschbacher RM, Long WB, Gebhart JH *et al.* (2004) Pressure Ulcer Prevention. *Journal of Long-Term Effects of Medical Implants.* **14** (4): 285–304.
Hatfield A (2014) *The Complete Recovery Book*, 5th ed. Oxford, Oxford University Press.
Neighbors M, Green-Nigro CJ, Sands JK, Marek JF and Monahan FD (2006) *Phipps Medical Surgical Nursing: Health and Illness Perspectives*, 8th ed. St Louis, Elsevier – Health Sciences Division.
Pearce CA (1996) Intraoperative Pressure Sore Prevention. *British Journal of Theatre Nursing* **6** (4): 31.
Price MC, Whitney JD, King CA and Doughty D (2005) Development of a Risk Assessment Tool for Intraoperative Pressure Ulcers. *Journal of Wound, Ostomy and Continence Nursing* **32** (1): 19–30.
Sanders W and Allen RD (2006) Pressure Management in the Operating Room: Problems and Solutions. *Managing Infection Control Journal* **6** (9): 63–72.

Further Reading

Dziedzic ME (2014) *Fast Facts about Pressure Ulcer Care for Nurses*. New York, Springer.
Lyder CH and Ayello EA (2008) Pressure Ulcers: A Patient Safety Issue. In *Patient Safety and Quality: An Evidence-Based Handbook for Nurses*. Available at http://www.ncbi.nlm.nih.gov/books/NBK2650/ (accessed 26 March 2015)
Thomas DR and Compton GA (2013) *Pressure Ulcers in the Aging Population*. Totowa NJ, Humana Press.

Websites

Pressure Ulcers: http://www.rcn.org.uk/development/practice/clinicalguidelines/pressure_ulcers (accessed 26 March 2015)
Pressure Ulcers: http://www.patient.co.uk/doctor/pressure-ulcers-pro (accessed 26 March 2015)
Pressure Ulcers: Prevention and Management of Pressure Ulcers: https://www.nice.org.uk/guidance/cg179 (accessed 26 March 2015)

Videos

Caring for Pressure Ulcers: https://www.youtube.com/watch?v=QvcjH98ipeU (accessed 26 March 2015)
Pressure Ulcer Prevention: https://www.youtube.com/watch?v=wyicm4dBH8M (accessed 26 March 2015)
Pressure Ulcer Prevention (PUPP) Competency Demo: https://www.youtube.com/watch?v=qTVM74sRdhY (accessed 26 March 2015)
Pressure Ulcers (Sores) – Treatments: https://www.youtube.com/watch?v=5_sRHSJsr1U (accessed 26 March 2015)
Preventing Pressure Ulcers – a SKIN Bundle Approach for Community Carers: https://www.youtube.com/watch?v=rkBWclrJnK8 (accessed 26 March 2015)

90. Managing Diabetes in Perioperative Patients

References

Banasch M and McConachie I (2014) Diabetes. In McConachie I (ed) *Anesthesia and Perioperative Care of the High Risk Patient*. Cambridge, Cambridge University Press.

Dagogo-Jack S and Alberti GMM (2002) Management of Diabetes Mellitus in Surgical Patients. *Diabetes Spectrum Journal* **15** (1): 44–48. Available at http://spectrum.diabetesjournals.org/content/15/1/44.full (accessed 27 March 2015)

Dhatariya K, Flanagan D, Hilton L, Kilvert A, Levy N, Rayman G and Watson B (2011) Management of Adults with Diabetes Undergoing Surgery and Elective Procedures. London, NHS Diabetes.

Hatfield A (2014) *The Complete Recovery Book*, 5th ed. Oxford, Oxford University Press.

National Patient Safety Agency (2009) Safety in Doses: Improving the Use of Medicines in the NHS. Available at http://www.nrls.npsa.nhs.uk/resources/patient-safety-topics/medication-safety/?entryid45=61625andq=0%C2%ACsafety+in+doses%C2%AC (accessed 29 March 2015)

Plodkowski RA and Edelman SV (2001) Pre-Surgical Evaluation of Diabetic Patients. *Clinical Diabetes Journal* **19** (2): 92–95. Available at http://clinical.diabetesjournals.org/content/19/2/92.full (accessed 27 March 2015)

Rubino F, Moo TA, Rosen DJ, Dakin GF and Pomp A (2009) Diabetes Surgery: A New Approach to an Old Disease. *Diabetes Care* **32** (Suppl. 2): S368–S372. Available at http://www.ncbi.nlm.nih.gov/pmc/articles/PMC2811475/ (accessed 27 March 2015)

Further Reading

Flanagan D, Ellis J, Baggot A, Grimsehl K and English P (2010) Diabetes Management of Elective Hospital Admissions. *Diabetic Medicine Journal* **27**: 1289–1294.

Frisch A, Chandra P, Smiley D, Peng L, Rizzo M, Gatcliffe C *et al.* (2010) Prevalence and Clinical Outcome of Hyperglycemia in the Perioperative Period in Noncardiac Surgery. *Diabetes Care Journal* **33**: 1783–1788.

Joslin Diabetes Center (2009) Inpatient Management of Surgical Patients with Diabetes. Available at https://www.joslin.org/docs/Inpatient_Guideline_10-02-09.pdf (accessed 27 March 2015)

Whitlock J (2014) Diabetes and Surgery – How to Improve Your Chance of a Great Outcome. Available at http://surgery.about.com/od/beforesurgery/ss/DiabetesSurgery.htm (accessed 27 March 2015)

Websites

Clinical Guidelines for the Management of Adult Patients Diabetes Mellitus during Surgery: http://www.rcht.nhs.uk/GET/d10154878 (accessed 27 March 2015)

Perioperative Management of the Diabetic Patient: http://emedicine.medscape.com/article/284451-overview (accessed 27 March 2015)

Precautions with Patients with Diabetes Undergoing Surgery: http://www.patient.co.uk/doctor/precautions-with-patients-with-diabetes-undergoing-surgery (accessed 27 March 2015)

Videos

Diabetes – Causes, Symptoms, Diagnosis and Treatment: https://www.youtube.com/watch?v=rxG4t2wZ60s (accessed 27 March 2015)

Diabetes Metabolic Surgery: https://www.youtube.com/watch?v=o-I7elwgFY8 (accessed 27 March 2015)

Diabetes Surgery: https://www.youtube.com/watch?v=q9aWhsakTHM (accessed 27 March 2015)

Effective Use of the Diabetes Health Team: https://www.youtube.com/watch?v=6O2hKC0sRq4 (accessed 27 March 2015)

91. Smoking, Alcohol and Drug Abuse

References

Bourhenne C (2007) *Fitness and Long Life Manual: Smoking Drinking and Drugs*. Rolling Hills CA, Writer's Guild of America. Available at http://www.longestlife.com/ebook/drugs.html (accessed 31 March 2015)

Drinkaware.co.uk (2015) Alcohol Unit Guidelines. Available at https://www.drinkaware.co.uk/check-the-facts/what-is-alcohol/alcohol-unit-guidelines/ (accessed 31 March 2015)

Evans G (2014) Smoking, Alcohol and Recreational Drug Abuse. In McConachie I (2014) *Anesthesia and Perioperative Care of the High Risk Patient*. Cambridge, Cambridge University Press.

NHS Choices (2015) Cannabis: The Facts. Available at http://www.nhs.uk/Livewell/drugs/Pages/cannabis-facts.aspx (accessed 31 March 2015)

Vizcaychipi MP (2013) A Descriptive Review of Magnesium in Homeostasis. *Journal of Operating Department Practice* **1** (1): 40–45.

Further Reading

Harmful Effects of Medication, Alcohol, Drugs and Addiction. Available at http://cte.unt.edu/content/files/_HS/curriculum/Harmful_Effects_of_Medication_alcohol_drugs.ppt (accessed 31 March 2015)

Lidya AT (2015) Effects of Smoking, Alcohol, and Drugs on the Body. Available at http://www.slideshare.net/angel_lello/effects-of-smoking-alcohol-and-drugs-on-the-body (accessed 31 March 2015)

Mangerud WL, Bjerkeset O, Holmen TL, Lydersen S and Indredavik MS (2014) Smoking, Alcohol Consumption, and Drug Use among Adolescents with Psychiatric Disorders Compared with a Population Based Sample. *Journal of Adolescence* **37** (7): 1189–1199. Available at http://www.sciencedirect.com/science/article/pii/S0140197114001420 (accessed 31 March 2015)

Tønnesen H, Nielson PR, Lauritzen JB and Møller AM (2009) Smoking and Alcohol Intervention before Surgery: Evidence for Best Practice. *British Journal of Anaesthesia* **102** (3): 297–306.

Websites

Drinking and Alcohol: http://www.nhs.uk/LiveWell/Alcohol/Pages/Alcoholhome.aspx (accessed 31 March 2015)

How Smoking Affects the Way You Look: http://ash.org.uk/files/documents/ASH_115.pdf (accessed 31 March 2015)

Stop Smoking: http://www.nhs.uk/LiveWell/Smoking/Pages/stopsmokingnewhome.aspx (accessed 31 March 2015)

Students: Smoking, Alcohol and Drugs: http://www.nhs.uk/livewell/studenthealth/pages/smoking, alcoholanddrugs.aspx (accessed 31 March 2015)

Videos

Danger Drugs Alcohol Smoking Addicted Kevin Rehab: https://www.youtube.com/watch?v=Z0szxE2-FAo (accessed 31 March 2015)

Danger Drugs Alcohol Smoking Addicted Klea Rehab: https://www.youtube.com/watch?v=ikP-UPjJ0B8 (accessed 31 March 2015)

Danger Drugs Alcohol Smoking Dr. G. Maria Death: https://www.youtube.com/watch?v=yw8_AnW4_ls (accessed 31 March 2015)

Stop Drinking, Stop Smoking, Stop Doing Drugs: https://www.youtube.com/watch?v=FdhlDt7hLeY (accessed 31 March 2015)

92. Perioperative Care of the Elderly Patient

References

Association of Anaesthetists of Great Britain and Ireland (AAGBI) (2014) *Peri-operative Care of the Elderly 2014*. London, AAGBI. Available at http://www.aagbi.org/sites/default/files/perioperative_care_of_the_elderly_2014.pdf (accessed 1 April 2015)

Dodds C, Foo I, Jones K, Singh SK, Waldmann C (2013) Peri-operative Care of Elderly Patients – an Urgent Need for Change: A Consensus Statement to Provide Guidance for Specialist and Non-specialist Anaesthetists. *Perioperative Medicine Journal* **2** (1): 6. Available at http://www.perioperativemedicinejournal.com/content/2/1/6 (accessed 1 April 2015)

Malcolm C (2015) Acute Pain Management in the Older Person. *Journal of Perioperative Practice* **25** (7–8): 134–139

Office for National Statistics (2012). *Population Ageing in the United Kingdom, its Constituent Countries and the European Union*. Available at http://www.ons.gov.uk/ons/dcp171776_258607.pdf (accessed 1 April 2015)

Sharma PT, Sieber FE, Zakriya KJ, Pauldine RW, Gerold KB, Hang Jand Smith TH (2005) Recovery Room Delirium Predicts Postoperative Delirium after Hip-Fracture Repair. *Anesthesia and Analgesia Journal* **101**: 1215–1220.

Shippee-Rice RV, Fetzer SJ and Long JV (2012) *Gerioperative Nursing Care: Principles and Practices of Surgical Care for the Older Adult*. New York, Springer.

Sieber FE, Zakriya KJ, Gottschalk A, Blute MR, Lee HB, Rosenberg PB and Mears SC (2010) Sedation Depth during Spinal Anesthesia and the Development of Postoperative Delirium in Elderly Patients Undergoing Hip Fracture Repair. *Mayo Clinic Proceedings Journal* **85** (1): 18–26.

Vizcaychipi MP (2013) A Descriptive Review of Magnesium in Homeostasis. *Journal of Operating Department Practitioners* **1** (1): 40–45.

Further Reading

Brown NA and Zenilman ME (2010) The Impact of Frailty in the Elderly on the Outcome of Surgery in the Aged. *Advanced Surgery Journal* **44**: 229–249.

Dodds C, Kumar CM and Servin F (2007) *Oxford Anaesthesia Library: Anaesthesia for the Elderly Patient*. Oxford, Oxford University Press.

Harari D, Hopper A, Dhesi J, Babic-Illman G, Lockwood L and Martin F (2007) Proactive Care of Older People Undergoing Surgery ('POPS'): Designing, Embedding, Evaluating and Funding a Comprehensive Geriatric Assessment Service for Older Elective Surgical Patients. *Age Ageing Journal* **36**: 190–196.

Shepperd S, Lannin NA, Clemson LM, McCluskey A, Cameron ID and Barras SL (2013). Discharge Planning from Hospital to Home. *Cochrane Database of Systematic Reviews*. **1**: CD000313.

Websites

Optimal Preoperative Assessment of the Geriatric Surgical Patient: http://www.guysandstthomas.nhs.uk/resources/our-services/acute-medicine-gi-surgery/elderly-care/optimal-preoperative-assessment-of-the-geriatric.pdf (accessed 1 April 2015)

Peri-operative Care for Older Patients Undergoing Surgery: http://www.bgs.org.uk/index.php/topresources/publicationfind/goodpractice/2402-bpg-pops (accessed 1 April 2015)

Perioperative Management of the Geriatric Patient: http://emedicine.medscape.com/article/285433-overview (accessed 1 April 2015)

Safer Surgery and Anaesthesia in Older People: http://patientsafety.health.org.uk/area-of-care/frail-older-people/safer-surgery-and-anaesthesia-older-people (accessed 1 April 2015)

Videos

Care for Older People with Mental Health – Nursing Care: https://www.youtube.com/watch?v=LBRJq4vGB78 (accessed 1 April 2015)

Health-Related Quality of Life after Cardiac Surgery in the Elderly Patient: https://www.youtube.com/watch?v=fhHR-9aUC2U (accessed 1 April 2015)

How to Recognize Delirium: https://www.youtube.com/watch?v=hwz9M2jZi_o (accessed 1 April 2015)

Preparing to Care for Aging Patients – NICHE: https://www.youtube.com/watch?v=QWGU5iK5c8Q (accessed 1 April 2015)

93. Anaemia, Coagulopathy and Bleeding

References

Cave A (2014) Anemia, Blood Transfusion and Coagulopathy. In McConachie I (ed) *Anesthesia and Perioperative Care of the High-Risk Patient*. Cambridge, Cambridge University Press.

Chant C, Wilson G, Friedrich JO (2006) Anemia, Transfusion, and Phlebotomy Practices in Critically Ill Patients with Prolonged ICU Length of Stay: A Cohort Study. *Critical Care Journal* **10** (5): R140.

Corwin HL, Parsonnet KC and Gettinger A (1995) RBC Transfusion in the ICU: Is There a Reason? *Chest Journal* **108** (3): 767–771.

Goodnough LT (2012) Iron Deficiency Syndromes and Iron-Restricted Erythropoiesis (CME). *Transfusion Journal* **52** (7): 1584–1592.

Hayden SJ, Albert TJ, Watkins TR and Swenson ER (2012) Anemia in Critical Illness: Insights into Etiology, Consequences, and Management. *American Journal of Respiratory and Critical Care Medicine* **185** (10): 1049–1057.

Marik PE and Corwin HL (2008) Efficacy of Red Blood Cell Transfusion in the Critically Ill: A Systematic Review of the Literature. *Critical Care Medicine Journal* **36** (9): 2667–2674.

Murphy N (2010) Bleeding and Clotting Disorders. In Smith FG and Yeung J (eds) *Core Topics in Critical Care Medicine*. Cambridge, Cambridge University Press.

Nissenson AR, Wade S, Goodnough T, Knight K and Dubois RW (2005) Economic Burden of Anemia in an Insured Population. *Journal of Managed Care Pharmacy* **11** (7): 565–574.

Okam MM, Mandell E, Hevelone N, Wentz R, Ross A and Abel GA (2012) Comparative Rates of Adverse Events with Different Formulations of Intravenous Iron. *American Journal of Hematology* **87**(11): E123–E124.

Shippee-Rice RV, Fetzer SJ and Long JV (2012) *Gerioperative Nursing Care*. New York, Springer.

Thomas J, Jensen L, Nahirniak S and Gibney RT (2010) Anemia and Blood Transfusion Practices in the Critically Ill: A Prospective Cohort Review. *Heart Lung* **39** (3): 217–225.

Woodman R, Ferrucci L and Guralnik J (2005) Anemia in Older Adults. *Current Opinion in Hematology Journal* **12** (2): 123–128.

Further Reading

Drews RE (2003) Critical Issues in Hematology: Anemia, Thrombocytopenia, Coagulopathy, and Blood Product Transfusions in Critically Ill Patients. *Clinics in Chest Medicine Journal* **24**: 607–622.

Greinacher A and Selleng K (2010) Thrombocytopenia in the Intensive Care Unit Patient. *American Society of Hematology* **2010** (1): 135–143. Available at http://asheducationbook.hematologylibrary.org/content/2010/1/135.full (accessed 5 April 2015)

Spahn DR, Bouillon B, Cerny V, Coats TJ, Duranteau J, Fernández-Mondéjar E *et al.* (2013) Management of Bleeding and Coagulopathy following Major Trauma: An Updated European Guideline. *Critical Care Journal* **17**: R76.

Websites

Anaemia Due to Excessive Bleeding: http://www.merckmanuals.com/home/blood_disorders/anemia/anemia_due_to_excessive_bleeding.html (accessed 5 April 2015)

Bleeding Disorders: http://www.ihtc.org/patient/blood-disorders/bleeding-disorders/ (accessed 5 April 2015)

Blood Disorders (Anaemia, Leukopenia, and Thrombocytopenia): http://www.lef.org/Protocols/Heart-Circulatory/Blood-Disorders/Page-01 (accessed 5 April 2015)

Coagulation Abnormalities in Critically Ill Patients: http://ccforum.com/content/10/4/222 (accessed 5 April 2015)

Videos

Anaemia: https://www.youtube.com/watch?v=cP72MVAcpC4 (accessed 5 April 2015)

Blood Disorders | Anaemia, Allergies, Haemophilia, and Autoimmunity: https://www.youtube.com/watch?v=s-AJGlnGlrE (accessed 5 April 2015)

Iron Deficiency Anaemia: https://www.youtube.com/watch?v=Q6C2UTuC_p0 (accessed 5 April 2015)

Transfusion of Blood and Blood Products: https://www.youtube.com/watch?v=FHJZqL7wxJA (accessed 8 April 2015)

94. Care of the Morbidly Obese Patient

References

Al-Benna S (2011) Perioperative Management of Morbid Obesity. *Journal of Perioperative Practice* **21** (7): 225–233.

Brette M (2015) The Moving and Handling of Bariatric Patients in the Perioperative Environment. *Journal of Operating Department Practitioners* **3** (2): 67–71.

Cobbold A and Lord S (2012) Treatment and Management of Obesity: Is Surgical Intervention the Answer? *Journal of Perioperative Practice* **22** (4): 114–121.

Dybec RB (2004) Intraoperative Positioning and Care of the Obese Patient. *Plastic Surgery Nursing Journal* **24** (3): 118–122.

Garza SF (2004) Perioperative Care of the Morbidly Obese. Available at http://www.modernmedicine.com/modern-medicine/content/periop-care-morbidly-obese?page=full (accessed 6 April 2015)

Green D, Ervine M and White S (2003) *Fundamentals of Perioperative Medicine*. London, Greenwich Medical Media.

Singh PM, Ludwig N, McConachie I and Sinha AC (2014) The Obese or Thin Patient. In McConachie I (ed) *Anesthesia and Perioperative Care of the High Risk Patient*. Cambridge, Cambridge University Press.

Smedley P (2014) First Class Care for the Obese Patient. Available at http://www.rcn.org.uk/__data/assets/pdf_file/0006/596634/Pat_Smedley.pdf (accessed 7 April 2015)

Further Reading

Apau D (2014) Considering Bariatric Surgery Interventions. *Journal of Operating Department Practitioners* **2** (3): 130–135.

Busetto L, Segato GS, De Luca M *et al.* (2005) Weight Loss and Postoperative Complications in Morbidly Obese Patients with Binge Eating Disorder Treated by Laparoscopic Adjustable Gastric Banding. *Obesity Surgery Journal* **15** (2): 195–201.

Freeman AL, Pendleton RC and Rondina MT (2010) Prevention of Venous Thromboembolism in Obesity. *Expert Review of Cardiovascular Therapy Journal* **8** (12): 1711–1721.

Stamou SC, Nussbaum M, Stiegel RM *et al.* (2011) Effect of Body Mass Index on Outcomes after Cardiac Surgery: Is There an Obesity Paradox? *Annals of Thoracic Surgery* **91** (1): 42–47.

Zajacova A, Dowd JB and Burgard SA (2011) Overweight Adults May Have the Lowest Mortality – Do They Have the Best Health? *American Journal of Epidemiology* **173** (4): 430–437.

Websites

Perioperative Care for Morbid Obese Patient Undergoing Bariatric Surgery: Challenges for Nurses: http://www.scielo.br/scielo.php?pid=S0103-21002009000500004andscript=sci_arttextandtlng=en (accessed 11 April 2015)

Positioning of the Obese Patient: http://www.ispcop.org/index.php/component/content/article/42-publications/67-dr-j-brodsky-positioning-the-morbidly-obese-patient-for-surgery (accessed 11 April 2015)

Thinner People after Surgery: http://healthland.time.com/2011/11/22/why-are-thinner-people-more-likely-to-die-after-surgery/ (accessed 11 April 2015)

Thin People at Much Higher Risk of Death after Surgery: http://www.livescience.com/17134-surgery-risk-death-obesity.html (accessed 11 April 2015)

Videos

Care of the Morbidly Obese Trauma Patient: https://www.youtube.com/watch?v=0SD3GOqISWQ (accessed 11 April 2015)

Lap Sleeve Gastrectomy with Hiatal Repair in a Morbidly Obese Patient: https://www.youtube.com/watch?v=Oly85o-qcU0 (accessed 11 April 2015)

Totaltrack: Morbid Obese Patient 191 Kg: https://www.youtube.com/watch?v=vIPjYfGRbfI Accessed: 11/4/15

Ventral Hernia in the Morbidly Obese Patient: https://www.youtube.com/watch?v=VhpcA6Cgzt8 (accessed 11 April 2015)

Index

Rapid Perioperative Care, First Edition. Paul Wicker and Sara Dalby.

Printed and bound by CPI Group (UK) Ltd, Croydon, CR0 4YY

10/06/2025

14686692-0001

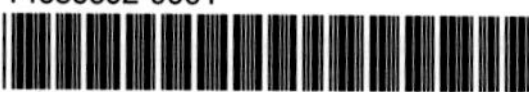